MEDICAL RADIOLOGY

Diagnostic Imaging and Radiation Oncology

Interventional Neuroradiology

Contributors

H. Alvarez · A. Berenstein · I. S. Choi · G. M. Debrun · J. M. Eskridge
G. Fabris · R. Garcia-Monaco · G. Guglielmi · V. V. Halbach
P. Lasjaunias · A. Lavaroni · M. Leonardi · G. Rodesch
A. Setton · A. Valavanis · S. M. Wolpert · F. Zanella · H. Zeumer

Edited by
Anton Valavanis

Foreword by
Martin W. Donner and Friedrich Heuck

With 86 Figures and 26 Tables

Springer-Verlag
Berlin Heidelberg New York London Paris
Tokyo Hong Kong Barcelona Budapest

ANTON VALAVANIS, M. D., Professor
Abteilung für Neuroradiologie
Departement Medizinische Radiologie
Universitätsspital Zürich
Frauenklinikstrasse 10
8091 Zürich, Switzerland

MEDICAL RADIOLOGY · Diagnostic Imaging and Radiation Oncology

Continuation of
Handbuch der medizinischen Radiologie
Encyclopedia of Medical Radiology

ISBN-13: 978-3-642-84436-2 e-ISBN-13: 978-3-642-84434-8
DOI: 10.1007/978-3-642-84434-8

Library of Congress Cataloging-in-Publication Data
Interventional neuroradiology/contributors, A. Berenstein ... [et al.]; edited by Anton Valavanis; foreword by Martin W. Donner and Friedrich Heuck. p. cm. – (Medical radiology) Includes bibliographical references and index.

1. Nervous system-Interventional radiology. I. Berenstein, Alex, 1947– . II. Valavanis, A. (Anton), 1952– . III. Series. [DNLM: 1. Central Nervous System Diseases-radiotherapy. 2. Neuroradiography. 3. Radiography, Interventional. WL300 I635 1993] RD594.15.I6 1993 617.4'8059-dc20 DNLM/DLC 93-12634

Softcover reprint of the hardcover 1st edition 1993

Reproduction of the illustrations: G. Dreher, Württembergische Graphische Kunstanstalt GmbH, Stuttgart
Typesetting: Best-set Typesetter Ltd., Hong Kong

21/3130-543210 – Printed on acid-free paper

Foreword

The methods of interventional neuroradiology represent a distinct and difficult branch within the new field of interventional radiology. The editor of this volume, Anton Valavanis, is a pioneer in this area, and one of the outstanding neuroradiologists in the world. Furthermore, he has brought together the foremost scientists and clinical neuroradiologists in the field to present the individual chapters.

The book gives an overview of the state of the art in interventional neuroradiology. Each of the 12 chapters is devoted to a disease which can be treated by interventional neuroradiological techniques. Pertinent information is provided on anatomical detail, technical background, and clinical aspects; in each case a detailed description of the indications, techniques, and possible complications of interventional neuroradiology is provided. Due consideration is given to the endovascular and nonvascular applications of the techniques.

This book is the first comprehensive update of interventional neuroradiology and will acquaint the reader with well-established facts, recent advances, and future perspectives within this new discipline. It will be of special value to those working in neuroradiology but will also prove very helpful for neurosurgeons, neurologists, and ophthalmologists, as well as all physicians and researchers in the clinical neurosciences.

We hope that the book will meet with the reception and success that it undoubtedly merits.

Baltimore/Stuttgart

Martin W. Donner (†)
Friedrich Heuck

Preface

In an evolving, complex, "surgical" field such as interventional neuroradiology neither a book nor a series of didactic books can replace proper training. With this in mind, this volume was conceived primarily to inform its readers on the current state of the art in interventional neuroradiology, which initially evolved from an endovascular occlusive technique based on craniocerebral and spinal angiography. The aim of this endovascular technique was to occlude arteries feeding vascular malformations, carrying aneurysms, or supplying neoplasms in the head and neck area, the brain, and the spinal cord. Despite some success in achieving this goal, the endovascular approach was generally far inferior to direct surgical elimination of such lesions and neither the concept of endovascular treatment nor the endovascular techniques employed at that time were widely accepted or popular during this initial period of development in the 1960s and early 1970s.

During the 1970s and early 1980s there were significant break-throughs, which influenced and determined the further evolution and growth in the field. These include the introduction of flow-guided, detachable and nondetachable microballoons for occlusions of vessels, obliteration of arteriovenous fistulas, endovascular obliteration of certain aneurysms, and for achieving flow control and performing functional hemodynamic testing; the production, experimental evaluation, and clinical application of a wide variety of embolic agents and materials for obliteration of vascular malformations, devascularization of tumors, and occlusion of arteries, such as microparticulate agents, polymerizing and nonpolymerizing fluid materials, and devices such as microcoils and seeds; and the development of highly flexible, flow-dependent or steerable microcatheters for superselective navigation within the arterial and venous vascular territories of the central nervous system and the head and neck area.

A further important contribution to the growing field was the introduction of the concept of functional vascular anatomy, which provided the theoretical framework for the practice of interventional neuroradiology. This concept helped to better understand the composition of vascular lesions, to identify selective targets for endovascular obliteration, to diagnose potentially dangerous vessels, to detect weak angioarchitectural points within vascular malformations, and to develop specific endovascular protocols for the endovascular exploration and embolization of the various diseases amenable to endovascular treatment. This functional approach based on sound anatomic knowledge greatly contributed to reducing morbidity and mortality and in increasing the efficiency of interventional neuroradiology.

During the 1980s and early 1990s the activities and scope of interventional neuroradiology expanded. The initially occlusive endovascular techniques were modified to be applicable as recanalizing endovascular techniques. Ballon angioplasty became available for treating certain atherosclerotic and other stenotic lesions of the brachiocephalic arteries and for treating vasospasm of intracranial arteries. In addition to this, the endovascular approach has been used to deliver selectively into the vascular system chemotherapeutic agents for the treatment of cerebral malignancies, fibrinolytic agents for the treatment of acute thrombotic occlusions of the vertebrobasilar, carotid, and, recently, ophthalmic arterial systems and of major dural venous sinuses; and vasodilating agents for the treatment of vasospasm. These evolving techniques need to be further defined in terms of indications, timing of the procedure, and long-lasting efficiency.

At the same time interventional neuroradiology also found extravascular applications. Percutaneous approaches under direct imaging control have been developed for the management of spinal disk and degenerative disease as well as for stereotactic purposes.

Finally, in the early 1990s the technique of endovascular electrothrombosis using electrolytically detachable microcoils was developed and experimentally tested and is already being applied in the treatment of intracranial aneurysms. Besides opening new avenues in the treatment of aneurysms, this technique may well find other endovascular applications in the future such as in vascular malformations, arteriovenous fistulas, and acute hemorrhagic conditions, comparable to bipolar coagulation in neurosurgery.

Based on this progress, interventional neuroradiology gained increasing acceptance in the fields of neurosurgery, head and neck surgery, and other related specialties. Interventional neuroradiologic techniques are now being applied preoperatively, to transform inoperable lesions into operable ones and to facilitate surgery, curatively, to treat a number of lesions definitively, and palliatively, to improve the natural history of diseases which cannot be cured by any of the techniques available.

Several centers for interventional neuroradiology around the world have already been established and others will be created in the near future as a response to the need for such an activity. Their scope is to provide an adequate patient care, to perform experimental and clinical research necessary for the advancement of the field, to evaluate continuously and critically the results obtained by endovascular treatment and to train individuals who have decided to devote their professional activity to this fascinating but also cumbersome discipline.

This volume aims to inform interested physicians of the concepts governing the current practice of interventional neuroradiology and of the various techniques currently available, with their advantages, disadvantages, and limitations. It is the hope of the editor and the authors that it will also provide insight into the established and often critical role of interventional neuroradiology among neurosurgeons, head and neck surgeons, and other clinical and basic neuroscientists challenged to understand and treat the diseases described in this book.

Zurich, June 1993 ANTON VALAVANIS

Contents

1 Embolization of Vascular Lesions of the Head and Neck

RICARDO GARCIA-MONACO, PIERRE LASJAUNIAS, HORTENSIA ALVAREZ, and GEORGES RODESCH

CONTENTS

Vascular lesions of the head and neck are rich in clinical and therapeutic features and their management usually requires a multidisciplinary approach. Head and neck surgeons, stomatologists, plastic surgeons, neurosurgeons, orthodontists, pediatricians, and radiologists are often involved in their management. Radiologists performing endovascular therapy not only should be comfortable with catheter techniques and embolic materials, but also should have a thorough clinical and anatomic knowledge of this region. This allows adequate patient selection with precise definition of therapeutic goals and avoids potential complications. We will therefore discuss some general principles of functional vascular anatomy and embolization techniques in the head and neck region, as well as specific pathologies amenable to endovascular therapy, i.e., vascular malformations, vascular proliferations, and traumatic lesions.

RICARDO GARCIA-MONACO, M.D.; PIERRE LASJAUNIAS, M.D., Ph.D., Professor of Radiology and Neurosurgery; HORTENSIA ALVAREZ, M.D.; GEORGES RODESCH, M.D.; Unité de Neuroradiologie Vasculaire Diagnostique et Thérapeutique, Hôpital Bicêtre, Université Paris Sud, 78, Rue du Général Leclerc, 94275 Kremlin-Bicêtre, France

1.1 Functional Vascular Anatomy

In general, the external carotid artery (ECA) supplies all the structures of the head and neck area, except for the central nervous system and optic nerves. Traditionally the ECA system and its branches are described as one arterial tree that divides into multiple branches. However, this description is not appropriate in all situations and gives an erroneous impression of consistency in the anatomy of this system and also of reliability in its branching pattern. In fact, the ECA and its primary branches are extremely variable, and their embryologic origins are multiple (LASJAUNIAS and CHOI 1986; LASJAUNIAS and BERENSTEIN 1987). The standard anatomic appearance of this arterial system can be represented by a schematic drawing, allowing for the fact that it represents a frozen and predetermined picture of an inherently variable arterial network (Fig. 1.1).

Knowledge of the anatomy of the ECA system and an understanding of its variations improve the reliability and safety of endovascular therapeutic procedures. Indeed, the main danger in embolization lies in a lack of familiarity with the anatomic arrangement. The transosseous (emissary) vessels at the base of the skull are of utmost concern. These arteries form the arterial anastomoses between the ECA and either the internal carotid artery (ICA) or the vertebral artery (Figs. 1.2, 1.3).

Embryologically, the ICA-ECA anastomoses represent remnants of the arterial feeders to the neural crest. Their role in the supply to the cranial and upper cervical nerves remains important in adults (Table 1.1). Similarly, the ECA to vertebral artery anastomoses correspond to the remnants of the metameric arterial feeders in the embryo. Their role in the supply of the upper cervical nerves also persists in the adult, with patency of the arterial anastomoses at the corresponding interspaces (LASJAUNIAS and BERENSTEIN 1987).

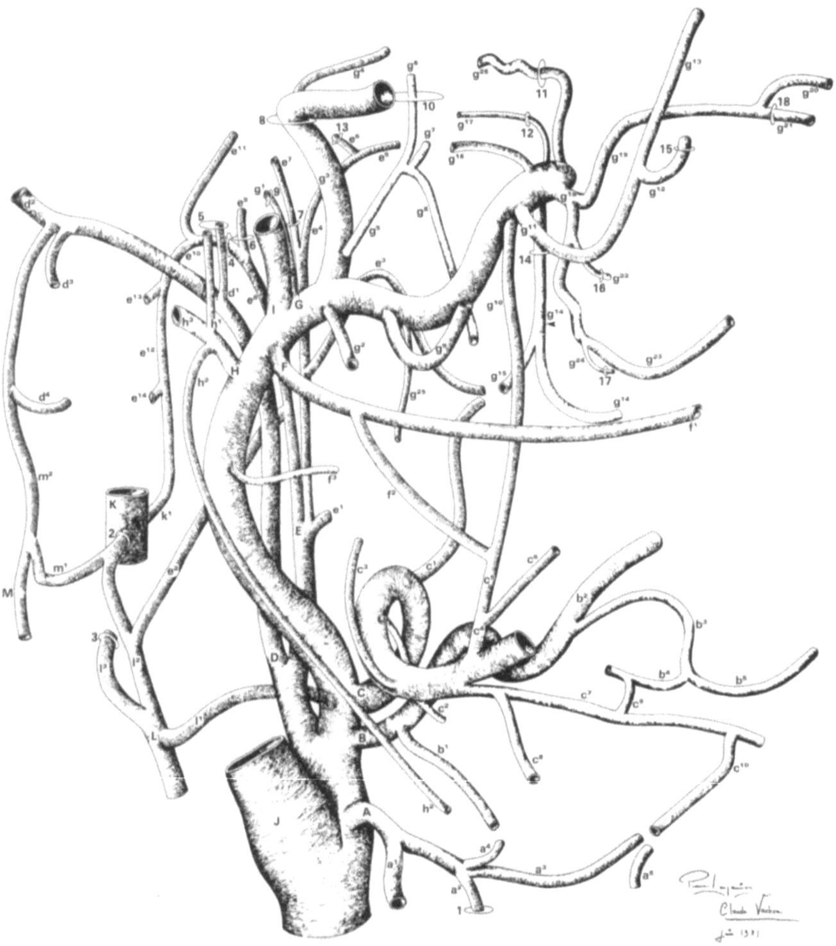

Fig. 1.1. Schematic drawing of the external carotid artery. (Lasjaunias and Choi 1986)

A. *Superior Thyroidal Artery*
a^1 Posterior branch (glandular)
a^2 Superior laryngeal artery
a^3 Anterior anastomotic branch
a^4 Hyoidian branch
a^5 Thyrohyoidian branch

B. *Lingual Artery*
b^1 Hyoidian branch
b^2 Distal lingual artery
b^3 Sublingual artery
b^4 Sublingual anastomosis
b^5 Medial mandibular artery

C. *Facial Artery*
c^1 Ascending palatine artery
c^2 Submandibular artery
c^3 Inferior masseteric artery
c^4 Buccojugal trunk
c^5 Buccal artery
c^6 Posterior jugal artery
c^7 Submental artery
c^8 Posterior hyoidian branch
c^9 Sublingual anastomosis
c^{10} Anterior hyoidian branch

D. *Occipital Artery*
d^1 Stylomastoid artery
d^2 Cutaneous branch
d^3 C1 occipitovertebral anastomosis
d^4 C2 occipitovertebral anastomosis

E. *Ascending Pharyngeal Artery*
e^1 Inferior pharyngeal branch
e^2 Musculospinal branch
e^3 Middle pharyngeal branch
e^4 Superior pharyngeal branch
e^5 Inferior eustachian tube artery
e^6 Mandibular anastomosis
e^7 Inferior tympanic artery
e^8 Neuromeningeal trunk
e^9 Jugular branch
e^{10} Hypoglossal branch
e^{11} Clival branch
e^{12} Odontoid arterial arch system
e^{13} Epidural branch (C1)
e^{14} Epidural branch (C2)

F. *Transverse Facial Artery*
f^1 Jugal branch
f^2 Superior masseteric artery
f^3 Middle masseteric artery

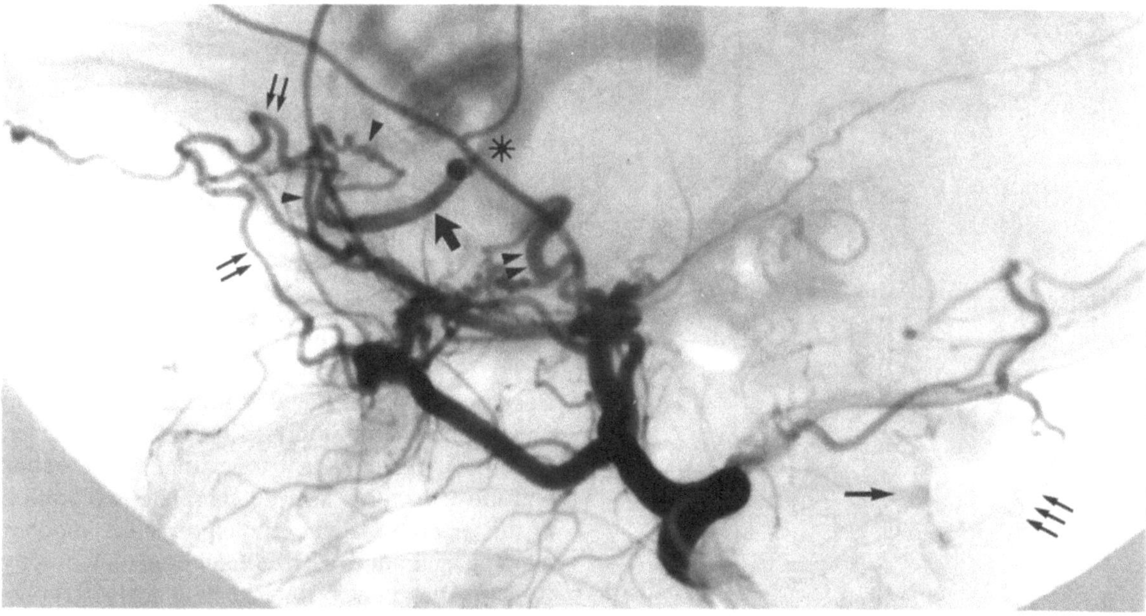

Fig. 1.2. Selective injection of the distal ECA in a child shows filling of the ophthalmic (*thick arrow*), internal carotid (*asterisk*), and vertebral (*thin arrow*) arteries through extracranial–intracranial anastomoses: anterior deep temporal–lacrimal artery (*double arrow*), orbital branch of the middle meningeal artery (*arrowhead*), inferolateral trunk (*double arrowhead*), and artery of the C2 space (*triple arrows*)

◁ **Fig. 1.1** (*continued*)

G. Internal Maxillary Artery
g^{1} Anterior tympanic artery
g^{2} Inferior dental artery
g^{3} Middle meningeal artery
g^{4} Cavernous branch
g^{5} Accessory meningeal artery
g^{6} Cavernous branch
g^{7} Eustachian tube branch
g^{8} Palatine branch
g^{9} Middle deep temporal artery
g^{10} Buccal artery
g^{11} Anterior deep temporal artery
g^{12} Orbital branch
g^{13} Musculocutaneous branch
g^{14} Greater palatine artery
g^{15} Pterygoid branch
g^{16} Pterygovaginal artery
g^{17} Vidian artery
g^{18} Infraorbital/superior alveolar trunk
g^{19} Infraorbital artery
g^{20} Orbital branch
g^{21} Jugal branch
g^{22} Antral branch
g^{23} Jugal branch
g^{24} Alveolar branch
g^{25} Deep masseteric artery
g^{26} Artery of the foramen rotundum

H. Posterior Auricular Artery
h^{1} Stylomastoid artery
h^{2} Stylomuscular artery
h^{3} Cutaneous branch

I. Superficial Temporal Artery

J. Internal Carotid Artery

K. Vertebral Artery
k^{1} Odontoid arterial arch system

L. Ascending Cervical Artery
l^{1} C4 collateral
l^{2} Anterior anastomotic artery (C3)
l^{3} Anterior anastomotic artery (C4)

M. Deep Cervical Artery
m^{1} Posterior anastomotic artery (C3)
m^{2} Posterior longitudinal anastomosis

1. Foramen of the thyrohyoidian membrane
2. Foramen transversarium (third cervical space)
3. Foramen transversarium (fourth cervical space)
4. Hypoglossal canal
5. Stylomastoid foramen
6. Jugular foramen
7. Jacobson's canal
8. Foramen spinosum
9. Anterior tympanic canal
10. Foramen ovale
11. Foramen rotundum
12. Vidian canal
13. Foramen lacerum
14. Posterior palatine canal
15. Malar bone foramen
16. Antral foramen
17. Superior alveolar (dental) canal
18. Infraorbital canal

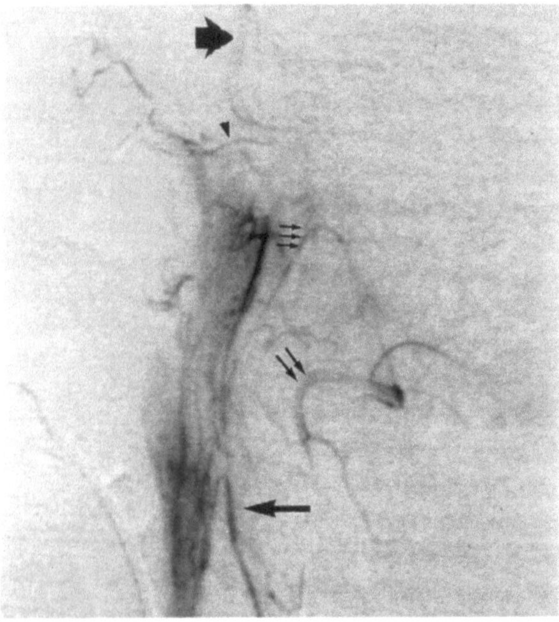

Fig. 1.3. Selective injection of the ascending pharyngeal artery (*arrow*). There is filling of the vertebral artery (*double arrows*) through the anastomoses of the C3 space and odontoid arc system and of the ICA (*thick arrow*) through the mandibular artery (*arrow-head*). Note also the vascular supply to the IXth, Xth, and XIth cranial nerves (*triple arrows*)

In addition, in some rare arrangements, the ECA system supplies further sensitive territories (Table 1.2); inferiorly the larynx (superior laryngeal artery) and posteriorly the cervical spinal cord (spinal artery) should not be overlooked (LASJAUNIAS and BERENSTEIN 1987).

The aforementioned "dangerous" arterial branches do not in themselves represent a strict contraindication to therapeutic angiography but should limit the use of certain embolic materials when recognized (even if they are only partially visualized). They also emphasize the need for a precise anatomic analysis of the information provided by superselective angiograms. Attention must also be paid to the possibility of flow reversal from extracerebral to intracerebral anastomoses during the actual embolization procedure, even if these anastomoses were not visualized during the preembolization study.

There are also some areas that become dangerous when using certain types of embolic agents. The unexpected response is due to the acute ischemic effect produced by the embolization. For example, muscle appears particularly vulnerable to anoxia. Therefore, before undertaking therapeutic angiography in the lingual, temporal, or masseteric arteries, one must bear in mind the fact that the response observed following distal vascular occlusion of these vessels can be more intense than in other territories. However, only normal territories are painful; strict embolization of a vascular malformation or tumor is painless (except in the case of the use of alcohol, and then for the time of injection only).

1.2 Technical Principles of Embolization

Because of the detailed knowledge needed to understand the anatomy of the ECA in a given patient, it is necessary to change prior habits and move towards a more complete exploration of this arterial system. In daily practice, modern imaging techniques such as computed tomography (CT) and magnetic resonance imaging (MRI) provide an accurate topographic diagnosis. The vascular study is indicated to answer the specific questions that may arise as each treatment alternative is considered. For therapeutic angiography one has to examine the arteries of the surrounding healthy tissue, the dangerous arrangements or anastomoses, the possibility of flow control, and the arterial supply to the adjacent cranial nerves. Therefore superselective injections should be performed and topographic protocols of angiographic explorations designed for each case (LASJAUNIAS and BERENSTEIN 1987).

1.2.1 Catheters and Embolic Materials

Therapeutic procedures in the head and neck are best performed under general anesthesia, except when patient cooperation is required, as in carotid or vertebral occlusions. We routinely use femoral puncture and 4F catheters (LASJAUNIAS' catheter, Ingenor, Paris, France) or coaxial systems (5F/ 2.5F microcatheters, Minitorquer, Ingenor, Paris, France or Tracker, Target Therapeutics, California, USA) depending on the embolic material and the therapeutic goals.

The choice of the embolic agent depends on the goal of the procedure, the selectivity accomplished, and the vascular anatomy of the pathologic territory. The following are the commonly used embolic materials for embolization in the head and neck.

Table 1.1. Dangerous vessels of the external carotid system

Arterial trunk (external carotid)	Specific dangerous branch	Specific course	Peripheral nervous system supply	Region (intracranial anastomoses)
Internal maxillary	Infraorbital (orbital branch)	Inferior orbital fissure		Orbit/ophthalmic artery branches
	MMA (meningo-ophthalmic)	Superior orbital fissure	VIth	
	MMA (recurrent meningeal)			
	Anterior deep temporal (orbital branch)	Transmalar		
Internal maxillary	MMA (cavernous ramus)	Foramen spinosum	GG, V2th	Parasellar region: internal carotid siphon
	Accessory meningeal (cavernous ramus)	Foramen ovale or Vesalii	V3th, Vmth, V2th	
	Artery of the foramen rotundum	Foramen rotundum	V2th	
Ascending pharyngeal	Superior pharyngeal (carotid branch)	Foramen lacerum	GG, PPP	
	Jugular branch (lateral clival)	Jugular foramen	VIth, IXth, Xth, XIth	
	Hypoglossal branch (medial clival)	Hypoglossal foramen	XIIth	
Internal maxillary	MMA (petrosal branch)	Petrosal canal	VIIth	Temporal bone/ intrapetrous internal carotid artery
	Anterior tympanic	Anterior tympanic canal	Chorda tympani	
	Vidian artery	Vidian canal	Vidian nerve	
Ascending pharyngeal	Superior pharyngeal (mandibular anastomosis)	Foramen lacerum		
	Inferior tympanic	Jacobson's canal	Jacobson's nerve	
Posterior auricular or occipital	Stylomastoid branch	Facial canal	VIIth	
Occipital	C1 anastomotic branch	First cervical space	C1	Upper cervical spaces/ vertebral artery
	C2 anastomotic branch	Second cervical space	C2	
Ascending pharyngeal	Hypoglossal (odontoid arterial arch)	Third cervical space and hypoglossal foramen	C3 XIIth	
	Musculospinal artery	Third and fourth cervical spaces anastomoses	C3, C4, XIth	

MMA, middle meningeal artery; GG, gasserian ganglion; PPP, pericarotid parasympathetic plexus; Vm, mesenteric branch of Vth.

Table 1.2. Major dangerous unusual normal congenital arrangements and their additional territory. (Lasjaunias and Berenstein 1987a)

Middle meningeal origin of the ophthalmic artery (IInd)
Accessory meningeal dominance to the cavernous sinus region (IIIrd, IVth, Vth, VIth, VIIth)
Accessory meningeal origin of the ophthalmic artery and anterior cerebral artery
Hypoglossal artery persistence (brain stem)
Pharyngocerebellar artery (ascending pharyngeal origin of PICA) (cerebellum)
Proatlantal artery persistence (brain stem)

Polyvinyl Alcohol Foam (PVA). PVA is a nonabsorbable biocompatible sponge material. A particulate form is used on most occasions. Particulate PVA varies in size from 150 to 1000 μm (150–250, 250–600, and 600–1000 μm). These particles can be easily injected and penetrate into the vascular bed. Various concentrations of PVA suspensions can be used depending upon the flow rate and vascularity of a given lesion.

Gelfoam. Gelfoam is available in powder form with particle sizes of 40–60 μm. These particles penetrate into the capillary beds, producing perivascular necrosis. However, they are smaller than the caliber of the dangerous anastomoses and certain AV shunts. Large strips can be used for proximal embolization if a similar (but transient) effect to surgical ligation of an artery is desired (traumatic vascular injury, protection of dangerous vessels, etc).

In general microparticles of PVA are preferred for a presurgical embolization (in patients with a tumor or vascular malformation) to decrease intraoperative blood loss and facilitate surgery. Embolization with small particles is also recommended when the goal of the procedure is to reduce the mass volume and to provide an an-

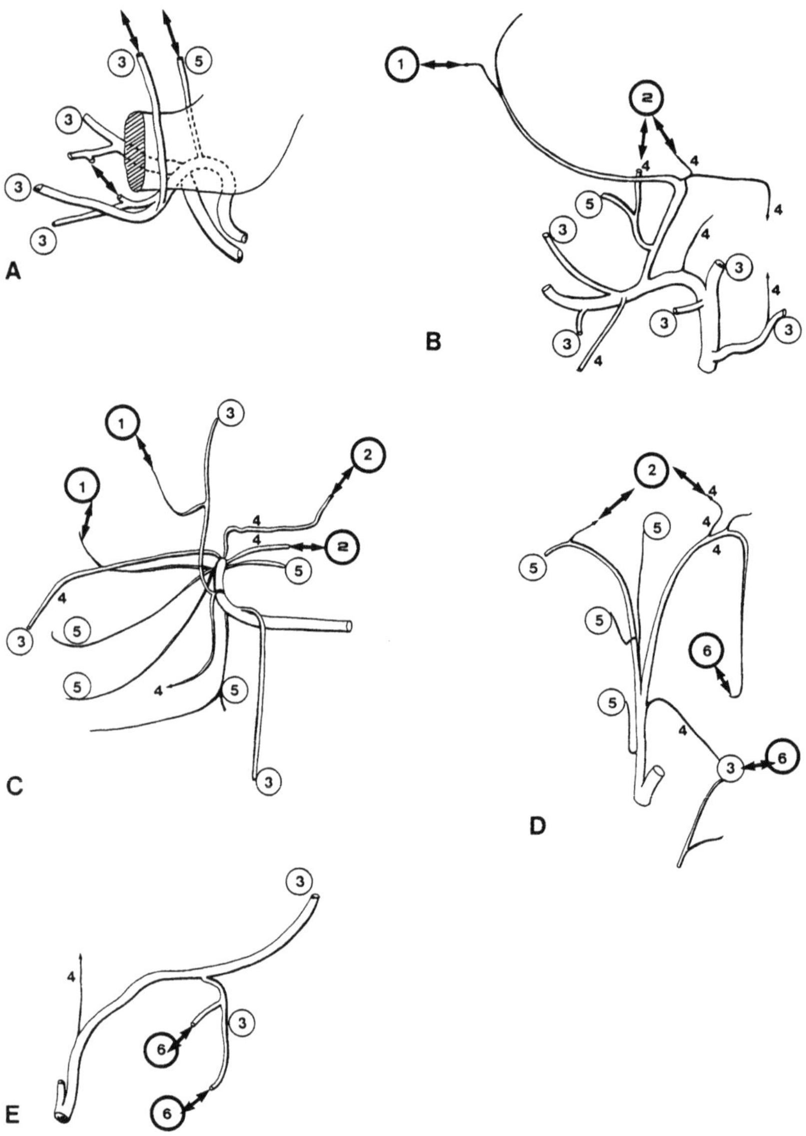

algesic or antihemorrhagic effect. However, one has to bear in mind that particle embolization is always temporary.

n-Butyl-cyanoacrylate (NBCA). This is a low viscosity liquid which polymerizes quickly when in contact with protons or changes in Ph. It has tissue-adhesive properties and causes an inflammatory reaction of the vascular wall.

Polymerization time can be delayed by adding Lipiodol so that the distal vessels can be reached. NBCA is seldom used in head and neck embolization, usually being indicated when a permanent result of embolization is desired, as in some cases of arteriovenous malformation or fistula.

Fig. 1.4 A–E. Diagrammatic representation of the various territories of the ECA and the bidirectional flow through the collateral circulation. **A** Lingual and facial arteries; **B** proximal internal maxillary artery; **C** distal internal maxillary artery; **D** ascending pharyngeal and cervical arteries; **E** occipital artery. ① Ophthalmic system anastomosis; ② intracavernous and intrapetrous ICA anastomosis; ③ musculocutaneous territories; ④ peripheral nervous system territories; ⑤ mucosal territories; ⑥ vertebral anastomosis. (Lasjaunias and Berenstein 1987b)

Ethyl Alcohol. The potent sclerosing effect of ethyl alcohol in the endothelium makes it an effective embolic material. However, if inadvertently perfused into normal tissue, serious complications can occur. It can also cause extensive skin necrosis if it reaches cutaneous branches.

Therefore, we limit the use of ethyl alcohol to the treatment of certain types of extracranial venous malformation.

Detachable Balloons. These are the agent of choice for most cases of direct single hole arteriovenous fistula or for carotid or vertebral artery occlusion. Detachable balloons are provided by various companies and are made of either latex or Silastic. We personally prefer the latex balloons (gold valve balloon, Ingenor, Paris, France).

Coils. Coils are small pieces of guidewire from which the inner core has been removed and a foreign body such as cotton or Dacron added to promote thrombosis. They have very little use in head and neck embolization. They are easily introduced with the assistance of a conventional guidewire and are of various gauges and lengths. They can be used to protect normal vessels or anastomoses (see later).

Ethilbloc. This is a promaline corn zen protein mixed with 60% ethanol which solidifies in 10–15 min. It is used by several teams to treat venous malformations (RICHE et al. 1983). We have no experience with this embolic agent.

1.2.2 Embolization Technique

In our analysis of the functional anatomy of the head and neck we have illustrated the various anastomoses between the neighbouring territories (Figs. 1.2–1.4). Although anastomoses do not represent a contraindication to embolization, their presence requires that care be taken to ensure that endovascular therapy is carried out safely and properly.

When flow-directed particles (PVA) are used for devascularization, a careful analysis of the distal sump effect reduction must be done. Dangerous anastomoses not visualized previously may now fill. In this situation one can follow the distal washout and the behavior of the anastomosis as the flow slows. If very small particles are used and no gross change is seen in the abnormality after multiple injections, one can increase the particle concentration accordingly. A high concentration usually results in faster devascularization but probably with less penetration.

An obvious safety measure to avoid dangerous anastomoses would be catheterization beyond the "dangerous" point but this is not always possible with 4F catheters. Microcatheters can achieve this goal but they also increase the complexity and cost of the procedure since heparin and coaxial and flushing systems become mandatory.

A more simple way to ensure protection from dangerous anastomoses is to occlude them mechanically. This can be done with a large strip of Gelfoam or with coils. After the anastomosis is controlled, embolization can be carried out with microparticles or other embolic agents. If this is not accomplished, flow reversal techniques can be used. Reversal of flow can be achieved with an occlusive balloon catheter proximal to the anastomosis or with a wedged catheter. The aim is to impose a craniofugal flow to the anastomosis, redirecting flow away from the dangerous territory (the vertebral artery, for example) and towards the "nondangerous" distal target. This reversed flow will assist or "push" the embolic material towards the lesion. Prior to injection of embolic material, various hand test injections are done with contrast alone to determine the tolerance and/or pressure needed not to fill the anastomosis. As the embolization begins, the contrast and emboli mixture is gently injected during systole and monitored as the nonopacified reversed blood flow (away from the vertebral) washes the emboli distally toward the desired territory. As the embolization progresses, the washout slows and more careful injections are required. When the flow is significantly slowed, the embolization is stopped. The artery proximal to the anastomosis should be washed carefully before restoring the flow into it.

When using particles it is important to rotate continuously or to change the syringe position to prevent sedimentation and/or aggregation of the particles at any one part of the syringe (which may result in catheter occlusion). Prior to reuse, catheters full of embolic material should be thoroughly backflushed and rinsed to ensure that they are free of the material; only then may the rest of the angiographic procedure be continued.

1.2.3 Special Considerations in Pediatric Populations

Arterial embolization presents some distinctive features when performed in newborns and infants (BURROWS et al. 1987; GARCIA-MONACO et al. 1990, 1991; LASJAUNIAS and BERENSTEIN 1987a,b).

The small size of femoral arteries necessitates the use of small catheters to perform angiographic examinations and embolizations. The procedure should be performed as fast as possible to reduce the catheterization time. Postintervention femoral patency is essential to allow staged embolization, if needed, and future normal growth of the lower limbs. We routinely puncture the femoral artery with a 20G Teflon needle and place a 4F sheath before selective catheterization. A 4F catheter is used for angiography and embolization in most of the cases. If a thinner catheter is necessary to achieve distal catheterization in infants under 2 years old, we do not use a coaxial system but rather a direct approach with a Minitorquer (Ingenor, Paris, France) (GARCIA-MONACO et al. 1990). This avoids the need for heparin and coaxial perfusion. Contrast material is a limiting factor in babies weighing only a few kilograms because of the danger of volume overload. Fortunately this is of less concern since the introduction of new low osmotic contrast material. Nevertheless, we try not to use more than 6–7 ml contrast (Hexabrix, Guerbet, Paris, France) per kilogram body weight. Accurate hemodynamic balance should be maintained during the procedure, especially in infants with congestive heart failure. Special attention should be paid when injecting the embolic agent in the ECA since anastomoses with the ICA and vertebral artery are widely open in infants (see Fig. 1.2).

1.2.4 Indications for Embolization

Embolization has proven to be of benefit in the treatment of various head and neck lesions. Thus it is of use (a) for total cure or stabilization of vascular lesions (e.g. arteriovenous malformations or fistulas), (b) for presurgical devascularization of tumors (e.g. paragangliomas), (c) to arrest acute hemorrhagic episodes that cannot be arrested by simpler techniques (e.g. epistaxis, bleeding due to laryngopharyngeal tumors, trauma), (d) to provide an analgesic effect (e.g. in the case of metastases), (e) for reduction of tumor volume, and (f) for mass effect relief (e.g. in the case of subglottic hemangioma).

In the following sections we describe the specific role of embolization in head and neck lesions, with the exception of skull base tumors and epistaxis which will be discussed in separate chapters.

1.3 Head and Neck Lesions Amenable to Embolization

Head and neck pathologies amenable to endovascular therapy can be grouped into vascular malformations, vascular proliferations, and traumatic lesions. The descriptions of craniofacial vascular lesions in the literature and the nomenclature employed are complex and confusing. The majority of classifications are descriptive, based on clinical macroscopic appearances and/or histologic features, and are not useful in clinical practice. In addition, the term "angioma" is widely used in the literature to refer to different types of lesion. A practical and clinicobiologic classification was proposed by MULLIKEN and GLOWACKI (1982), who differentiated two types of vascular lesion: vascular malformations and vascular tumors (Table 1.3). The predictable differences in clinical behavior in these two major categories of vascular lesion, malformations and hemangiomas, dictate entirely different therapeutic approaches.

The treatment strategy that we propose is based on our experience with vascular malformations and hemangiomas in different parts of the body. Each territory carries specific therapeutic risks which will affect the choice between conservative management and the search for a complete cure.

1.3.1 Vascular Malformations

Vascular malformations are inborn errors of vascular morphogenesis. They may be formed by any combination of abnormal capillary, arterial, venous, or lymphatic channels with or without shunt. Their clinical behavior varies according to the morphology of the channel abnormalities, their secondary hemodynamic effects, and their

Table 1.3. Craniofacial vascular lesions. [Modified from MULLIKEN and GLOWACKI (1982)]

Vascular malformations	Vascular proliferations
Arterial with or without fistula	Hemangiomas
	Capillary in children (potentially involutive)
Capillary	
Capillarovenous	Cavernous in adults (noninvolutive)
Venous	Hemangiopericytoma
Lymphatic	Hemangioendothelioma
Venolymphatic	Kaposi's sarcoma
	Angiosarcoma

Table 1.4. Dormant AVM clinical manifestations. (LASJAUNIAS and BERENSTEIN 1987b)

Mass effect
Facial deformity (cosmetic)
Functional disturbance
(swallowing, breathing, vision, mastication)
Maxillofacial growth disturbance
Teeth eruption disturbance
Skin discoloration

Table 1.5. Factors triggering or aggravating maxillofacial AVMs. (LASJAUNIAS and BERENSTEIN 1987b)

Direct trauma
Mouth hygiene
Feeding
Blunt
Iatrogenic (biopsy, surgery, tooth extraction, oral prosthesis, proximal ligations, or embolizations)
Regional infections
Teeth eruption
Hormones and contraceptives
Psychological stress
Venous and arterial hypertension
Excessive sun exposure

location. They differ significantly from hemangiomas because of the absence of proliferative and involutive potential. Certain lesions may exist in a dormant state (Table 1.4), until stimulated to expand by a triggering factor (Table 1.5). The majority enlarge gradually in proportion to the growth of the patient. Their effects vary from minor cosmetic blemishes to major deformity or functional impairments. The treatment of these complex lesions requires careful planning by a multidisciplinary team. In general, treatment of vascular malformations in children should be conservative in the absence of significant function impairment or life-threatening complications. In adults the aggressiveness of the therapeutic approach may depend more on the team skills and cultural environment (as it relates to the goal of treatment and possible complications) than on the characteristics of the vascular malformation. As shown in Table 1.3, vascular malformations are classified according to the type of abnormal vessels involved.

1.3.1.1 Arteriovenous Malformations

Maxillofacial arteriovenous malformations (AVMs) pose specific problems related to their location. They have a major psychological impact related to the magnitude of the cosmetic problem. In addition, as the oral cavity in children represents the pivotal area of maxillofacial growth, the interference of a vascular malformation may result in abnormal mandibular development (micrognathia, prognathism) (LASJAUNIAS et al. 1985; LASJAUNIAS and BERENSTEIN 1987b).

Symptomatic lesions may involve hemorrhage, musculocutaneous ischemic ulceration, or pain. Secondary functional disturbances such as trismus, speech problems, or difficulties in swallowing may be quite disabling. Typically, maxillofacial AVMs present as a reddish discoloration with visible subcutaneous or submucosal dilated vessels. Strong pulsations, thrills, and bruits that can be auscultated are usually found. Although the diagnosis is clinical, angiography is necessary for therapeutic planning. CT is of value in establishing whether bone involvement is present.

In general, maxillofacial AVMs are most effectively treated by complete surgical excision following embolization after skeletal maturity has been achieved (LASJAUNIAS and BERENSTEIN 1987a; LEIKENSOHN et al. 1981; MULLIKEN and YOUNG 1988) (Fig. 1.5). Hemorrhagic complications may require emergency intervention prior to the time for optimal surgical therapy. In the case of maxillary or mandibular lesions, bleeding usually occurs with dental eruption or loosening and may be life threatening. Aggressive embolization combined with prophylactic dental extractions is preferable to hemimandibulectomy or maxillectomy, which may be the only alternative to obtain hemostasis. Extraction of the teeth involved in the local hemorrhage should be undertaken within a few days following embolization (BURROWS et al. 1987; LASJAUNIAS and BERENSTEIN 1987b).

Technically, embolization of oral lesions must be carried out bilaterally in most cases. The tongue represents a difficult territory because of its muscular nature and particularly sensitive response to ischemia; therefore, we prefer the use of particles rather than NBCA.

If complete cure can be obtained by embolization alone, or if radical surgery is not feasible, embolization with liquid agents is indicated. NBCA is preferable to PVA if such an approach is used to treat maxillofacial, subcutaneous, or scalp AVMs. PVA or other particles may reach normal territories since repetitive injection alters progressively the protective sump effect of the AVM. In addition, recanalization is likely to occur

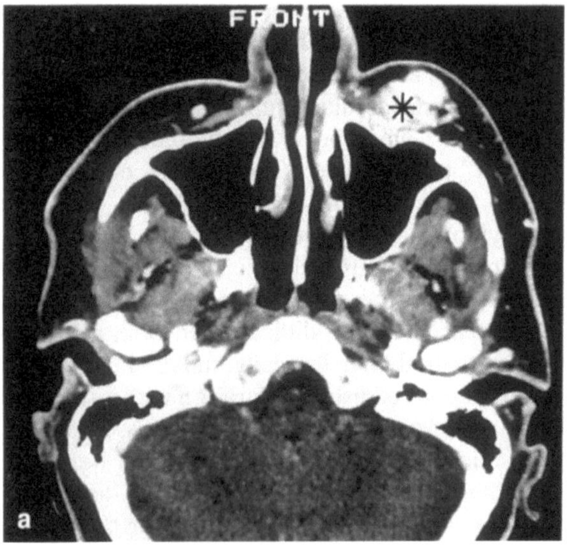

Fig. 1.5. **a** CT scan shows a subcutaneous AVM (*asterisk*) in the malar region without bony involvement. Ipsilateral facial angiography (**b** lateral and **c** anteroposterior view) shows the vascular supply through the anterior and middle jugal arteries. There is venous drainage to the angular vein (*V*). **d** Injection of the superficial temporal artery demonstrates additional vascular supply through the malar branches of the zygomatic–orbital (*arrow*) and transverse facial (*double arrow*) arteries. **e** Early and **f** late phase of carotid angiography after presurgical embolization with microparticles of all the above-mentioned pedicles. Devascularization of the middle and inferior compartment. The remaining compartment is supplied by the infraorbital artery (*arrow*), which also receives sources from the alveoantral (*double arrow*) and the inferior muscular (*arrowhead*) arteries. The maxillary artery was embolized years before in another institution; therefore supply to those vessels is through collaterals from the inferolateral trunk (*crossed arrow*), superior pharyngeal artery (*double arrowheads*), and ascending palatine artery (*triple arrow*).

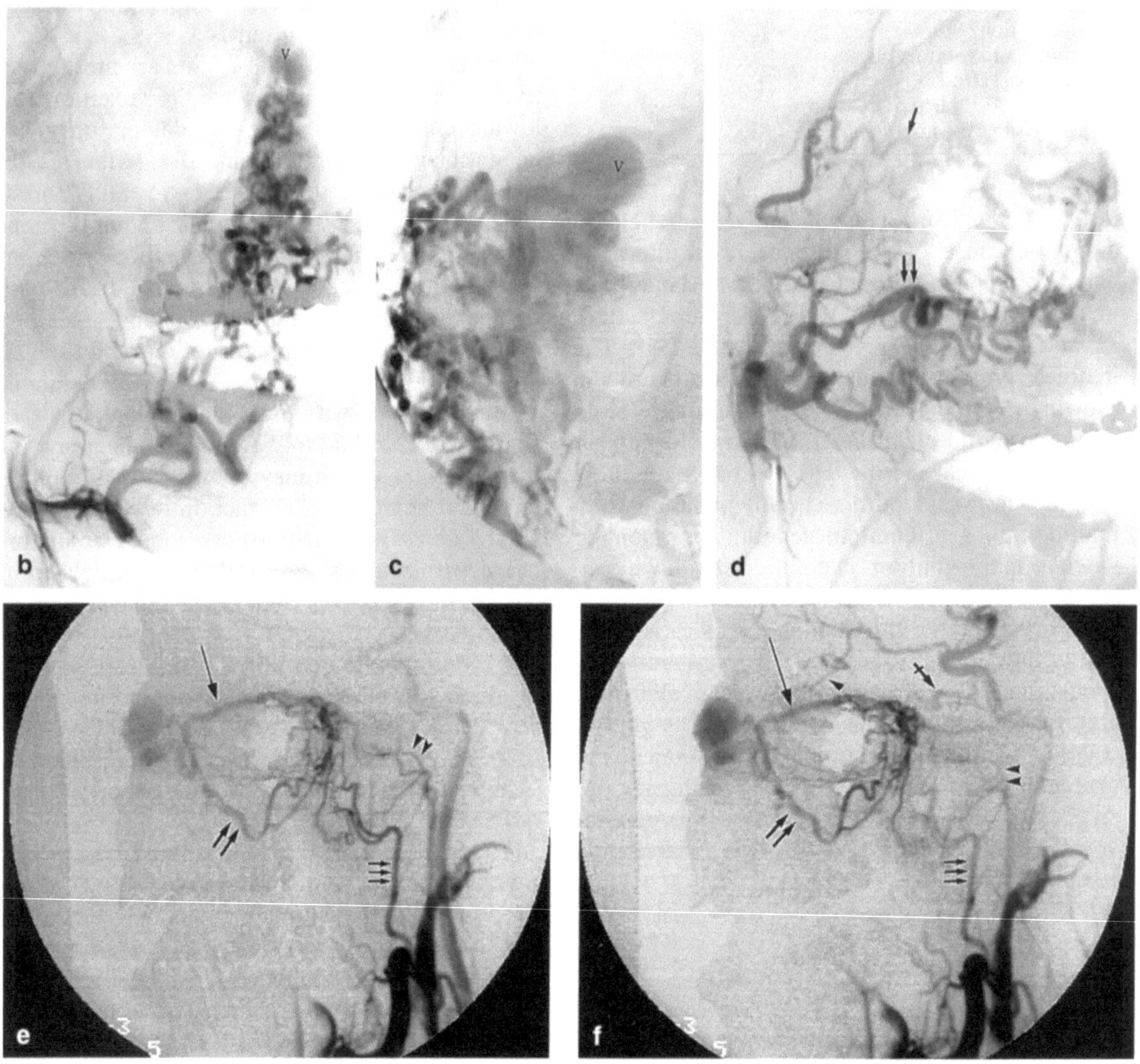

◁ **Fig. 1.5** (*continued*). Complete surgical excision was performed 3 days after embolization with minimal blood loss. The extracranial portion of the infraorbital artery was easily controlled by the surgeon at the level of the external infraorbital foramen

after PVA embolization. It should be stressed that there is no indication for partial treatment of AVMs when complete cure can be obtained by single or combined techniques.

Palpebral AVMs are potentially supplied by ophthalmic artery branches. Therefore a careful anatomic analysis should be done to embolize the lesion distal to the normal vascularization of the retina. Embolization from or distal to the second portion of the ophthalmic artery is necessary to avoid the retina and optic nerve supply (ALVAREZ et al. 1990).

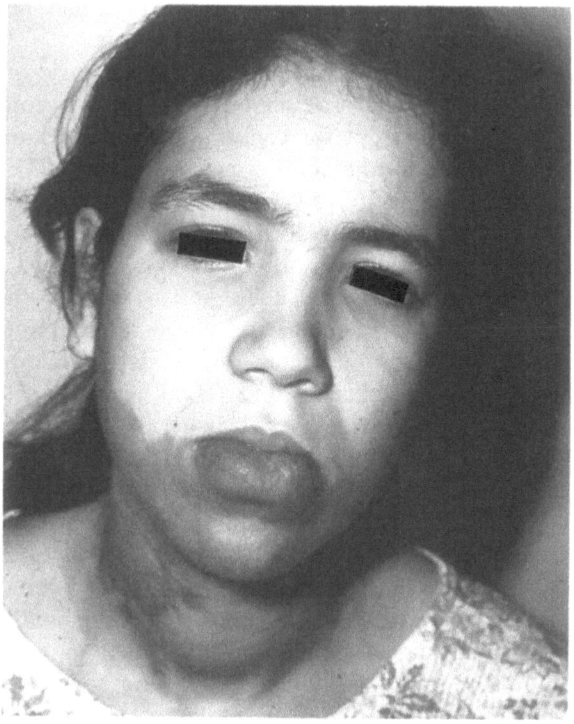

Fig. 1.6. Port wine stain in the territory of V2 and V3 nerves combined with a labial venolymphatic malformation. No venous anomaly was found in the intracranial study

1.3.1.2 Capillary and Capillarovenous Malformations

Capillary and capillarovenous malformations are slow flow lesions presenting vascular lakes of small size visualized in the late capillary–venous phase of angiograms. They usually present in young patients, in whom they produce facial asymmetry in relation to the mass effect without bony involvement. The skin or mucous membranes are usually not involved. No abnormal pulsations, thrills, or bruits can be palpated or auscultated. Symptomatic lesions may fluctuate, with periods of increased swelling associated with pain or tenderness; they occasionally have minor bleedings that stop spontaneously or after manual compression. When present in the growing face or mouth they may interfere with normal growth of the maxillofacial area, inducing secondary function impairments and dysmorphism. Angiography demonstrates feeding arteries of normal caliber, displacement, and hypervascularity in the mid and late capillary phase. A dense blush and vascular lakes are seen in the venous phase. Indications for treatment are primarily related to complications (major functional disturbances, bleeding, psychological problems). Treatment is by a combined endovascular and surgical approach.

Among these types of vascular lesion is the so-called port wine stain. This is a vascular malformation that consists of small venular channels located within the dermis. Port wine stains are frequently present in the mesodermal dysplastic syndromes and, when isolated in the face, may represent a minor expression of Sturge-Weber syndrome (Fig. 1.6). Angiography usually fails to demonstrate any vascularization and embolization has little indication.

1.3.1.3 Venous Malformations

Purely venous vascular malformations develop on the venous side of the vascular tree. They do not have any connection with the arterial capillary system and cannot be visualized through it by conventional angiography. They are constituted by large communicating or septated venous spaces.

Patients usually consult for cosmetic problems. Typically the lesions present as a bluish decoloration of the skin and/or mucous surface. They are soft and easily compressible. One can empty the venous pouch by manual compression; refilling occurs in seconds. They increase in size as a result of maneuvers that raise the venous pressure, such as use of the "head down" position or the Valsalva maneuver. No abnormal pulsations, thrill, or bruit can be found. Phleboliths are almost always found in radiologic examinations. In addition to cosmetic problems, episodic pain may be observed secondary to phlebothrombosis.

The diagnosis can be made on the basis of a purely clinical assessment, and the decision on whether to opt for conservative observation or therapeutic intervention can be easily taken without angiography. CT scan before and after contrast enhancement demonstrates the extension of the lesion (Fig. 1.7a). Special attention has to be paid to whether there is compromise of the airway and alimentary passages. If treatment is needed, direct percutaneous puncture of the malformation is carried out (Boxt et al. 1983) (Fig. 1.7b). Provided that the lesion does not communicate widely with normal veins, treatment is carried out with local injection of 95% ethyl alcohol inside the venous pouch. The lesion usually thromboses immediately and produces a painless swelling. Some weeks later shrinking of the venous pouch and improvement in both symptoms and cosmetic results are usually noted. However, many lesions have different compartments separated by septae, either spontaneously or after previous unsuccessful surgery, and several therapeutic sessions then may be required to achieve good results.

Although technically simple, intralesional treatment with ethyl alcohol is not risk free. Indeed, if the ethyl alcohol migrates to normal veins (facial, intracranial, spinal) there may be disastrous consequences. In addition, local injection of alcohol or other sclerosing agents may not provide complete and stable disappearance of the malformation in every instance (Lasjaunias and Berenstein 1987b).

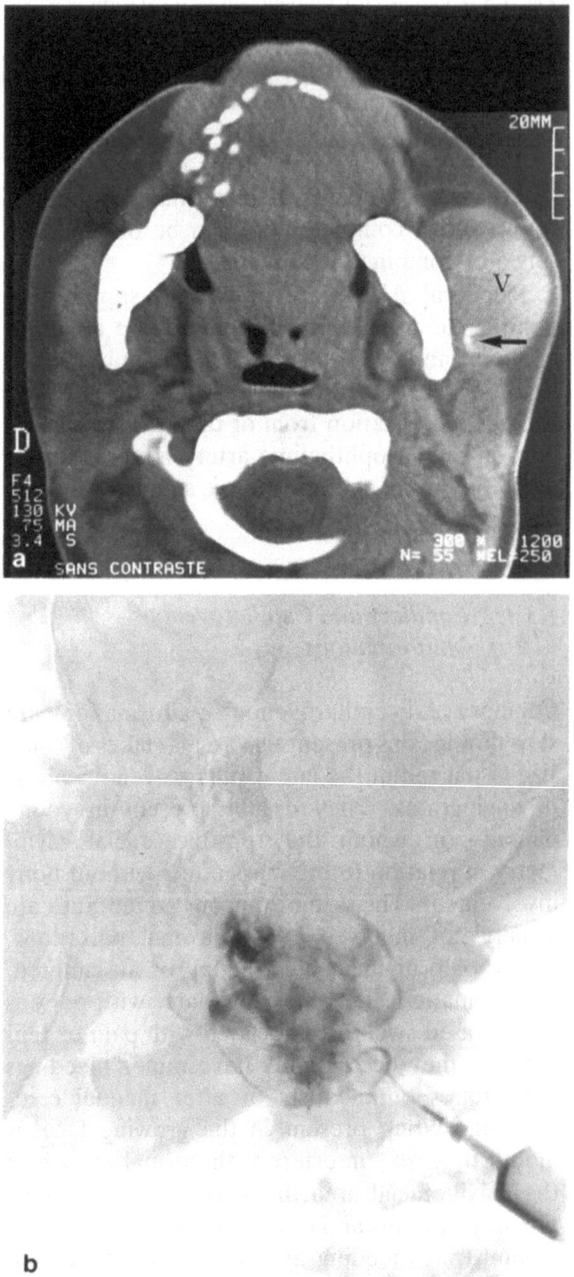

Fig. 1.7. **a** CT scan shows a venous malformation (*V*) in the left masseteric region. A phlebolith is clearly seen (*arrow*). **b** Percutaneous direct injection of contrast material into the malformation prior to in situ injection of 95% ethyl alcohol

1.3.1.4 Lymphatic Malformations

Head and neck "lymphangiomas" are lymphatic malformations and should not be considered true neoplasms (Batsakis 1979). They often communicate with adjacent systemic veins and may be combined with venous malformations (the so-called hemolymphangiomas) (Fig. 1.8). Lymphatic malformations of the cheek can also be associated with port wine stains, particularly in cases of Sturge-Weber syndrome.

Purely lymphatic lesions or cystic ones are usually asymptomatic but are of concern due to the cosmetic problems that they cause. Mixed venolymphatic lesions of the face and of the tongue are different as they usually present earlier in children and evolve by acute swelling episodes; after local infections they may show partial regression under antiseptic and anti-inflammatory medication. In the tongue area, the mucosa becomes dark and the mouth is permanently opened (Fig. 1.9); bleeding may occur following des-

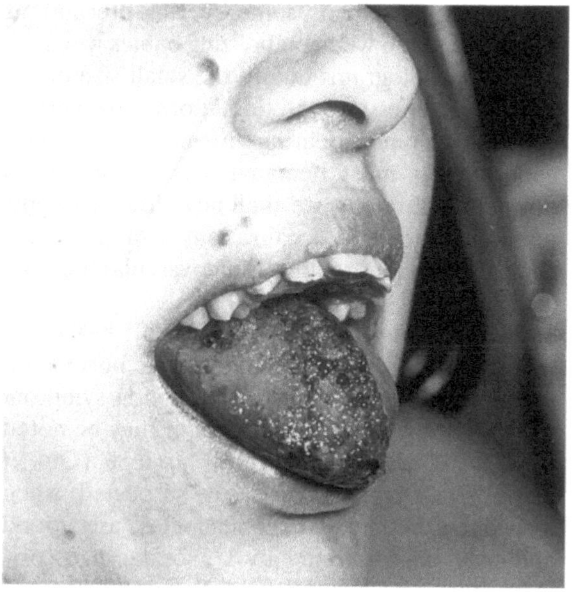

Fig. 1.8. Typical aspect of a venous lymphatic malformation (so-called hemolymphangioma) of the tongue

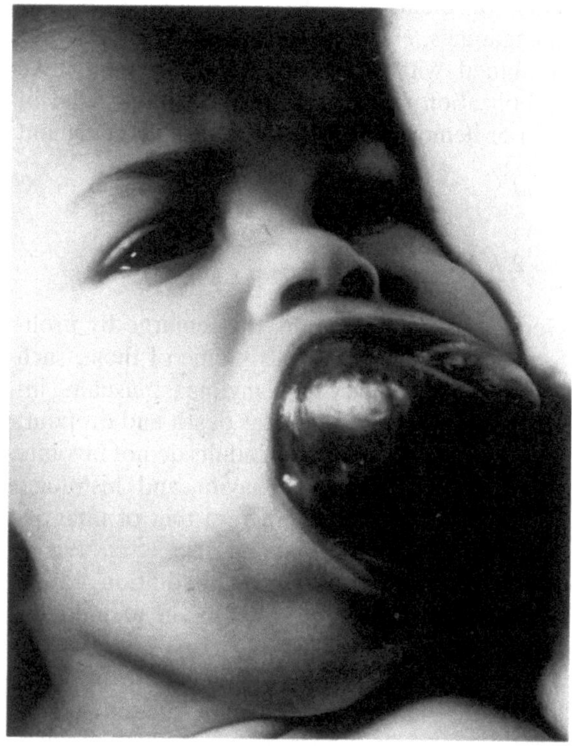

▷ **Fig. 1.9.** Acute swelling of an venolymphatic malformation (hemolymphangioma) of the tongue

quamation of the permanently protruding dry tongue. Extensive lesions compromise the airway or alimentary tract and may require intubation or tracheostomy.

These acute episodes are frequently corticosteroid resistant. In the acute phase of swelling embolization can be useful. In our experience, complete resolution of swelling and stabilization can be obtained after embolization with PVA. Moderate shrinkage of the tongue lesions can usually be followed by conservative treatment with orthodontic assistance.

It seems to us that particularly in the tongue, bilateral embolization with particles must be considered when glossectomy, even cuneiform, appears to be the only alternative. Pure lymphatic malformations of the tongue are clinically different as they present with a permanent mass but with a normal pinkish, pale appearance of the mucosae (Fig. 1.10). In our experience embolization is not effective in this type of lesion.

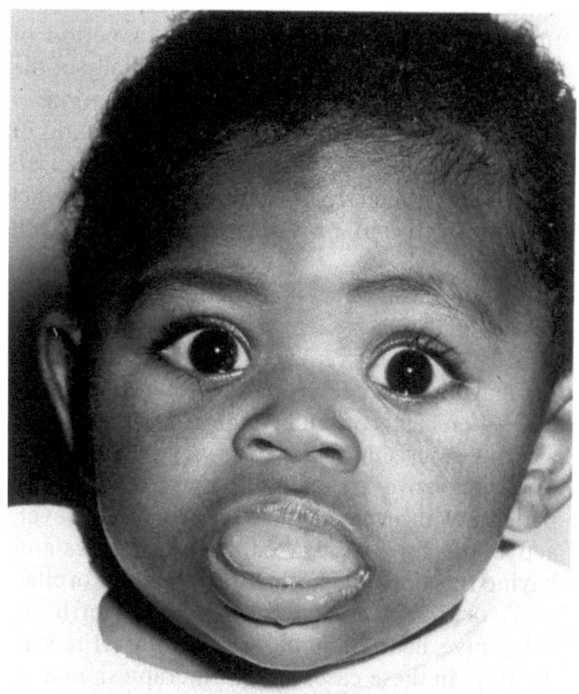

Fig. 1.10. Pure cystic lymphangioma of the tongue causing macroglossia and protrusion of the tongue. Embolization is useless in this case

1.3.2 Vascular Proliferations

Definitive treatment of most types of head and neck tumors is surgical. However, embolization plays an important role in the management of some of them, such as hemangiomas or paragangliomas, either as a sole treatment option or combined with surgery. In addition, palliative embolization may provide symptomatic relief of pain or hemorrhage in some uncurable malignant lesions.

1.3.2.1 Hemangiomas

Hemangiomas are tumors that enlarge by proliferation of endothelial cells. Some of them, such as infantile capillary hemangiomas, usually involute by progressive cellular death and dropout. Cavernous hemangiomas of adults do not involute and present a clinical behavior and histologic appearance quite different from that of infantile hemangiomas (LASJAUNIAS and BERENSTEIN 1987b; MULLIKEN and YOUNG 1988). In addition, cavernous hemangiomas are rare in the head and neck area.

Infantile capillary hemangiomas are frequent lesions that have a strong female predominance. They are present at birth in only approximatively 30% of patients; the majority appear in the first 3 months of life as a red or bluish cutaneous tumor. They typically demonstrate a period of rapid growth (proliferation phase), usually in the first 6 months of life, followed by a period of gradual involution, starting at about 12 months of age and completing by 7 years (PITANGUY et al. 1984). Unfortunately, it is not possible to predict the rare occasions on which involution will not occur.

The diagnosis of capillary hemangioma is easy, based on its macroscopic characteristics and typical clinical history. Angiography is not needed for diagnosis; its features are similar to those of any other highly vascular tumor, with moderate arteriovenous shunting.

Conservative treatment is the rule for most patients with capillary hemangiomas. However, active therapy is indicated in selected patients having functional impairment (subglottic, orbital, oral) or complications (recurrent hemorrhage, congestive heart failure, Kasabach-Merritt syndrome). In these cases steroid therapy should be the initial treatment to accelerate the involution of the lesions. In the case of failure of medical therapy (resistance to or intolerance of corticosteroids), embolization with PVA particles is indicated to stabilize the proliferative phase and speed up the onset of tumoral involution. As previously described, some special precautions should be taken when embolizing babies weighing only a few kilograms due to the small size of the femoral arteries and the limitations in respect of contrast volume. Bearing in mind the general concept that most hemangiomas in infants do not need treatment, we shall now discuss specific features of certain localizations and particular clinical evolutions requiring endovascular therapy.

Subglottic Hemangiomas. Dyspnea before 6 months of age (usually following a normal interval after birth) is the most common symptom of subglottic hemangiomas. Stridor may be noted in 87% of cases and cyanosis in 16% (OHI et al. 1979). Diagnosis is easily suspected when associated cutaneous hemangiomas are found and may be confirmed by CT or laryngoscopy (MULLIKEN and YOUNG 1988). Subglottic hemangiomas are usually localized in the posterior or left lateral wall of the larynx and are constantly fed by branches of the inferior thyroid artery (Fig. 1.11). In spite of their small size, these lesions can cause asphyxia and require emergency therapy (endotracheal intubation or tracheostomy) to prevent airway obstruction. Even when these lesions begin to involute spontaneously, they may demonstrate rebound growth following infection or discontinuation of therapy.

Treatment should begin with steroids. If such treatment fails, embolization of the tumor through

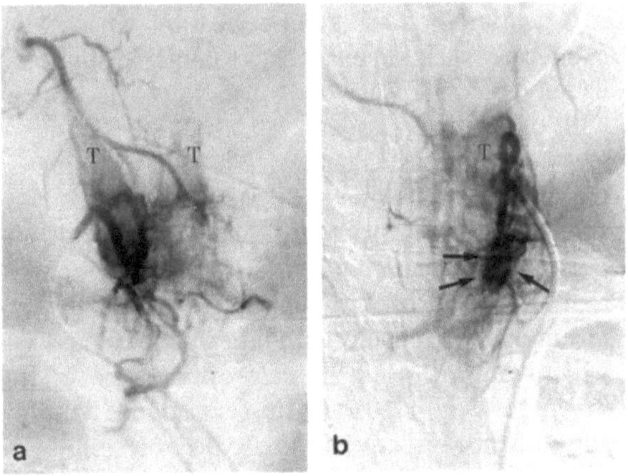

Fig. 1.11a,b. 5-month-old girl with a symptomatic subglottic hemangioma. Steroid therapy and intubation failed to stabilize the symptoms. **a** Right and **b** left inferior thyroid angiography prior to embolization of the subglottic hemangioma (*arrows*). Note the normal blush of the thyroid gland (*T*). Embolization with particles resolved the dyspnea and laryngeal stridor. The baby was extubated and no further treatment was needed

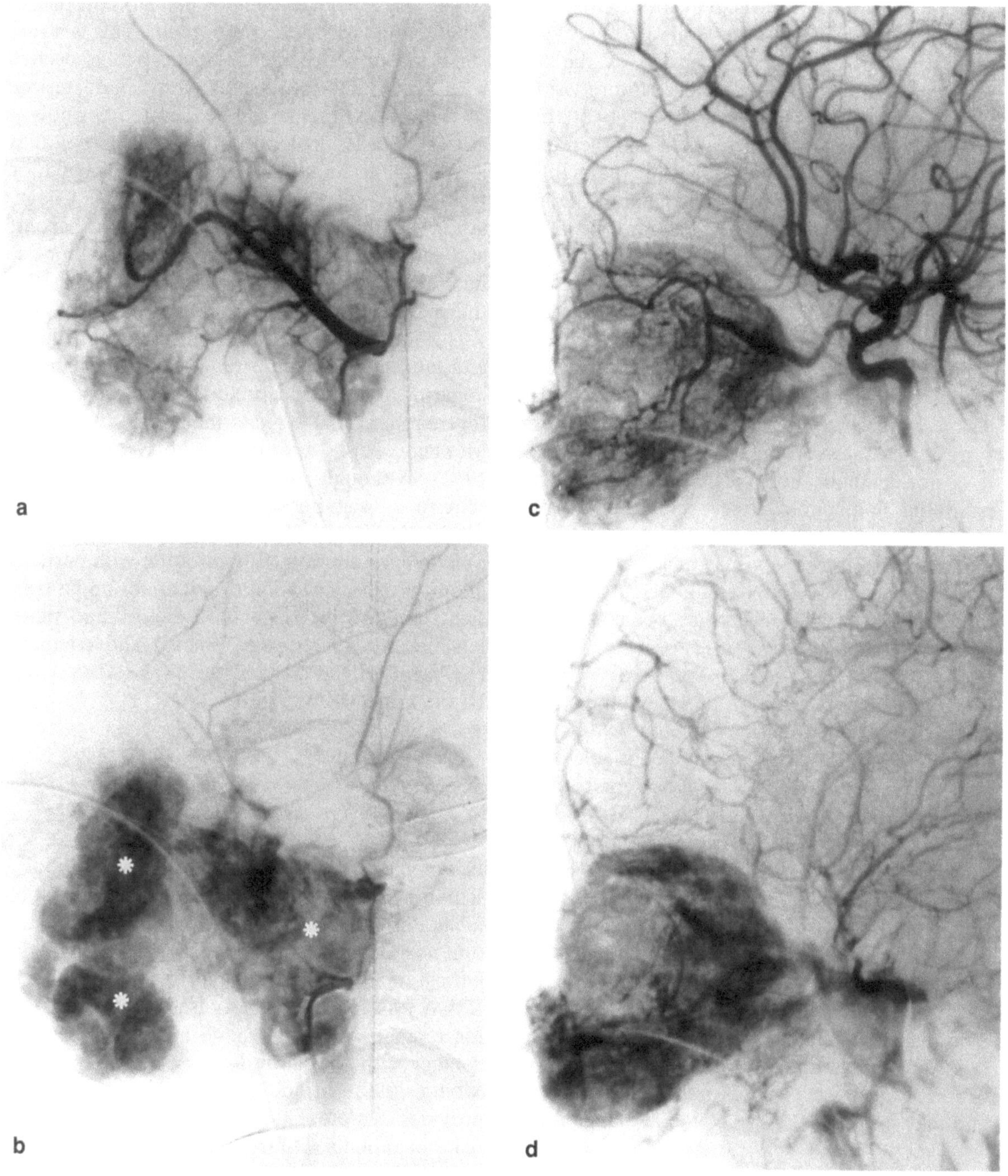

Fig. 1.12a–d. 3-month-old girl presenting orbital, labial, cheek, and parotid hemangiomas. **a** Early and **b** late phase of maxillary angiography shows the vascular supply and the multilobulated capillary blush of the hemangiomas (*asterisks*). **c** Early and **d** late phase of internal carotid angiography shows the main vascular supply of the orbital hemangioma through branches of the ophthalmic artery

the inferior thyroid artery has proven to be effective in dealing with the obstructive symptomatology of the hemangiomas (BOXT et al. 1983; LASJAUNIAS and BERENSTEIN 1987b). Tracheostomy can therefore be avoided.

Eyelid or Orbital Hemangiomas. Hemangiomas of the orbit (Fig. 1.12) or upper eyelid present a special problem because they are a potential cause of amblyopia or refractive errors (MULLIKEN and YOUNG 1988; THOMSON et al. 1979). Infants presenting with complete occlusion of the eye require rapid treatment to preserve future vision. It was reported by THOMSON et al. (1979) that blindness will follow 1–2 weeks of complete palpebral occlusion in young infants. Treatment is based on the clinical picture. The goal of therapy is to reduce the volume of the tumor to allow opening of the eye and reception of visual stimuli, thus avoiding loss of vision. Medical treatment should be discouraged in these cases since it may take weeks for a satisfactory response to occur. Embolization with particles allows shrinkage of the lesion within 2–4 days if at least 70% of the lesion is reached through the external carotid system (LASJAUNIAS and BERENSTEIN 1987b). If it is not, embolization of the branches arising from the ophthalmic artery should be carried out. Catheterization beyond the first portion is mandatory to preserve visual function (ALVAREZ et al. 1990). In cases of failure, intratumoral injection of corticosteroids has been suggested (MULLIKEN and YOUNG 1988).

Oral Hemangiomas. Oral hemangiomas rarely involve the bone but may present with rapid osseous deformity and spontaneous bleeding. Surgical treatment may be needed in combination with embolization (LASJAUNIAS and BERENSTEIN 1987b; MULLIKEN and YOUNG 1988). Soft tissue hemangiomas of the cheek are usually well tolerated; when necessary, embolization can expedite the involution to avoid any consequences for teeth eruption or psychological development.

In adults, hemangiomas of the tongue are usually of a cavernous type and may present with pain or mass syndromes. They are poorly vascularized at angiography; however, particle embolization produces stable relief of the pain syndromes and may decrease the size of the hemangioma.

Further Clinical Problems Associated with Hemangiomas. Diffuse hemangiomas may be responsible for congestive cardiac failure. In all cases symptoms develop in the proliferation phase; therefore they are absent at birth. Medical treatment with steroids should be adjunctive to classical treatment (diuretics, cardiotonics, fluid restriction) of cardiac failure. In cases where symptoms cannot be stabilized with these measures, embolization of the hemangiomas has been shown to control the cardiac failure (GARCIA-MONACO et al. 1991).

On rare occasions patients may present the so-called Kasabach-Merritt syndrome. This is a rare condition in which hemangiomas are associated with a consumption coagulopathy characterized by thrombocytopenia and accelerated fibrinolytic activity. Stasis of blood in the hemangioma may lead to an accumulation of activated coagulation factors and increased local fibrinolysis. Coagulation in the hemangioma may then become autocatalytic, resulting in thrombocytopenia and depletion of coagulation factors. In some patients the coagulopathy is mild and does not affect survival, but in others it can result in uncontrollable and fatal massive hemorrhages. Steroid therapy, heparin, and aminocaproic acid have been used for treatment (LASJAUNIAS and BERENSTEIN 1987b; MULLIKEN and YOUNG 1988; NEIDHART and ROACH 1982). Although reported to be effective, they require a long period of treatment unless the generic factor (i.e., the hemangioma) is corrected to stop consumption. Embolization with particles allows devascularization of the tumor and a transient increase in coagulation factors and platelets, permitting surgical removal and complete resolution of the coagulopathy (LASJAUNIAS and BERENSTEIN 1987b).

1.3.2.2 Other Types of Vascular and Non-vascular Proliferation

In other types of head and neck tumors endovascular therapy is sometimes needed. Embolization facilitates surgical excision of highly vascular tumors such as paragangliomas or hemangiopericytomas (LASJAUNIAS and BERENSTEIN 1987b; VALAVANIS 1986). It is also useful before surgery for a stage N3 lymph node metastasis in close contact with the carotid artery (GONZALEZ and MORET 1990). In addition, embolization usually provides symptomatic relief (of hemorrhage or pain) in patients with incurable malignant tumors.

Fig. 1.13. **a** Common carotid angiography demonstrates two paragangliomas (*asterisks*), one located at the carotid body and one in the exocranial stylomastoid region. **b** Catheterization of the ascending pharyngeal artery prior to embolization of the carotid body tumor (*asterisk*) through the musculospinal branch (*arrow*). **c** Catheterization of the stylomastoid artery (*arrow*) prior to embolization of the other tumor (*asterisk*). **d** Common carotid angiography after embolization with particles shows complete devascularization of the tumors and patency of normal vessels. Both paragangliomas were successfully excised 3 days later ▷

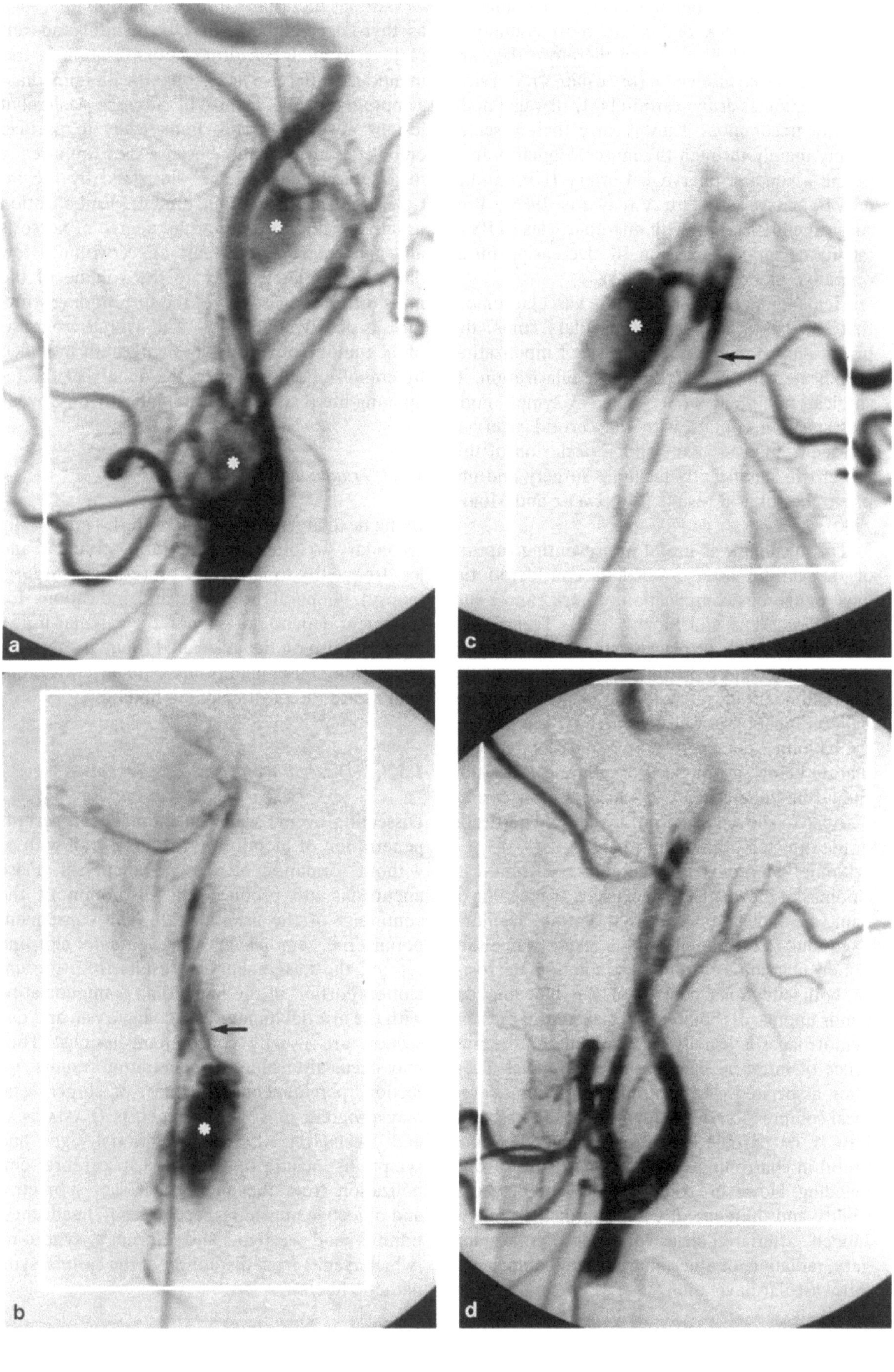
a
c
b
d

Paragangliomas and hemangiopericytomas in the head and neck region are most commonly located in the skull base and therefore they are better described elsewhere (see Chap. 4). Cervical paragangliomas at the carotid body or vagal node are not uncommon. They receive their vascular supply mainly through the musculospinal branch of the ascending pharyngeal artery (Lasjaunias and Berenstein 1987b; Valavanis 1986). Presurgical embolization with microparticles of PVA facilitates surgical excision by decreasing intraoperative blood loss (Fig. 1.13).

Hemangiopericytomas are rare vascular tumors that can be located in the maxillary sinus, the oral cavity, or the nasal fossa. Embolization is indicated for presurgical devascularization. If surgical treatment of a stage N3 lymph node metastasis in contact with the carotid artery is foreseen, endovascular balloon occlusion of this vessel will significantly facilitate surgery and improve the surgical results (Gonzalez and Moret 1990).

This technique is useful in preventing rupture of the carotid artery, which is considered the most dangerous complication of neck cancer surgery (Gonzalez and Moret 1990). Technically, the balloon should be placed in the internal carotid artery immediately proximal to the origin of the ophthalmic artery. If a 20-min occlusion test by balloon inflation is well tolerated by the patient, the balloon is detached. A second balloon may be placed below it for security. Surgical excision should be done at least 15–20 days after carotid sacrifice to allow normalization of blood perfusion in the affected brain hemisphere.

Some symptoms of incurable recurrent carcinomas of the head and neck, such as bleeding or pain, are indications for embolization. Hemorrhages due to arterial ulceration result from either tumor invasion or from postradiation necrosis. In both situations control of the bleeding depends upon accessibility. Surgical control of these hemorrhages is usually very difficult. In the presence of intraoral bleeding due to lingual ulceration associated with postradiation trismus, even local compression of the involved area is difficult. NBCA or particle embolization may be quite useful in controlling oncologic acute and chronic bleeding. However, results will depend on accessibility and the general condition of the patient. Indeed, arterial changes following previous surgery, radiation, or atheromatosis may compromise intravascular navigation.

Osseous metastasis from vascular tumors, such as thyroid carcinoma, may be painful and refractory to analgesic drugs. Embolization is tremendously effective against pain, with immediate symptomatic relief in most of the cases. Malignant lesions always respond dramatically to particle embolization, probably because they are already in a subischemic state as illustrated by the intralesional necrosis often present. Embolization usually produces an important degree of necrosis and a decrease in the mass effect within a few days. Pain related either to the volume of the mass or to "congestion" of the surrounding structures is poorly understood. The overall prognosis of the tumor is obviously not significantly modified by embolization; however, the quality of the remaining life is sometimes dramatically improved.

1.3.3 Traumatic Vascular Lesions

In the head and neck, vascular injuries are usually secondary to blunt or penetrating trauma, and less frequently to iatrogenic procedures (surgery, biopsy). General prognosis and indications for treatment depend not only on the vascular injury itself but also on the associated traumatic lesions. Dissection, false aneurysms, and arteriovenous fistulas are the most common findings.

1.3.3.1 Dissection and False Aneurysms

Dissection occurs when an intimal tear permits penetration of blood into the vessel wall with or without formation of a pseudoaneurysm. False aneurysms are produced by disruption of the continuity of the arterial wall. The consequent periarterial hemorrhage will eventually clot and retract; the false aneurysm results from the unclotted portion of the hematoma communicating with the arterial lumen. Pseudoaneurysm and dissection are usually concomitant lesions. They may occur after blunt or penetrating trauma, infection, percutaneous puncture, or surgery and may progress to vessel thrombosis (Lasjaunias and Berenstein 1987a). Additional signs and symptoms include those related to cerebral embolization from the aneurysmal sac, subjective and objective murmurs, cervical pain, headaches, tinnitus and vertigo, and Horner's syndrome (which results from disruption of the carotid sympathetic fibers).

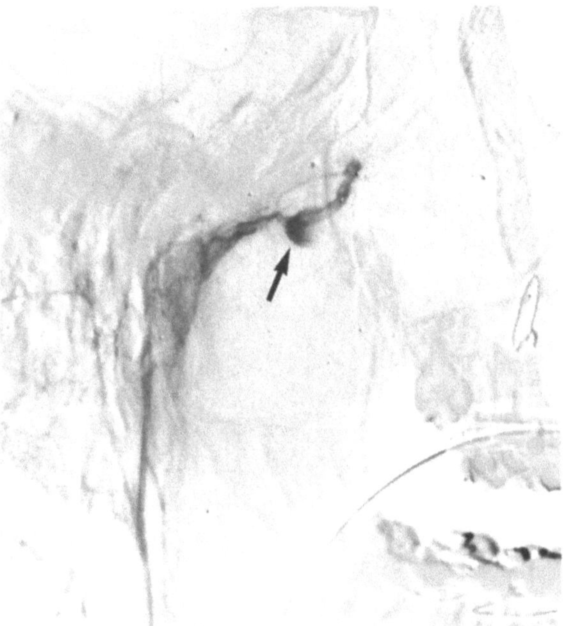

Fig. 1.14. 20-year-old male with uncontrollable epistaxis after plastic surgery (anterior maxillofacial traction) to correct superior maxillary hypoplasia. Catheterization of the ascending pharyngeal artery shows the site of bleeding and a false arterial aneurysm (*arrow*). Embolization with a strip of Gelfoam resulted in complete and permanent hemostasis

If patients are hemodynamically stable (i.e., without major hemorrhage), conservative treatment is sufficient. Endovascular therapy is not indicated in these cases. Angiographic follow-up will demonstrate spontaneous resolution of the vascular lesion.

In contradistinction, an acute false aneurysm causing a massive and life-threatening hemorrhage (Fig. 1.14) should immediately be treated by endovascular occlusion of the parent vessel, if possible. Wedge catheterization and superselective contrast injection should be avoided since a consequent increase in endoluminal pressure may aggravate the hemorrhage by causing pseudoaneurysmal rupture.

1.3.3.2 Arteriovenous Fistulas

A traumatic arteriovenous fistula is an abnormal communication between an artery and a vein secondary to vessel laceration. The consequences of this acute hemodynamic change can occur at the site of the fistula or distal to it, producing secondary venous hypertension. Locally the presentation is as a pulsatile mass with thrill. A subjective or objective cranial bruit is usually perceived. There is frequently a delay between the traumatic insult and the clinical manifestations.

Extracranial arteriovenous fistulas may develop from the vertebral or external carotid systems. Trauma is not the only etiology of extracranial arteriovenous fistulas; they may also occur spontaneously as a consequence of fibromuscular dysplasia, neurofibromatosis, Ehler-Danlos disease, etc.

Endovascular embolization is the treatment of choice; it has a cure rate of over 95% and entails very little risk and significantly less morbidity and hospitalization than any other form of treatment (Lasjaunias and Berenstein 1987b). The choice of the embolic agent depends upon the location of the fistula and its flow characteristics. In most cases a permanent agent should be used, a possible exception being those traumatic fistulas where there is no intrinsic vascular pathology. In general, particulate agents are not suitable since they tend to pass through the large arteriovenous connections of these lesions. The goal of embolization is occlusion of the fistula itself rather than occlusion of the feeding pedicles. Due to the vast collateral network in the head and neck, the fistulas will recur if only proximal embolization is performed (as evidenced by the surgical experience).

Detachable balloons are the preferred embolic agent and are usually best in large arteriovenous fistulas in the proximal portion of external carotid artery branches. The high flow aids in guiding the balloon to the site of fistula. Balloons can usually be placed directly at the site of the abnormal arteriovenous communication (Fig. 1.15). However, occasionally precise placement of the balloon at the fistula site may be difficult, as the high flow may push the balloon into the venous side with significant force.

Arteriovenous fistulas developing in the vertebral system are usually high flow lesions. Patients may be asymptomatic or complain of pulsatile tinnitus. Exceptionally they may have additional symptoms such as hemisensory deficit or motor dysfunction (Lasjaunias and Berenstein 1987b).

Pretherapeutic angiographic examination is essential to determine the normal blood supply to the cord and especially the exact localization of the fistula, i.e., whether it is in the vertebral artery or in the anastomosis of the cervical spaces.

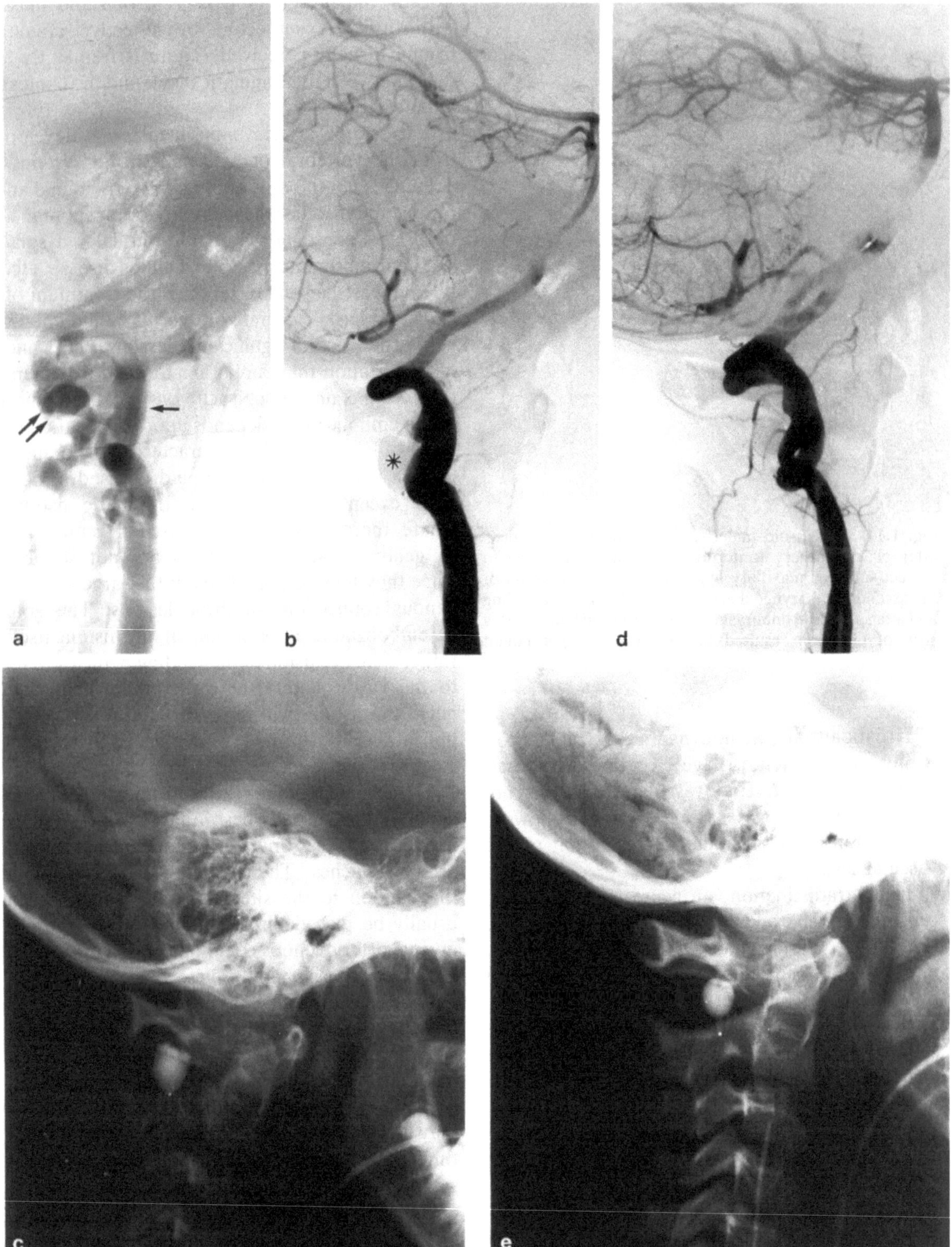

Fig. 1.15. **a** Vertebral injection shows a traumatic arteriovenous vertebral fistula. *Arrow*, vertebral artery; *double arrows*, vertebral plexus. **b** Immediate angiographic control after endovascular treatment with a detachable balloon (*asterisk*) shows complete occlusion of the arteriovenous fistula. **c** Standard roentgenogram shows exact position of the detached balloon filled with contrast medium (GV no. 16, Ingenor, filled with Hexabrix 160 mg/liter). **d** Control angiography performed 6 months later is normal. Notice the decrease in size of the vertebral artery compared to figures **a** and **b**. **e** Standard roentgenogram at the time of the angiographic control shows the balloon still inflated

Although endovascular balloon occlusion of the fistula with preservation of the vertebral artery is ideal, in the former localization a balloon trapping is adequate to cure the lesion. In contradistinction, in a fistula at the level of the cervical anastomoses, vertebral occlusion is useless since the fistula will receive its vascular supply from other sources (occipital, dorsal, or ascending cervical arteries, depending on the localization). Therefore, in this case occlusion of the fistula itself is mandatory.

Fistulas of the external carotid main trunk are uncommon. Collateral circulation analysis may be useful to localize the fistula. However, if complete transection of the main trunk occurs, the proximal segment may be difficult to visualize. The arteriovenous fistula is usually located at the site of an abrupt change in caliber between the artery and the vein. Endovascular occlusion with a balloon or glue is the treatment of choice.

1.4 Emergency Embolization

Clinical indications for embolization on an emergency basis, or within 24–48 h of consultation, include life-threatening hemorrhage, progressive respiratory obstruction, occular occlusion in an infant, high output cardiac failure, and platelet depletion coagulopathy (Kasabach-Merritt syndrome).

Major hemorrhage is the most frequent indication for emergency embolization in the head and neck region. As previously described, acute vascular trauma, maxillary AVMs, carcinomas eroding blood vessels, or consumption coagulopathy in giant hemangiomas may be responsible for the bleeding. Embolization is rewarding for symptom control and hemodynamic stabilization. Later prognosis will depend directly on the etiology of the primary or associated lesions.

Respiratory obstruction may be the primary indication for emergency embolization in patients with subglottic hemangiomas, lingual capillary malformations, cervical–oral hemolymphangiomas, or venous malformations compromising the airway tract. Embolization usually reduces the volume and mass effect of the lesions, allowing endotracheal extubation and avoiding the need for tracheostomy (Burrows et al. 1987; Lasjaunias and Berenstein 1987b).

Palpebral occlusion in infants with hemangiomas should be treated without delay to avoid amblyopia. In cases of failure, intratumoral injection of corticosteroids has been suggested (Mulliken and Young 1988).

Cardiac failure is a rare clinical situation in infants with hemangiomas or arteriovenous fistulas. If medical treatment (digitalis or diuretics) fails to control the cardiac manifestations, embolization will rapidly improve the clinical situation by decreasing intratumoral vascular flow and cardiac overload (Garcia-Monaco et al. 1991).

1.5 Complications and Precautions

State of the art external carotid embolization can, in skilled hands, have a permanent morbidity below 1% and no mortality.

Major complications, such as stroke, occur when the embolic agent passes unintentionally to the intracranial vessels due to reflux or with the opening of the anastomoses. Both complications can be avoided using a cautious technique and with knowledge of vascular anatomy. In cases where preoperative carotid balloon occlusion has been done, a 2- to 3-week delay before surgery is recommended to normalize cerebral hemodynamics and avoid delayed ischemic complications (Gonzalez and Moret 1990). If surgery has to be done earlier, attention should be paid to maintaining normal pressure during surgical anesthesia in order to preserve collateral circulation at the circle of Willis.

Peripheral cranial nerve palsy is of concern in embolization of vascular pedicles of a lesion that also supply cranial nerves. Fortunately, this complication is rare and usually transient. Aggressive agents such as Gelfoam powder or NBCA are more likely to produce cranial nerve palsy since they reach the distal capillary network supplying the peripheral nerves.

Tissue ischemia secondary to embolization is responsible for some minor complications (trismus, pain) and more important ones such as cutaneous necrosis. Postembolization trismus is related to arterial ischemia induced by embolization of the normal muscular vascular territory and is always transient. Pain is a frequent but transient symptom after maxillofacial embolization, and is usually well controlled by analgesic medication.

The same arterial mechanism of ischemia is involved when ectopic emboli reach the capillary level of a cutaneous territory (distal to the last possible collateral channel) and produces cutaneous necrosis. It is therefore important to take the surgical approach into account when performing a presurgical embolization to ensure normal cicatrization of the surgical incision. Special attention is also necessary in bilateral tongue embolization since this mucosal territory is quite sensitive to ischemia and ulceration. Aggressive agents such as Gelfoam powder or NBCA should be avoided in these territories.

Some special precautions should be taken when performing angiography and embolization in babies weighing only a few kilograms owing to the small size of arteries and contrast material limitations. The small caliber of the arteries requires the use of small catheters (maximum 4F) to preserve vessel patency. This is essential to allow staged embolization and to ensure normal limb growth. Contrast material is a minor concern since the introduction of low osmotic or nonionic contrast media. However, injection of fluids should be carefully controlled and monitored to avoid systemic complications.

1.6 Conclusion

Embolization of vascular malformations, vascular tumors, and traumatic injuries has been definitively incorporated into the multidisciplinary therapeutic strategy for head and neck lesions. Clinical and anatomic knowledge of head and neck pathologies, as well as experience with embolization, is the basis for therapeutic success. Clinical knowledge will lead to adequate patient selection. Thorough anatomic knowledge and mastery of endovascular techniques will avoid predictable complications. Provided these conditions are met, embolization in the head and neck yields rewarding therapeutic and clinical results.

References

Alvarez H, Rodesch G, Garcia-Monaco R, Lasjaunias P (1990) Embolization of the ophthalmic artery branches distal to its visual supply. Surg Radiol Anat 12:293–297

Batsakis JG (1979) Tumors of the head and neck, clinical and pathological considerations, 2nd edn. Williams & Wilkins, Baltimore, pp 296–301

Boxt L, Lenin D, Fellows K (1983) Direct puncture angiography in congenital venous malformations AJR 140:135

Burrows P, Lasjaunias P, TerBrugge K, Flodmark O (1987) Urgent and emergent embolization of lesions of the head and neck in children: indication and results. Pediatrics 80:386–394

Garcia-Monaco R, Alvarez H, Lasjaunias P (1990) Utilization of the Minitorquer in cerebral arteriovenous malformations of the newborn and infants. Diagn Intervent Radiol 2:123–124

Garcia-Monaco R, de Victor D, Mann C, Hannedouche A, TerBrugge K, Lasjaunias P (1991) Congestive cardiac manifestations from cerebrocranial arteriovenous shunts. Endovascular management in 30 children. Childs Nerv Syst 7:48–52

Gonzalez C, Moret J (1990) Balloon occlusion of the carotid artery prior to surgery for neck tumors. AJNR 11:649–652

Lasjaunias P, Choi I (1986) The external carotid artery: functional anatomy. In: Taveras JM and Ferruci JT (eds) Radiology. Lippincott, Philadelphia, Chap 99, pp 1–7

Lasjaunias P, Berenstein A (1987a) Surgical neuroangiography, vol 1. Functional anatomy of craniofacial arteries. Springer, Berlin Heidelberg New York

Lasjaunias P, Berenstein A (1987b) Surgical neuroangiography, vol 2. Endovascular treatment of craniofacial lesions. Springer, Berlin Heidelberg New York

Lasjaunias P, Deffez JP, Fellus P, Huard JL, Franchi-Deffez I (1985) Les malformations vasculaires linguales, leurs conséquences sur la croissance de l'étage inférieur. Rev Stomatol Chir Maxillofac 86:99–102

Leikensohn U, Epsdein L, Vasquez L (1981) Superselective embolization and surgery of noninvoluting hemangiomas and A-V malformations. Plast Reconstr Surg 68:143

Mulliken JB, Glowacki J (1982) Hemangiomas and vascular malformations in infants and children: a classification based on endothelial characteristics. Plast Reconstr Surg 69:412–420

Mulliken B, Young A (1988) Vascular birthmarks: hemangiomas and malformations. Saunders, Philadelphia

Neidhart JA, Roach RW (1982) Successful treatment of skeletal hemangioma and Kasabach Merritt syndrome with aminocaproic acid; is fibrinolysis "defensive"? Am J Med 73:434–438

Ohi M, Sakakura Y, Nozaki S, Mitsui H, Yatani R, Moriwaki K (1979) Subglottic hemangioma: a case report and review of the literature. Mie Med J 2–3: 107–113

Pitanguy I, Cladeira AML, Calixto CA et al. (1984) Clinical evaluation and surgical treatment of hemangiomata. Head Neck Surg 7:47–59

Riche M, Hadjean E, Tran-Ba-Huy T, Merland J (1983) The treatment of capillary venous malformations using a new fibrosing agent. Plast Reconstr Surg 71:607–612

Thomson HG, Ward CM, Crawford JS, Stigmar G (1979) Hemangiomas of the eyelid: visual complications and prophylactic concepts. Plast Reconstr Surg 63:641–647

Valavanis A (1986) Preoperative embolization of the head and neck: indications, patient selection, goals and precautions. AJNR 7:943

2 Endovascular Management of Carotid Cavernous Fistulas

GERARD M. DEBRUN

CONTENTS

2.1 Classification of Carotid Cavernous Fistulas

The management of carotid cavernous fistulas (CCFs) depends on their physiopathology. The classification into traumatic and spontaneous CCFs is usually considered obsolete; it is, however, the first question that we ask when a patient with a CCF is referred to us. Knowing that a fistula is traumatic immediately tells us that we have a 95% chance of treating this fistula with a detachable balloon and with preservation of the carotid blood flow (CBF). Similarly, knowing that there is no history of trauma, one may conclude that a middle-aged patient with a red eye and a sixth nerve palsy probably has a spontaneous fistula of the dural type, while in the case of an older patient with this presentation one must consider the possibility of a ruptured preexisting cavernous aneurysm. Therefore, the age of the patient and the presence or absence of a history of trauma are important in the classification of CCFs.

With regard to therapy, however, the most important task is to classify the fistula as a fast flow or a slow flow fistula. The fast flow fistulas include the traumatic cases and the rare cases of ruptured cavernous aneurysms. The external carotid artery (ECA) is usually not involved in this type of fistula. The slow flow fistulas include most of the dural type CCFs. The ECA is almost always involved in this type of fistula, often from both sides, and the internal carotid artery (ICA) is frequently involved, at least on the ipsilateral side.

We will adhere to this classification throughout the chapter, referring to two types of CCF – type A and type B (DEBRUN et al. 1988b).

2.1.1 Type A CCFs

Type A CCFs are fast flow fistulas, which means that there is a sufficiently large tear between the ICA and the cavernous sinus (CS) to allow the passage of a balloon through the tear. The treatment for these fistulas consists in use of the detachable balloon technique, via the endarterial route. Other treatment modalities are considered only when the endarterial route fails. The ECA usually does not participate in the filling of the CS. As already mentioned, traumatic CCFs and ruptured cavernous aneurysms are type A CCFs.

2.1.2 Type B CCFs

Type B CCFs are slow flow fistulas. The communications between the ICA and the CS involve, when they exist, the small branches of the carotid siphon to the dura of the CS. They are too small to allow the passage of any type of balloon, with the consequence that this technique has no indication in most of these fistulas. It would in fact be an unacceptable mistake to occlude permanently the ICA with a balloon in this type of fistula. The potential risks of permanent occlusion of the ICA are unjustifiable in a disease which is usually benign, which has a substantial percentage of spontaneous cure, and which often involves both sides, simultaneously or sequentially.

GERARD M. DEBRUN, M.D., Professor of Radiology and Neurological Surgery, Director of Interventional Neuroradiology, Department of Radiology, Neuroradiological Section, The Johns Hopkins University Medical Institutions, Meyer Building #8-140, 600 North Wolfe Street, Baltimore, MD 21205, USA

The ECA is almost always involved in slow flow fistulas. According to the balance between the participation of the ECA and the ICA, three subgroups can be identified:

Type B1 involves only the ICA. It is exceptional. The relatively substantial number of these cases in certain reports is probably due to the fact that the cases in question were studied before the era of superselective catheterization of the ECA branches, causing the participation of the ECA to be overlooked.

Type B2 involves only the ECA branches. This type is relatively frequent and can be treated and cured with embolization of the ECA feeders only.

Type B3 involves both the ICA and the ECA. It is the most frequent type and represents 90% of the slow flow fistulas of the dural type. The treatment consists in embolizing the ECA feeders in the first stage. When the fistula is incompletely cured or recurs, the CS can be reached through the venous route, via either the inferior petrosal sinus (IPS) or the superior ophthalmic vein (SOV). The material used for embolization will typically be either solid particles or liquid polymerizing agents or coils but rarely detachable balloons introduced through the venous route (the IPS or SOV).

2.2 Traumatic Carotid Cavernous Fistulas

2.2.1 Clinical Presentation

Patients with traumatic CCFs develop an ipsilateral severe cavernous syndrome a few days or weeks after a major head injury. The fistula will rarely occur after a direct injury through the orbit or as a complication of rhizotomy, of transsphenoidal pituitary surgery, or of embolectomy of the carotid siphon with a Fogarty catheter (Eggers et al. 1979; Flandroy et al. 1988; Fuentes et al. 1985; Sekhar et al. 1979). It is amazing how often these fistulas are diagnosed late. The symptomatology is in fact obvious but is sometimes neglected among the multiple injuries that these patients suffer from their trauma. If it were standard practice to auscultate the eyes of patients who develop any ocular symptom after a trauma, CCFs would be detected early.

The proptosis and chemosis are usually impressive. The cranial nerves are frequently involved, the sixth more often than the third. The vision is preserved unless the optic nerve is damaged by a fracture of the optic canal. The ocular pressure has to be checked by a neuro-ophthalmologist and the treatment should be performed rapidly if the ocular pressure rises to more than 40 mmHg. Even when the ocular pressure remains lower, the arterialization of the orbital veins induces a hypertensive venous retinopathy which sooner or later will cause vision to deteriorate (Kupersmith et al. 1986).

2.2.2 Angiographic Workup

The angiographic workup (Figs. 2.1–2.4) must provide the following information:

- Status of the carotid bifurcation
- Existence or not of atheroma at the origin of the ICA
- Presence of a loop of the ICA below the base of the skull
- Size of the CS and its relation to the subarachnoid space and the sphenoid sinus
- Existence or not of a complete steal
- Type of venous drainage of the CS
- Presence or absence of cortical venous drainage
- Location of the fistula on the carotid siphon
- Quality of the circle of Willis
- Absence (in most cases) of ECA contribution

This information will be provided by performing:

- Ipsilateral common carotid angiography
- Ipsilateral internal carotid angiography
- Ipsilateral external carotid angiography
- Contralateral common carotid angiography; posteroanterior view of the arterial phase only with rectangular collimation over the orbits. This procedure typically can be carried out without ipsilateral compression of the ICA: such compression is reserved for cases in which there is no cross-flow through the anterior communicating artery
- Vertebral angiography (usually on the left side) with ipsilateral compression of the ICA. The lateral view is the most important one. It will show whether the posterior communicating artery is patent and will demonstrate the size and location of the fistula on the carotid siphon.

Let us analyze the aforementioned items of information (Figs. 2.1–2.4):

1. The status of the carotid bifurcation is of great importance for the strategy of the treatment via the endarterial route. Sometimes there is a

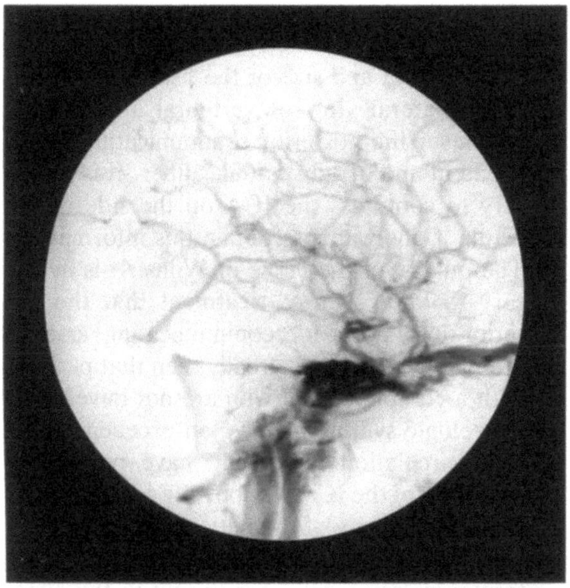

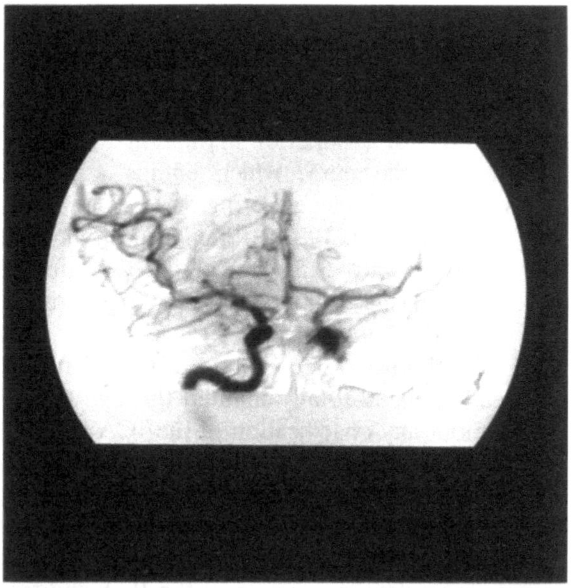

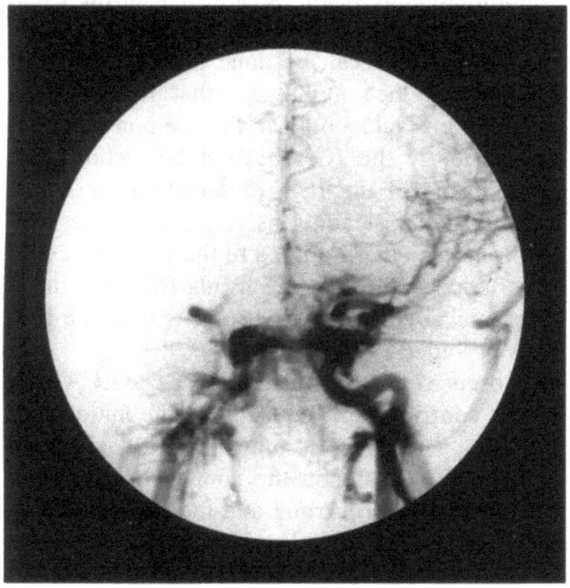

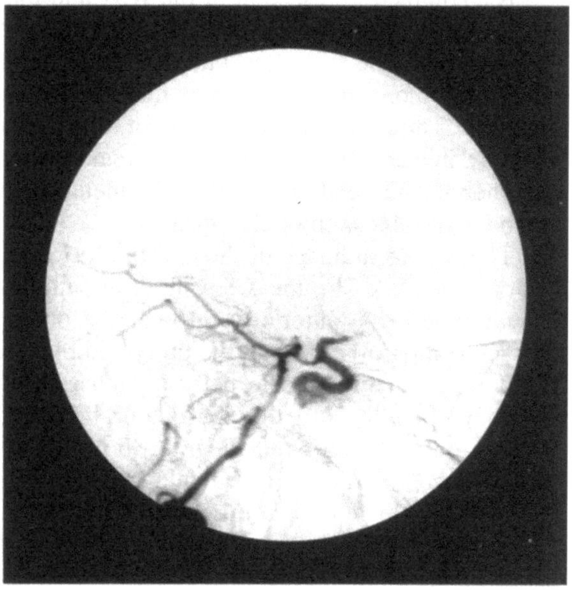

Fig. 2.1 (*upper left*). Angiography in a patient with traumatic CCF. Ipsilateral ICA – lateral view. Partial steal. There is massive and early filling of the CS, and it is impossible to localize the fistula precisely. Venous drainage is through the SOV, pterygoid plexus, and petrosal sinuses

Fig. 2.2 (*lower left*). Same case as in Fig. 2.1. Ipsilateral ICA – AP view. There is massive contralateral venous drainage with filling of both SOVs

Fig. 2.3 (*upper right*). Same case as in Figs. 2.1 and 2.2. Contralateral ICA – AP view. Good cross-flow is evident

Fig. 2.4 (*lower right*). Vertebral angiography. Lateral view, with ipsilateral compression of ICA. There is patency of the posterior communicating artery, retrograde filling of the ICA, and precise localization of the fistula

large bulb at the origin of the ICA which originates at right angles from the common carotid artery. Rather than trying to position an 8F or 9F straight guiding catheter into the ICA, it is wiser in such cases to keep the guiding catheter in the common carotid artery and to advance into the ICA with the balloon catheter only. A similar decision would be made if there were an ulcerated plaque of atheroma narrowing the origin of the ICA. Angioplasty or endarterectomy of the ICA could even be considered before treatment of the CCF. Also, when there is a double kink or a 360° loop of the ICA in the cervical portion, the guiding catheter must be positioned proximal to the kink or loop.

2. The size and shape of the CS: It is important to look for a superior herniation of the CS through the dura, which entails a risk of subarachnoid bleed (DOHRHANN et al. 1985; HALBACH et al. 1987b). Similarly, an anterior and downward extension of the CS into the sphenoid sinus can induce a catastrophic bleed into the nasopharynx.
3. The existence of a complete steal: It is rare to see the blood totally shunted through the CS without any opacification of the ICA distal to the fistula. Such a steal has three major implications. First, it means that a neurologically asymptomatic patient has an excellent circle of Willis. Second, it does not mean that there is a complete transection of the ICA and that the ICA cannot be preserved. At the time of treatment one will often find that these cases are no more difficult to treat than any other case. Third, the acute closure of the fistula may induce a normal pressure breakthrough phenomenon and staging the treatment might be wise (HALBACH et al. 1987a).
4. The venous drainage of the CS: In most cases of type A CCF, the CS will drain into its multiple exits, anteriorly through the orbital veins, inferiorly through the pterygoid plexus, posteriorly through the petrosal sinuses, and contralaterally into the contralateral CS (on the anteroposterior angiogram both SOVs are frequently seen to be filling). The only nonphysiologic drainage is upstream into the sylvian and cortical veins. Any venous cortical drainage should be considered as increasing the risk of subarachnoid bleed. The venous drainage may be strongly predominant. For example, an almost exclusive anterior venous drainage through the orbital veins increases the ocular pressure and the risk of monocular blindness. However, the facial vein can be a major channel of drainage of the orbital veins and such cases may present with minimal ocular symptoms. The predominant posterior venous drainage through the petrosal sinuses can be an indication for performing the treatment through the jugular vein and IPS. However, this venous approach is more attractive in the case of slow flow fistulas of the dural type, where coils can be used, than in the fast flow fistulas, where the tear is too large and balloons should be used. It is easier to advance coils into the IPS than balloons.
5. The location and size of the fistula are shown in the lateral view of vertebral angiography whenever the posterior communicating artery is patent and of substantial caliber. It is necessary to compress the ICA on the side of the fistula if one wants to obtain this information.
6. The quality of the circle of Willis: It is necessary to know before treatment that the anterior and posterior communicating arteries are patent. We have already seen that patients with a complete steal who are not developing neurologic symptoms have an excellent collateral circulation and could have permanent occlusion of the ICA without any complication. But the majority of the patients have a partial steal and we do not know whether the collateral circulation will be sufficient in the event of complete occlusion of the ICA. A balloon occlusion test can be done during treatment. It should be emphasized that this test will have any value only if the balloon occludes transiently the ICA beyond the fistula. The occlusion of the ICA proximal to the fistula could be misleading as it could induce symptoms which are related to the fact that a steal is induced through the fistula from the intracranial circulation at the same time as the ICA is occluded.
7. Absence of ECA contributions: The ECA does not contribute to the fistula in the majority of cases. However, it may be involved if the trauma has opened the connections between the inferolateral trunk and the internal maxillary artery. In cases in which the ICA has been trapped surgically many years previously, the ECA is almost always involved.

2.2.3 *Treatment*

2.2.3.1 *Endarterial Route*

The treatment for traumatic fast flow CCFs consists in inflating a balloon into the CS, which closes the fistula and preserves the CBF. This can be achieved through the endarterial route in the majority of cases. The venous route will be used in selected cases or when the arterial route has failed. The detachable balloon technique has been used for more than 16 years (SERBINENKO 1974) (DEBRUN et al. 1988b; HIGASHIDA et al. 1989).

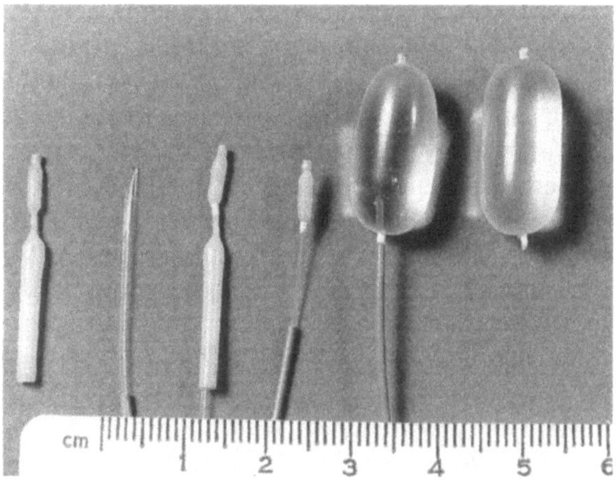

Fig. 2.5. Latex balloon tied and detached

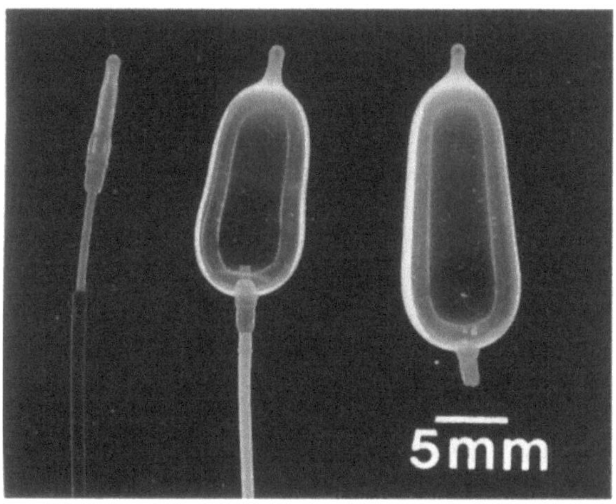

Fig. 2.6. Built-in valve latex balloon before and after detachment

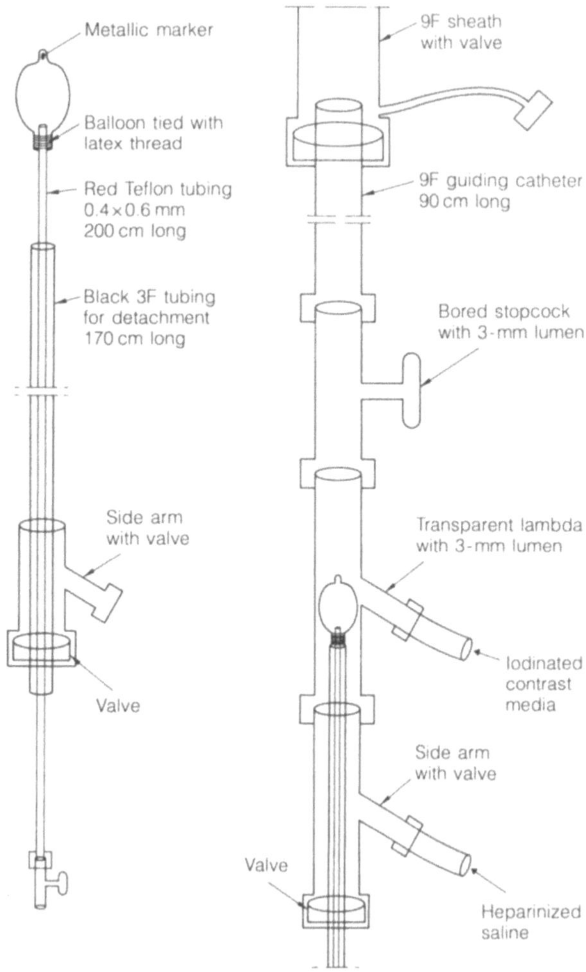

Fig. 2.7. *Left*: Latex tied balloon over a Teflon microcatheter with a coaxial polyethylene 3F catheter. *Right*: Coaxial detachable balloon catheter system through the 9F guiding catheter and 9F sheath with complete connection of accessories

There are now several types of detachable balloon on the market (Nycomed/Ingenor, Balt, ITC, Taki et al.; however, there is no ideal balloon which is totally safe. We have to understand that there is a compromise between a balloon strongly tied over the catheter, impossible to lose prematurely but difficult to detach, and a balloon lightly tied over the catheter, which will be easy to detach but will risk being lost prematurely. There are also latex and Silastic balloons. All Silastic balloons have a semipermeable membrane and a valve mechanism. Latex balloons are not permeable membrane balloons and can be either ligated with a latex thread over the catheter (strongly tied balloon) (Fig. 2.5) or purchased sterile and ready for use with a valve mechanism (Fig. 2.6). I prefer the strongly tied balloon that I ligate myself with a latex thread. The safety of the procedure is increased with this type of balloon. Certain people who are afraid of premature detachment of a built-in valve balloon have advised performing the treatment with a second balloon blocking the ICA transiently until the detachable balloon is inflated in good position in the CS.

The balloon catheter has to be advanced through a guiding catheter positioned in the cervical portion of the ICA (Fig. 2.7).

As large balloons sometimes need to be used, it is wise to position a 9F sheath in the femoral artery and to use a 9F guiding catheter. This catheter is straight or slightly bent at the tip. The quickest way to position it is to catheterize the

ICA with standard technique, to maintain an exchange guide in the ICA, and to advance the double 9F and 6F coaxial guiding catheters over the guide. The 6F catheter and the exchange guide are removed when the tip of the 9F catheter has reached the ICA. A tortuous ICA or severe atheromatous stenosis will preclude this maneuver and will increase the difficulties of the treatment as the guiding catheter will be positioned in the common carotid artery.

The latex balloons that I use for treatment are available in different sizes and capacities. They are designated by arbitrary numbers. The three most used are numbers 9, 12, and 16. The number 9 has a maximum capacity of 1 ml and an inflated size of 7 × 15 mm to 8 × 20 mm. The number 12 is the largest, with a maximum capacity of 2 ml and a size of 15 × 20–25 mm. The number 16 has a sausage form with a maximum capacity of 0.6 ml and a size of 5 mm × 20 mm. These balloons have a metallic marker in the tip (numbers 9 and 16) or inside the balloon (number 12). They are available (Nycomed/Ingenor) either without or with a built-in valve. I use those that I tie myself with a latex thread (12–14 half turns followed by three knots) over a red Teflon tubing of 0.4 inner × 0.6 outer diameter. This 2F tubing slides inside a 3F black polyethylene tubing which will be used for detachment of the balloon (Fig. 2.7). The black coaxial catheter is maintained inside the 9F guiding catheter until the balloon is ready to be detached. The red Teflon tubing is advanced with a slow pushing motion and the balloon slightly inflated whenever it stops advancing. The balloon is positioned at the estimated location of the fistula. It vibrates. It is inflated and a sudden change is seen in the position of the balloon, indicating that it has been sucked into the CS. The balloon is inflated to half its capacity and digital subtraction angiography performed. If the fistula is not closed, the balloon is inflated until total closure is achieved. If the balloon projects over the carotid siphon, one should check, by means of an orthogonal view, that the balloon is in the CS. It would be a mistake to detach a balloon which occludes the fistula but is still in the carotid siphon, because the balloon would not stay in this position after detachment; rather it would migrate and occlude the ICA termination. When it is considered that the balloon is in a good position in the CS, with the fistula totally closed and the CBF preserved, one gently pulls the red Teflon tubing and advances the black coaxial catheter until it reaches the balloon. During this procedure, permanent tension must be exerted on the red Teflon tubing, but the tension is reduced slightly when some friction of the black coaxial catheter is felt at the level of a curve of the ICA. This maneuver is delicate and needs experience. After detachment of the balloon, biplane angiography confirms the quality of the result. Probably 60% of traumatic CCFs can be effectively and easily treated by use of one balloon. However, the following technical problems require the strategy to be altered:

1. The balloon does not occlude the fistula when it is inflated to its maximum capacity. This happens when the CS is very large or when the tear of the fistula is large. Under these circumstances a larger balloon, a #12 balloon, may be tried. If the same thing happens, the first balloon should be detached and a second #12 balloon tried. If the fistula is not closed with the second large balloon, as many balloons as necessary should be detached until the fistula is closed. However, there is a risk that the last balloon will protrude through the fistula and stenose the ICA. If one considers that the CBF cannot be safely preserved, the decision may be taken to occlude the carotid artery permanently. In this scenario, one has to be sure that the carotid artery is trapped distal and proximal to the fistula. This can be achieved only if the patient has a good collateral circulation and tolerates the permanent occlusion of the ICA. The result ultimately will be excellent. In case treated with multiple balloons and preservation of CBF, the immediate follow-up can be complicated by severe transient pain and oculomotor nerve palsies as the CS will have been packed with multiple balloons. This situation occurs rarely but when it does, there is no option other than to occlude the ICA permanently. The venous route would not allow a better result as the last balloon would also protrude into the carotid siphon, and the CS is too large to be packed with anything other than balloons.
2. The fistula is closed with one balloon but the ICA is stenosed. Eventually, the CBF is completely interrupted when the fistula is totally closed. One may try using the largest balloon (#12) to see whether the CBF is thereby better preserved. If it is not, one again faces the choice of closing the fistula totally and occlu-

ding the ICA or of slightly deflating the balloon until the CBF is again restored. It is amazing that a few hundredths of a milliliter of inflation of the balloon can totally occlude the flow or restore it. Therefore one may choose to detach the balloon, knowing that the fistula is incompletely but almost totally closed. In this situation, the patient is followed up clinically. If the ocular symptoms subside rapidly and if no bruit is heard over the eye, the fistula has probably closed completely. This must be confirmed by angiography before the patient is discharged. If the patient remains symptomatic and if the bruit is still heard over the eye, a second treatment is necessary. It is, however, wise to wait 1 or 2 weeks. The first balloon will then probably have deflated a little, increasing the chances of entering the CS with a second balloon. If the procedure fails, other treatments should be considered before the ICA is permanently occluded.

3. The balloon does not enter the CS. The red Teflon tubing has some stiffness, and it can be softened by elongating it a little over its last 5 cm until it becomes 7 cm long. It must also be checked that the Teflon tubing has been pulled from inside the balloon as much as it can be. One can also try to deflate the balloon as much as possible when it is at the level of the fistula, as if wishing to create a vacuum (with a large Luer-Lok syringe of 50 ml). Sometimes, slightly inflating the balloon just distal to the fistula will cause the base of the balloon (which inflates first) to be sucked into the CS. Finally, if all these tricks fail, a smaller balloon should be tried. However, occasionally the tear is very small and no balloon will enter the CS (Fig. 2.8). In such instances other treatments via the venous route must be considered.
4. One or several balloons have been detached into the CS but the fistula is still not closed and the next balloon that one tries to position in the CS will not enter it because of the presence of the other balloons. Under such circumstances it is wise to abandon the procedure and to carry out a second treatment 1–2 weeks later.
5. The result looks perfect immediately after detachment of the balloon and there is no longer a bruit over the eye, but several hours later or on the next day the bruit is again heard. This may be because the balloon has deflated faster than it should (normally a balloon keeps the same volume for days), with partial reopening of the fistula. Alternatively the balloon may have been slightly underinflated and not strongly anchored into the CS by its partitions, causing the balloon to move slightly and the fistula to reopen. When this happens, a second treatment is necessary.
6. It may happen that the CCF is secondary to the tear of a persistant trigeminal artery (Debrun 1988a). Every effort should be made to enter the trigeminal artery with the balloon which is the best way to preserve the CBF. This is achieved after controlling that the vertebrobasilar circulation is preserved as well.

2.2.3.2 *Venous Route* (Debrun et al. 1989; Dowd et al. 1991; Halbach et al. 1988)

The chief indications for the venous route are (a) failure of the endarterial route and (b) previous trapping of the ICA, precluding access to it. Even in this latter situation, an attempt may be made to puncture the ICA above the point of ligation or clampage. One may also request the neurosurgeon to reanastomose the ICA in the neck. I think, however, that this surgical step should be kept as a last resort for the eventuality that the venous route proves unsuccessful. Another good indication for the venous route is exclusive venous drainage through the IPS.

The CS can be reached through the IPS, the SOV, or after surgical exposure. The tremendous improvements in our skill in reaching the CS via the venous approach have reduced the indications for surgical exposure of the CS to anecdotal cases.

2.2.3.3 *The IPS Approach*

It has already been mentioned that it is difficult to advance a detachable balloon catheter into the IPS and to reach the compartment of the CS which is in direct contact with the fistula. Great care should be taken not to occlude the posterior exit of the CS without also occluding the fistula. This could redirect the drainage of the CS toward the SOV and suddenly increase the ocular symptoms, prompting treatment through the SOV. It is much easier to reach the CS with a microcatheter without a detachable balloon at the tip. However, this type of fast flow fistula with a large CS cannot be treated with coils in the majority of cases. The

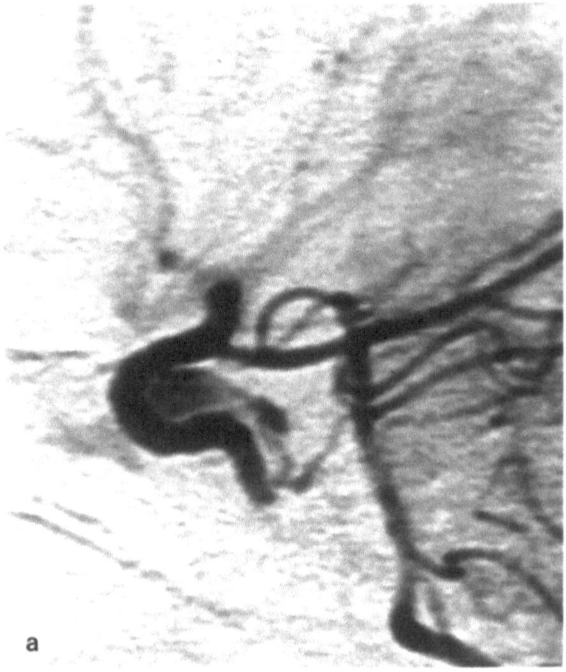

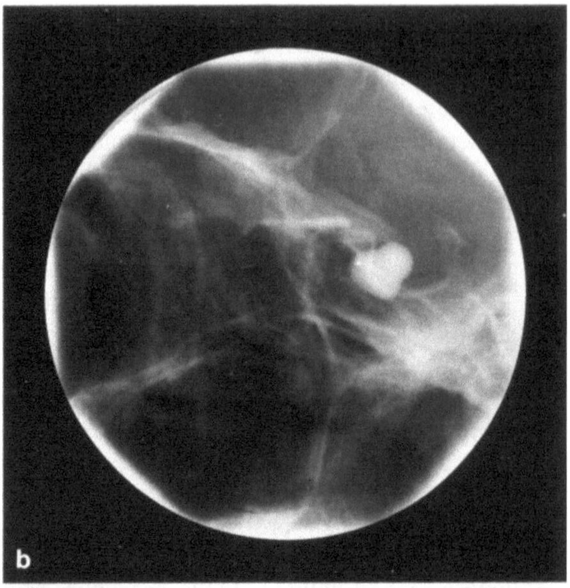

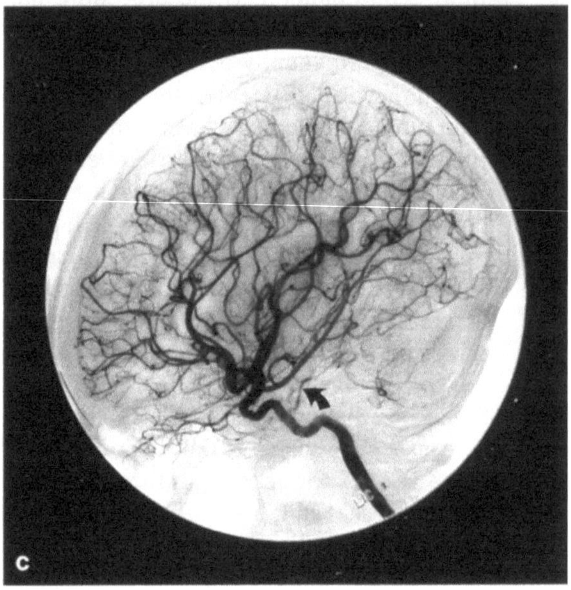

Fig. 2.8. **a** Traumatic CCF with a small tear which could not be catheterized with any balloon or microcatheter. No venous drainage into the IPS. Surgical exposure of the SOV was carried out and one balloon was detached into the CS (**b**) with complete cure. **c** Note that the access to the fistula was filling a cerebellar artery which was preserved by treatment (*arrow*)

injection of liquid polymerizing substance into the CS is risky and should be reserved for exceptional cases in which any other safe technique has failed or is not usable.

Injection of a liquid agent has the potential risk of reflux into the orbital veins, inducing extensive venous thrombosis and consequently monocular blindness. Also, the possibility of reflux of a liquid agent into the ICA through the tear of the fistula with catastrophic embolization of the middle cerebral artery territory should always be kept in mind. The risk can be decreased by inflating a balloon into the carotid siphon, when it is accessible by the endarterial route, at the level of the tear during the injection of a polymerizing substance.

2.2.3.4 Embolization Through the SOV

The SOV approach is a good way to reach the CS with a detachable balloon when the arterial route and the IPS route have failed. Cases have been reported in the literature (Teng et al. 1988) in which the SOV was punctured percutaneously at the medial angle of the orbit, or could be reached from the femoral vein through the external jugular vein and facial vein. However, most of these cases have been slow flow fistulas of the dural type and the SOV was catheterized with a microcatheter, allowing delivery of coils or liquid polymerizing agent but not a balloon. The percutaneous puncture of the SOV and the introduction of a catheter large enough to allow passage of detachable balloons does not seem to be safe and to give total control of any bleed which could occur. Therefore I prefer to expose the SOV surgically. This is done by our team comprising a vascular neurosurgeon and a neuro-ophthalmologist (DEBRUN et al. 1989; HANNEKEN et al. 1989). A meticulous and tedious microdissection of the vein allows the placing of two vessel loops around the SOV. This gives total control of the bleed through the small venotomy, which allows the balloon catheter to pass. This is done in the operating room with a C-arm and DSA equipment. A radiotransparent table permits the positioning of a catheter in the cerebral vessel at the same time through the femoral artery, enabling one to check whether the balloon inflated into the CS has closed the fistula before it is detached.

I have used the SOV approach in eight patients; in all eight the results have been excellent, without complications. Only two of these cases were traumatic CCFs: One of these was a CCF previously treated with surgical trapping of the ICA, without access to the CS through the IPS. The second case was one in which it was not possible to enter the CS with any balloon or microcatheter (Fig. 2.8).

2.2.4 Results of Treatment

I have personally been involved in the treatment of more than 150 traumatic CCFs. The endarterial route was used in 94% of the cases and the venous route in 6%. Preservation of the CBF was achieved in about 60% of the first 40 patients but is now achieved in 95% of cases (Fig. 2.9).

The cosmetic result is excellent in most cases. The proptosis and chemosis subside within a few weeks after complete closure of the fistula. The oculomotor nerve palsies that existed before treatment may take several weeks or months to subside. Those which occur in the hours or days following treatment are due to the compression of the nerves by the balloon. They almost invariably subside without permanent sequelae, even if their frequency can be as high as 30%. Angiography

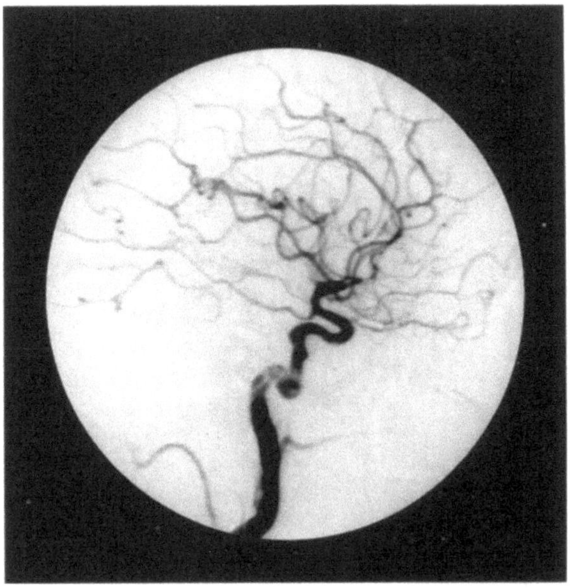

Fig. 2.9. Excellent result 6 months following treatment with one balloon. CBF is preserved, with a normal looking ICA

should be performed in every case between 3 and 6 months following treatment, even if the patient is asymptomatic. If I had not systematically controlled most of the cases that I treated, I would never have been able to demonstrate the frequency of "herniation" of the ICA into the CS at the level of the fistula. These venous pouches or pseudoaneurysms are frequent but remain asymptomatic in the majority of the cases (Fig. 2.10). A few patients have developed a large venous pouch a few days after treatment but they have been symptomatic at this time. All such patients have complained of severe trigeminal pain. The pulsations of arterial blood induced to this pouch are probably responsible for the fifth nerve neuralgia because the pain subsides very quickly after the closure of the pouch with a new detachable balloon or after permanent occlusion of the ICA when it was impossible to preserve the flow.

The mortality is extremely low. There have been only two deaths in this series which were directly related to a complication resulting from the treatment itself. In one case, the balloon was closing the fistula and was narrowing the ICA. Secondary thrombosis of the ICA was accompanied by a middle cerebral artery infarction and the patient finally died from iatrogenic complications in the intensive care unit. The second case was an 85-year-old woman who needed

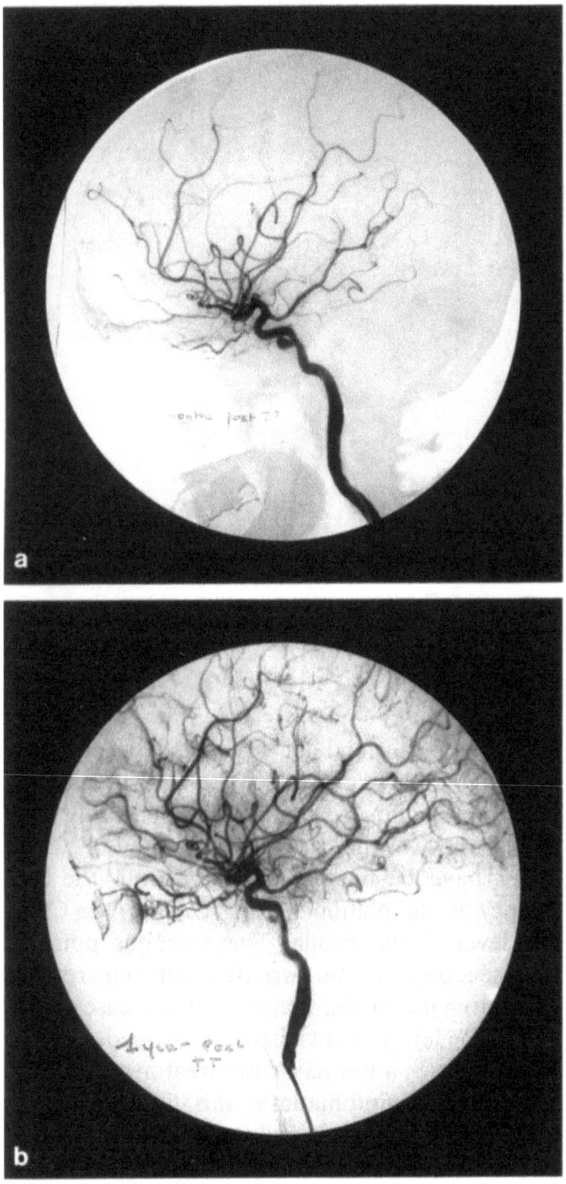

Fig. 2.10. a Venous pouch 3 months following treatment of a traumatic CCF. **b** Patient still asymptomatic 1 year later. The pouch is smaller

intracranial surgical ligation of the ICA and died several weeks later of a subdural empyema.

The morbidity is also low and should be kept lower than 5%. Technical problems related to the use of the detachable balloon technique are now exceptional. It is again necessary to emphasize that this rate can be different if other types of detachable balloon are used.

For example, I have never experienced premature balloon detachment during treatment of a CCF. Premature deflation or rupture of the balloon has occurred into the CS on a few occasions, but without any consequences.

Permanent occlusion of the ICA cannot be avoided in a small number of cases. The clinical outcome will be excellent in most cases, but one must be aware of the potential risk of complete occlusion of the ICA without complete closure of the fistula or with secondary reopening of the fistula.

Under these circumstances a patient who is old or has a borderline circle of Willis may become symptomatic as the fistula now steals blood from the circle of Willis and decompensates a precarious cerebral blood flow. Such patients have to be treated acutely and usually will need intracranial clipping of the ICA below the ophthalmic artery or clipping of the ICA and ligation of the origin of the ophthalmic artery. This does not entail a risk of monocular blindness as the external carotid circulation will take over the ophthalmic arterial supply. I have also treated one similar case in which I was able to navigate through the vertebral artery, posterior communicating artery, and ICA until I reached the remaining active fistula, which I closed with coils (Garcia-Cervigon et al. 1988).

I have not experienced any thromboembolic complications since I treat all patients under systemic heparinization with a bolus of 5000 units and an injection of 1000 units every hour, plus the amount of heparinized saline infused during the procedure. Most of the patients thus receive 7000–10000 units of heparin during the procedure, the heparinization being reversed by protamine sulfate before the sheath is removed from the groin. At this point it is appropriate to mention that the majority of these patients are now treated through the femoral artery. There are, however, exceptional cases where the tortuosity of the aortic arch and great vessels precludes easy placement of straight 8F or 9F tubing into the ICA. It is therefore necessary to be familiar with direct puncture of the carotid artery in the neck and positioning of an 8F sheath in the ICA. Experience and training are necessary to avoid any dissection or major damage to the ICA in advancing the dilator and sheath over the guide wire through the arterial wall of the carotid artery. This has to be done under fluoroscopic guidance. The introduction of the dilator into the artery over the guide wire is only safe if the puncture has been done obliquely. There is great risk of damage if the needle was at a 90° angle and if the guide wire is kinked (Fig. 2.11).

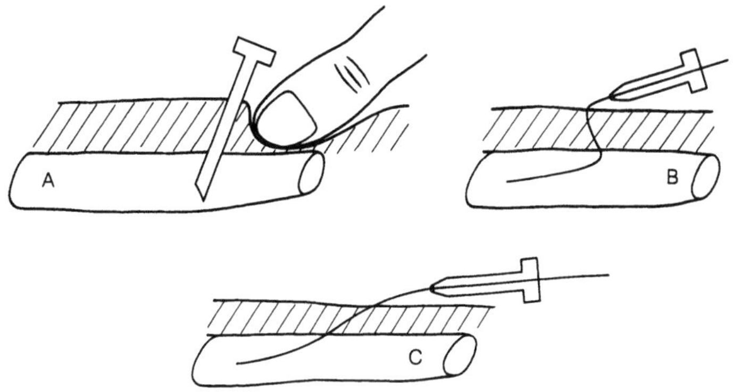

Fig. 2.11 A–C. Direct puncture of the carotid artery in the neck: risks of damage to the carotid artery when advancing the dilator with the sheath. **A** The finger of the operator depresses and stretches the soft tissues. If the needle is too perpendicular to the artery, as here, the guide wire usually can be introduced but, **B** after withdrawal of the needle the soft tissues return to their baseline position and the guide wire makes a zig-zag. The dilator will not perforate the artery but will increase the kink of the guide wire. **C** Good oblique position of the guide wire allowing safe advancement of the dilator and sheath

I would like to conclude by emphasizing that the detachable balloon technique is the ideal way to treat a traumatic CCF. The principle looks so easy and so elegant that it will seem pretentious to say that it is in fact a technique which should be concentrated in a few centers. The infinite multiplication of centers which consider that their reputation justifies the execution of interventional procedures has in fact increased the number of major complications associated with the technique. If it is true that approximately 50% of traumatic CCFs can be easily closed with one balloon, it is also true that 50% of them are difficult cases, in which lack of experience of the therapist will put the patient at risk.

The management of type B indirect slow flow fistulas is developed in Dr. HALBACH's chapter on treatment of dural AVMs (Chap. 3).

References

Debrun GM, Davis KR, Nauta HJ, Heros RE, Ahn HS (1988a) Treatment of carotid cavernous fistulae or cavernous aneurysms associated with a persistent trigeminal artery: report of three cases. AJNR 9: 749–755

Debrun GM, Vinuela F, Fox AJ, Davis KR, Ahn HS (1988b) Indications for treatment and classification of 132 carotid-cavernous fistulas. Neurosurgery 22: 285–289

Debrun GM, Nauta HJ, Miller NR, Drake CG, Heros RC, Ahn HS (1989) Combining the detachable balloon technique and surgery in imaging carotid cavernous fistulae. Surg Neurol 32:3–10

Dohrmann PJ, Batjer HH, Samson D, Suss RA (1985) Recurrent subarachnoid hemorrhage complicating a traumatic carotid-cavernous fistula. Neurosurgery 17: 480–483

Dowd CF, Halbach VV, Higashida RT, Barnwell SL, Hieshima GB (1991) Occlusion of the anterior superior ophthalmic vein in carotid-cavernous fistulae acutely aggravating visual symptoms. Neuroradiology [Suppl] 33:142–143

Eggers F, Lukin R, Chambers AA, Tomsick TA, Sawaya R (1979) Iatrogenic carotid-cavernous fistula following Fogarty catheter thromboendarterectomy. Case report. J Neurosurg 51:543–545

Flandroy P, Lenelle J, Collignon J, Stevenaert A (1988) Carotid cavernous fistula associated with Fogarty catheter angioplasty. AJNR 9:1242–1242

Fuentes JM, Benezech J, Joyeux A, Vlahovitch B, Thevenet A, Vavdin F (1985) Iatrogenic carotid-cavernous fistulas, complications of carotid thrombectomy. Neurochirurgie 31:265–270

Garcia-Cervigon E, Bien S, Laurent A, Weitzner I, Jr, Biondi A, Merland JJ (1988) Treatment of a recurrent traumatic carotid-cavernous fistula: vertebro-basilar approach after surgical occlusion of the internal carotid artery. Neuroradiology 30:355–357

Halbach VV, Higashida RT, Hieshima GB, Norman D (1987a) Normal perfusion pressure breakthrough occurring during treatment of carotid and vertebral fistulas. AJNR 8:751–756

Halbach VV, Hieshima GB, Higashida RT, Reicher M (1987b) Carotid cavernous fistulae: indications for urgent treatment. AJR 149:587–593

Halbach VV, Higashida RT, Hieshima GB, Hardin CW, Yang PJ (1988) Transvenous embolization of direct carotid cavernous fistulas. AJNR 9:741–747

Hanneken AM, Miller NR, Debrun GM, Nauta HJ (1989) Treatment of carotid cavernous sinus fistulas using a detachable balloon catheter through the superior ophthalmic vein. Arch Ophthalmol 107:87–92

Higashida RT, Halbach VV, Tsai FY, Norman D, Pribram HF, Mehringer CM, Hieshima GB (1989) Interventional neurovascular treatment of traumatic carotid and vertebral artery lesions: results in 234 cases. AJR 153:577–582

Kupersmith MJ, Berenstein A, Flamm E, Ransohoff J (1986) Neuro-ophthalmologic abnormalities and intravascular therapy of traumatic carotid cavernous fistulas. Ophthalmology 93:906–912

Sekhar LN, Heros RC, Kerber CW (1979) Carotid-cavernous fistula following percutaneous retrogasserian procedures. Report of two cases. J Neurosurg 51:700–706

Serbinenko FA (1974) Balloon catheterization and occlusion of major cerebral vessels. J Neurosurg 41:125–145

Taki W, Handa H, Miyake H, Kobayashi A, Yonekawa Y, Yamamura K, Suzuki M, Ikada Y (1985) New detachable balloon technique for traumatic carotid cavernous sinus fistulae. AJNR 6:961–964

Teng MM, Guo WY, Huang CI, Wu CC, Chang T (1988) Occlusion of arteriovenous malformations of the cavernous sinus via the superior ophthalmic vein. AJNR 9:539–546

3 Embolization of Dural Arteriovenous Malformations

VAN V. HALBACH

CONTENTS

3.1 Introduction

Dural arteriovenous malformations (DAVMs) are foci of arteriovenous shunting that occur within the dura mater, most often located in the wall of a dural sinus or where a major draining vein enters a dural sinus. Earlier investigators suggested that these arteriovenous shunts were developmental, thereby popularizing the term dural arteriovenous *malformation*. Recent evidence has documented, however, that this disease is often acquired from a dural sinus thrombosis or traumatic etiology (HOUSER et al. 1979; CHAUDHARY et al. 1982; PICARD et al. 1987). The term *fistulas* (or *fistulae*) implies an acquired etiology usually involving multiple connections and therefore has increasingly been used to describe these dural arteriovenous shunts. Dural arteriovenous fistulas (DAVFs) are subclassified usually by the location of the involved dural sinus (e.g., cavernous DAVF) or the location of the arteriovenous shunting (e.g., ethmoidal groove DAVF).

VAN V. HALBACH, M.D., Associate Professor of Radiology and Neurological Surgery, Neurointerventional Radiology Section, Department of Radiology, University of California, 505 Parnassus Avenue, San Francisco, CA 94143-0628, USA

3.2 Transverse and Sigmoid Sinus Dural Arteriovenous Fistulas

3.2.1 Pathophysiology and Clinical Presentation

The transverse and sigmoid sinuses are the most common locations for dural fistulas (PICARD et al. 1987). These fistulas have been reported to occur following trauma, especially associated with a linear fracture traversing the course of the lateral sinuses. Additional associations have been reported following surgical procedures and in patients with hereditary hemorrhagic telangiectasia. However, the vast majority of patients with DAVFs in this location have no history of trauma, surgery, infection, or vascular disease. HOUSER et al. (1979) and CHAUDHARY et al. (1982) reported four cases where acquired dural sinus thrombosis promoted the development of a DAVF at the site of the thrombosis. They suggested that dural sinus thrombosis is the inciting event that either enlarges normally present microscopic shunts in the wall of the sinus or, through an undisclosed angiogenesis factor, promotes the development of these shunts.

The clinical symptoms related to dural fistulas located in the lateral sinuses depend on the direction and adequacy of venous drainage pathways, the amount of arteriovenous shunting, and the location of the fistula, particularly in reference to the proximity to the middle ear apparatus. Small fistulas or fistulas located near the occiput without cortical drainage may be entirely without clinical

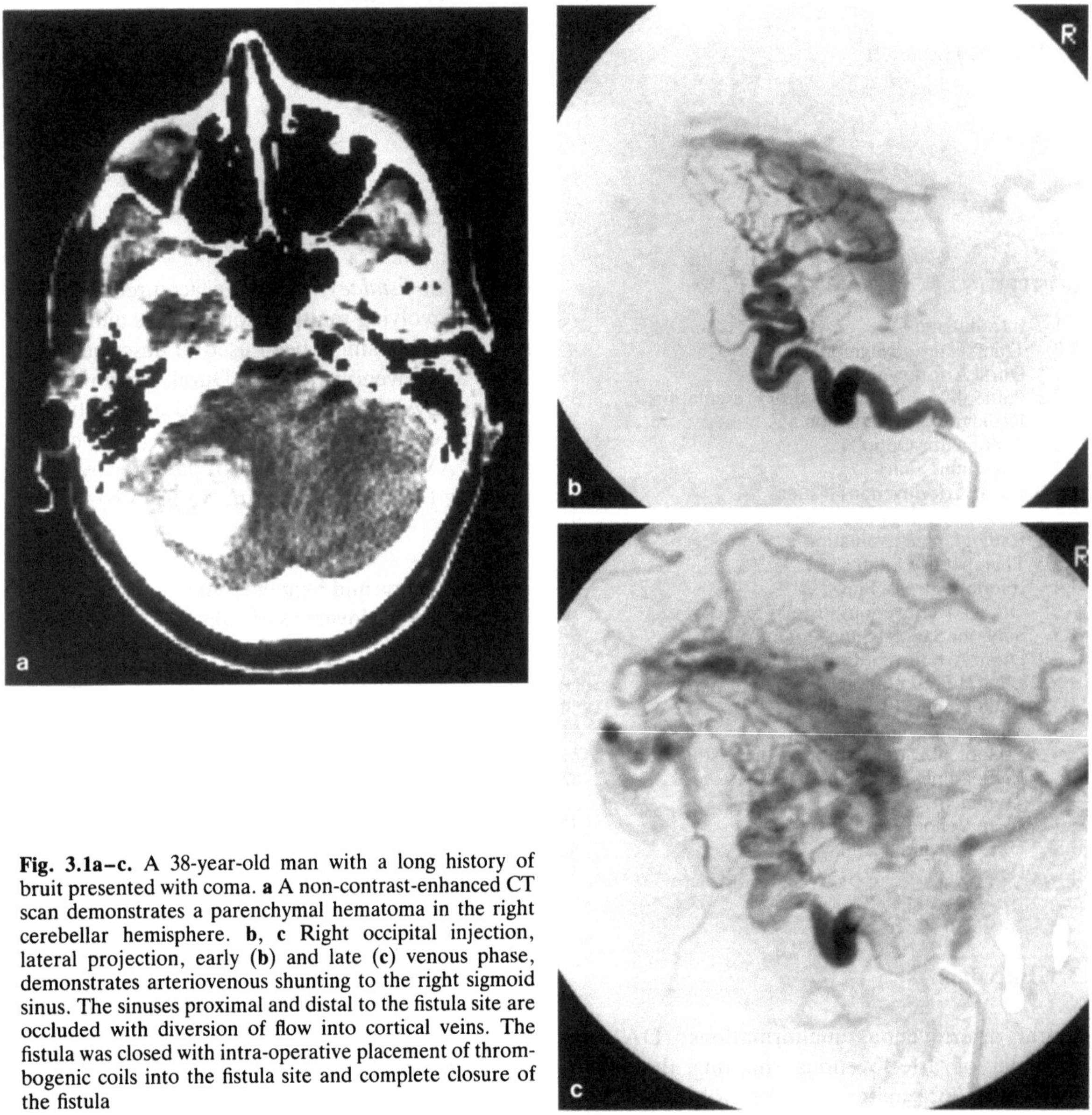

Fig. 3.1a–c. A 38-year-old man with a long history of bruit presented with coma. **a** A non-contrast-enhanced CT scan demonstrates a parenchymal hematoma in the right cerebellar hemisphere. **b**, **c** Right occipital injection, lateral projection, early (**b**) and late (**c**) venous phase, demonstrates arteriovenous shunting to the right sigmoid sinus. The sinuses proximal and distal to the fistula site are occluded with diversion of flow into cortical veins. The fistula was closed with intra-operative placement of thrombogenic coils into the fistula site and complete closure of the fistula

symptoms (Aminoff and Kendall 1973). One of the most common presenting symptoms is headache which can be aggravated by changes in head elevation, physical activity, or stress. Presumably these headaches are related to distention of the dural sinus or engorgement of venous collaterals, both of which are highly innervated structures. A pulse synchronous bruit is a commonly associated symptom, often high in pitch and aggravated by physical activity and positional changes. The turbulent flow through the arteriovenous shunt produces the pulse synchronous bruit which generally can be auscultated by a stethoscope positioned over the lateral sinus. Gentle compression of the jugular vein ipsilateral to the bruit usually produces only minimal changes in the character of the bruit. Digital compression of the common carotid artery ipsilateral to the bruit (Matas maneuver) may produce reduction or obliteration of the bruit. Similarly, digital compression of the occipital artery behind the mastoid may reduce or obliterate the fistula, particularly in dural fistulas located near the occiput or involving the transverse sinus. The bruit may change spontaneously in pitch. Diminution of the intensity of the bruit with increase in pitch is often associated with spontaneous closure of the fistulous site. However, similar findings can occur with pro-

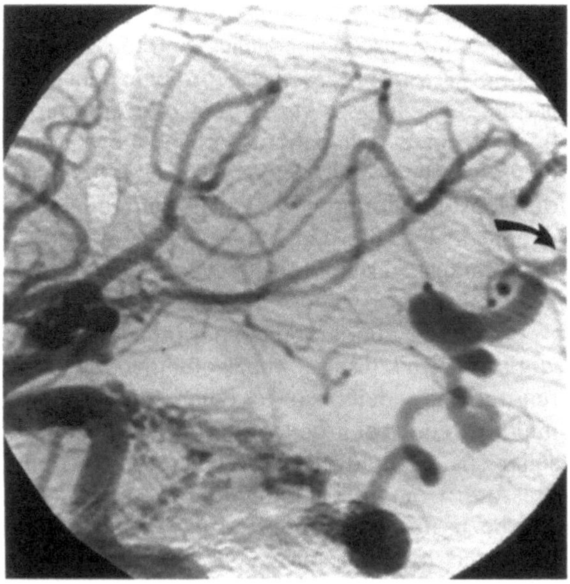

Fig. 3.2. A 59-year-old man presented with four episodes of subarachnoid hemorrhage within a 2-week period. Left internal carotid injection, lateral projection, demonstrates a DAVF located in the tentorium supplied by the meningohypophysial trunk. The venous drainage is by way of a cortical vein with a high-grade stenosis in the vein of Galen, where it enters the straight sinus, illustrated by a *curved arrow*

gressive narrowing and occlusion of the recipient dural sinus and alteration of the venous drainage to cortical venous structures. Cortical venous drainage or diversion of the arterialized blood towards the cerebral vasculature is an ominous finding and is often associated with intensification of headaches and production of both transient and permanent neurologic deficits. Therefore, any change in a patient's clinical symptoms, even reduction in the intensity of the bruit, should prompt repeat angiographic investigation looking for this ominous finding. Cortical venous drainage is associated with a high incidence of intradural hemorrhage, either subdural, subarachnoid, or intraparenchymal. Figure 3.1 is an example of a sigmoid sinus dural fistula with cortical drainage only that presented with a life-threatening posterior fossa hemorrhage. Repeated hemorrhages may occur in rapid succession (HALBACH et al. 1987c; ISHII et al. 1988; VINUELA et al. 1986; LASJAUNIAS et al. 1986). Figure 3.2 pertains to a patient who suffered four separate intraventricular hemorrhages in a 2-week period.

Neurologic deficits resulting from transverse and sigmoid dural AVFs are usually associated with cortical venous drainage. The primary mechanism for producing these deficits is by venous hypertension, venous infarction, or intradural hemorrhage (LASJAUNIAS 1986). Diffuse dural sinus hypertension can impair the reabsorption of cerebrospinal fluid, producing papilledema and/or a dementia-like picture. Rarely a varix or venous aneurysm in an arterialized draining vein can mechanically compress neural tissue, producing a deficit (VINUELA et al. 1986). Seizures can accompany this disease due to focal or diffuse neuronal dysfunction.

3.2.2 Radiographic Evaluation

Selective and superselective arteriography remain the gold standard for detection and characterization of dural fistulas involving the lateral sinuses. Complex logarithms have been developed for the evaluation of disease involving this area; they are beyond the scope of this chapter but have been well covered in other texts (LASJAUNIAS and BERENSTEIN 1987). The arterial supply to the arteriovenous shunt usually arises from branches of the external carotid artery. The most commonly involved arteries include transmastoid perforators arising from the occipital artery, the neuromeningeal division of the ascending pharyngeal artery, the posterior division of the middle meningeal artery, and perforating branches from the posterior auricular artery. Larger fistulas and fistulas that have undergone proximal occlusion of the external carotid branches will commonly recruit the posterior meningeal branch of the ipsilateral vertebral artery and marginal tentorial branches of the meningohypophysial trunk arising from the internal carotid artery. Very large fistulas can additionally recruit pial supply from the adjacent temporal and occipital lobes and cerebellar hemispheres. In addition to localizing the arterial supply, great care must be exercised in defining the direction of venous drainage, any associated downstream obstructions, and the presence of cortical venous drainage.

DJINDJIAN et al. (1973) differentiated dural fistulas in the lateral sinus into three different types. Type 1 fistulas drain via the ipsilateral sinus. In our experience these fistulas have a relatively low risk and usually present with bruit and headache and only rarely develop neurologic deficits and hemorrhage. We have seen one patient who developed diffuse dural sinus thrombosis with a type 1 fistula requiring emergent thrombolysis.

Type 2 fistulas drain toward the contralateral sinus, usually because of a stenosis or occlusion of the ipsilateral sinus inferior to the fistula site. In our experience, these fistulas are associated with more severe symptoms and can sometimes hemorrhage and develop increased intracranial pressure, particularly if the contralateral sinus is hypoplastic or stenotic.

Type 3 dural fistulas drain to cortical veins. These fistulas are the most ominous, have the highest risk, and frequently develop neurologic deficits, venous infarctions, and hemorrhage. In a review of dural fistulas, it was noted that 42% of fistulas with cortical venous drainage were associated with hemorrhage (Castaigne et al. 1975). Figure 3.1 is an example of a case of type 3 DAVF that presented with a parenchymal hemorrhage. In our own experience with 66 patients with dural fistulas in the lateral sinuses, over one-third presented with hemorrhage (Halbach et al. 1987c). In this group all but one demonstrated cortical venous drainage. In our experience the angiographic finding most predictive of repeated hemorrhage was cortical venous drainage in which a high-grade stenosis occurred in the draining vein downstream from the fistula site. This stenosis appears to occur frequently where a draining vein enters another dural sinus. Figure 3.2 demonstrates a DAVF with cortical drainage (type 3) with a high-grade stenosis where the draining veins enter the straight sinus. This stenosis can progress to complete occlusion and is often associated with severe repeated episodes of bleeding. Intraoperative observations and pathologic specimens have shown these lesions to demonstrate both intimal hyperplasia and subacute thrombosis.

Rarely, a high risk dural fistula can exist where a draining vein meets a dural sinus, but no connection exists between the vein and the neighboring dural sinus. This adjacent dural sinus may be widely patent and uninvolved with the dural fistula. These fistulas are best treated by intraoperative embolization or surgical excision of the fistula site. It is essential that the uninvolved adjacent sinus remains patent (Barnwell et al. 1991a).

In our experience dural fistulas can progress from a type 1 or low risk fistula to a higher risk type 2 or type 3 fistula spontaneously. The progression from a low risk to a high risk fistula can occur gradually or quite abruptly. Generally, this is associated with rapid changes in the patient's symptoms, usually a change or diminution in the bruit, an increase in headaches, and the development of new or progressive neurologic deficits. It is, therefore, important that repeat arteriography be performed if a patient with a known dural fistula involving the transverse or lateral sinuses develops an alteration in clinical symptoms. The patient in Fig. 3.1 had a long history of a bruit that diminished significantly several weeks before his hemorrhage.

Plain skull radiography is not indicated in the workup of this disease but if obtained for other reasons may demonstrate enlargement of the middle meningeal grooves and, in rare instances, sellar changes indicative of elevated intracranial pressure. Computed tomographic (CT) scanning can be useful for demonstrating edema related to venous hypertension, subarachnoid bleeding, subdural hematoma, and intraparenchymal hemorrhage. If iodated contrast material is administered, dilated cortical veins may be disclosed.

The role of magnetic resonance imaging (MRI) in the evaluation of dural fistulas is evolving as improved spatial resolution and newer pulse sequences permit evaluation of vascular structures. A recent review of the impact of MRI on patients with documented dural fistulas (DeMarco et al. 1990) has demonstrated that MRI is useful for disclosing the end-organ damage to the brain, effectively showing subdural and intraparenchymal hemorrhage. MRI is quite insensitive to subarachnoid hemorrhage, however. Areas of infarction and edema are well demonstrated. Low risk fistulas (Djindjian type 1) can escape detection on routine MR images. However, the dilated cortical veins draining a complex dural fistula (Djindjian type 3) are often disclosed on spin-echo imaging. Spin-echo imaging is most effective at depicting hemorrhage and edema. GRE imaging is sometimes useful in detecting areas of signal void corresponding to regions of sinus thrombosis highlighted by the increased signal in the adjacent patent sinus. Rarely, the arterial feeders and draining veins are also demonstrated on GRE images. Flow compensation gradients should not be utilized for the acquisition of T2-weighted images as the refocusing of laminar flow may increase signal in a dural sinus, obscuring or simulating dural sinus thrombosis and obscuring dilated cortical veins. The use of saturation bands may reduce intraluminal signal intensity on T1- and T2-weighted images and improve recognition of vascular structures. It must be emphasized, however, that both CT and MRI can completely miss some dural fistulas, especially Djindjian type 1, and should never be utilized as a screening technique for this disease.

3.2.3 Therapeutic Options

The decision whether to treat an individual patient and by which modality must be made with knowledge of the patient's symptoms, the projected risk of the disease, and the benefits and risks of the treatment modality. Fortunately the angiographic features, particularly diverted venous drainage, correlate quite well with the most severe sequelae of this disease, namely infarction and hemorrhage. Patients with visual loss, hemorrhage, or infarctions, as well as those with cortical venous drainage, demand prompt therapy. Since it is unknown whether subtotal occlusion of a dural fistula reduces the risk of hemorrhage or infarction, every attempt should be made to completely obliterate high risk fistulas (Djindjian type 3). At the other end of the spectrum, low risk fistulas (Djindjian type 1) can be followed clinically if the patient can tolerate the symptoms or can undergo safe transvascular embolization procedures. Patients who are followed conservatively without treatment should undergo repeated angiographic evaluation if their symptoms change. These patients should avoid medications such as aspirin and nonsteroidal anti-inflammatory drugs that could interfere with their clotting ability and prevent spontaneous closure.

3.2.3.1 Compression Therapy

Highly motivated patients with dural fistulas located in the posterior sigmoid or transverse sinus and who have the primary arterial supply arising from the occipital artery without severe symptoms or ominous angiographic anatomy can undergo compression therapy. These patients are instructed to manually compress the ipsilateral feeding occipital artery behind the mastoid for up to 30 min per compression. In our experience, this results in diminished arterial inflow and thrombosis in 27% of patients treated (Halbach et al. 1987b). The therapy seems most effective in small fistulas with the arterial supply arising entirely from the occipital artery.

3.2.3.2 Transarterial Embolization

Subselective catheterization and embolization of the feeding external carotid branches has emerged as an effective treatment modality. Knowledge of the vascular supply, anatomic variants, and dangerous anastomoses is essential for a safe treatment; these topics lie beyond the scope of this chapter but are well described in other texts (Lasjaunias and Berenstein 1987). The overall results of embolization of the external carotid feeding vessels have shown a lower cure rate for transverse and sigmoid sinus DAVFs than for their counterparts involving the cavernous sinus. Picard et al. (1987) reported on the treatment of 32 patients of whom 23 (70%) were cured clinically. However, only seven had angiographic documentation. Our own early results in 26 patients have shown a complete angiographic and clinical cure in 50%, with 38% having subtotal occlusion and improvement in symptoms (Halbach et al. 1987b). Subsequent development of smaller microcatheters has improved the effectiveness of transarterial embolization; however, some DAVFs remain patent despite repeated aggressive therapy.

Our current technique usually involves selective catheterization of the individual feeding vessels supplying the dural fistula with a 5F or 7F catheter. Digital subtraction angiography is performed to evaluate the arterial anatomy to the fistula as well as to delineate the presence of any dangerous anastomoses. It must be underscored that such anastomoses may not be demonstrable angiographically, but may indeed be present, and the alterations in flow that occur during embolization can allow inadvertent passage of embolic material to the intracranial circulation. Prior to subselective catheterization of the feeding vessel, topical nitroglycerin is applied and/or sublingual calcium channel blockers administered to minimize spasm associated with catheterization. A small microcatheter (Tracker, Target Therapeutics, San Jose, California) with a flexible platinum wire is navigated coaxially through the guiding catheter distally into the branch supplying the fistula. The decision as to which embolic agent to utilize depends on the experience of the operator, the location of the catheter, and the goal of the embolization. In our experience particulate embolization of feeding vessels carries an exceptionally low morbidity if performed by an experienced neurovascular team; however, there is often recanalization with recurrence of the fistula and symptoms. Liquid adhesives, on the other hand, have a much higher cure rate but are more difficult and hazardous to use. Should the liquid adhesives pass inadvertently into the involved sinus, occlusion of the sinus can occur, resulting in conversion of a low risk fistula into one of high risk. Proximal occlusion of the feeding artery by any technique invariably results in recruitment of the supply to the fistula from alternate sources and should be avoided at all costs.

Proximal occlusion of the external carotid artery by coils invariably results in recruitment of arterial supply from collateral sources and should never be performed. Occasionally, a coil can be utilized to occlude a distal normal vascular territory to allow diversion of embolic material into a feeding vessel. Digital compression or use of compression devices can also produce transient occlusion of normal distal vessels. Prior to embolization, a provocative test with lidocaine can alert the endovascular surgeon to the presence of a dangerous pedicle that may supply a cranial nerve (Horton and Kerber 1986). As with all provocative tests, the anesthetic material may bypass the dangerous vessel, flowing preferentially to the low resistance shunt and producing a falsely negative test.

3.2.3.3 Transvenous Embolization

The technique of closing a dural fistula by placing thrombogenic material into the involved dural sinus was pioneered by Mullan (1979) and Hosobuchi (1975). We have modified the technique in utilizing embolic material that is positioned in the sinus from a femoral venous access and have also utilized fluoroscopic guidance to accurately deposit the radiopaque embolic material, usually platinum coils with thrombogenic fibers.

Patient selection is essential to accurately choose patients who can benefit from this technique. One must remember that occlusion of a normal cortical vein or dural sinus poses the risk of venous infarction and hemorrhage. In the presence of a large or longstanding fistula, especially one associated with venous occlusive disease (Djindjian types 2 and 3), the pressure in the involved dural sinus can be markedly elevated. If the flow and elevated pressure are sufficient, reversal of flow into veins normally draining towards the sinus can occur. These dilated veins carrying high pressure arterialized blood away from the fistula site can therefore be either sacrificed at their origin, as with surgical excision, or occluded at their origin by an embolic device. Similarly, if the pressure in the involved dural sinus is markedly elevated either because of a large amount of shunting or the presence of severe obstructive disease, then the remainder of the cerebral venous drainage is diverted to alternate pathways. Therefore, we only recommend transvenous embolization in patients who demonstrate cortical venous drainage from the segment of sinus involved with the fistula and whose segment of involved dural sinus is not being used as a conduit for the venous drainage of the remaining brain. Patients who have antegrade venous drainage towards the involved dural sinus or who have normal brain venous drainage through the sinus should not undergo this therapy. These criteria select for the highest risk dural fistulas (cortical venous drainage often with dural sinus occlusive disease or Djindjian type 3). In some instances a small area of arteriovenous shunting may be localized to a vein draining into a transverse or sigmoid sinus. In these cases, selective occlusion of this vein with preservation of the adjacent dural sinus can be achieved without sequelae.

The preferred technique for transvenous embolization involves placement of steel or platinum thrombogenic coils directly into the involved dural sinus or vein from either a transfemoral or an intra-operative approach (Halbach et al. 1989c). Figure 3.1 pertains to a patient with a high risk fistula (type 3) in whom no safe transfemoral pathway to the fistula site was present. Preoperative embolization of the external carotid artery feeders was followed by surgical exposure of the fistula site and placement of fibered coils into the involved dural sinus. The puncture was made through a small burr hole placed over the involved sinus. Complete closure was documented on a follow-up arteriogram. The development of newer and softer delivery catheters and thrombogenic coils often woven with Dacron or silk fibers has permitted access to many dural fistulas. Prior to transvenous embolization, arterial embolization of the accessible feeders is usually performed using particulate emboli. The largest feeder, however, is left patent to allow angiographic "roadmaps" of the region of arteriovenous shunting. Thrombogenic (fiber containing) platinum coils are preferable to steel coils in that they are very soft and nonferromagnetic, thus allowing follow-up MRI scans. Silk sutures can be injected to intertwine with platinum coils and promote thrombosis. It is important to choose the proper diameter of coils to ensure that coil migration does not occur. Generally, a metal washer of a known diameter is placed over the ipsilateral mastoid bone during angiographic evaluation to allow for determination of the size of the dural sinus. Because the dural sinus is quite compliant, a coil should be chosen that has a slightly larger unrestrained diameter than the sinus. It is preferable to intertwine the coils to reduce the risk of migration. For safe transvenous embolization it is essential to ensure that the entire sinus is occluded and no areas left patent. If a region of sinus is skipped, then the trapped segment can divert flow into cortical veins, producing or aggravating the risks of stroke and hemorrhage. To eliminate this risk, adequate packing of the sinus is essential as well as continuous roadmap evaluation to ensure that the sinus is completely thrombosed. Figure 3.3 relates to a patient with a high risk DAVF (type 3) that was cured by transfemoral transvenous embolization. Despite subsequent anticoagulation for an unrelated process the fistula remained closed, as confirmed on a 3-year follow-up angiogram.

3.2.3.4 Preoperative Embolization

Some dural fistulas involving the lateral sinus cannot be cured by transfermoral or intraoperative vascular techniques. Surgical excision of high risk dural distulas has been shown to be an effective therapy but can be associated with significant morbidity and mortality related to massive bleeding occurring during the surgical procedure (SUNDT and PIEPGRAS 1983). The combination of aggressive preoperative embolization and subsequent surgical excision of the dural fistula has been shown to be effective in the treatment of complex dural fistulas (BARNWELL et al. 1989). Particulate emboli, because of their lower morbidity, are generally utilized 1–2 days prior to surgical excision. Intraoperative arteriography can be helpful for localizing the exact fistula site and judging the effectiveness of the surgical procedure (BARNWELL et al. 1989; HIESHIMA et al. 1987). The patient who is the subject of Fig. 3.2 underwent preoperative embolization of the feeding arteries followed by successful surgical excision at the fistula site.

3.3 Cavernous Sinus Dural Arteriovenous Fistulas

3.3.1 Pathophysiology and Clinical Presentation

The majority of dural fistulas involving the cavernous sinus occur in females (NEWTON and HOYT 1970). The development of these fistulas may be a result of hormonal changes, as suggested by the fact that the majority occur in postmenopausal females (NEWTON and HOYT 1970) or during pregnancy (DOYON and METZGER 1973; TOYA et al. 1981).

The most common presenting symptoms of cavernous DAVFs, with the exception of bruit, are related to the venous drainage, usually towards the orbit. The elevated pressure in the venous pathways draining to the orbit produce orbital venous congestion. Transudation of interstitial fluid and the increased caliber of the venous structures produce proptosis, which is the most commonly reported presenting symptom (NEWTON and HOYT 1970; HALBACH et al. 1987b). Chemosis and conjunctival edema are commonly associated with larger cavernous dural fistulas or fistulas that have developed stenoses in the draining venous pathways such as occlusion of the inferior petrosal sinus or stenoses or occlusion of the anterior (proximal) superior ophthalmic vein. Figure 3.4 shows a typical appearance in a patient with a cavernous DAVF that demonstrates mild proptosis and conjunctival injection. The aqueous humor normally drains into the orbital veins through the canal of Schlemm. Elevated venous pressure therefore increases intraocular pressure. It can produce secondary glaucoma and, if markedly elevated, rapid and sometimes irreversible visual loss. The elevated episcleral venous pressure may be responsible for the production of papilledema, choroidal detachment, and central retinal venous thrombosis (JRGENSEN and GUTHOFF 1988).

In our experience patients with cavernous dural fistulas often have mild impairment of visual acuity which can be recovered if the fistula is closed. However, rarely, patients will develop severe visual decompensation to the point of absence of light perception. Rarely is visual function recovered in these cases even if definitive closure of the fistula occurs (HALBACH et al. 1987d). Patients with rapid visual loss therefore are candidates for aggressive and emergent therapy. Pharmacologic agents that lower intraocular pressure, such as topical β-blockers or Diamox, can

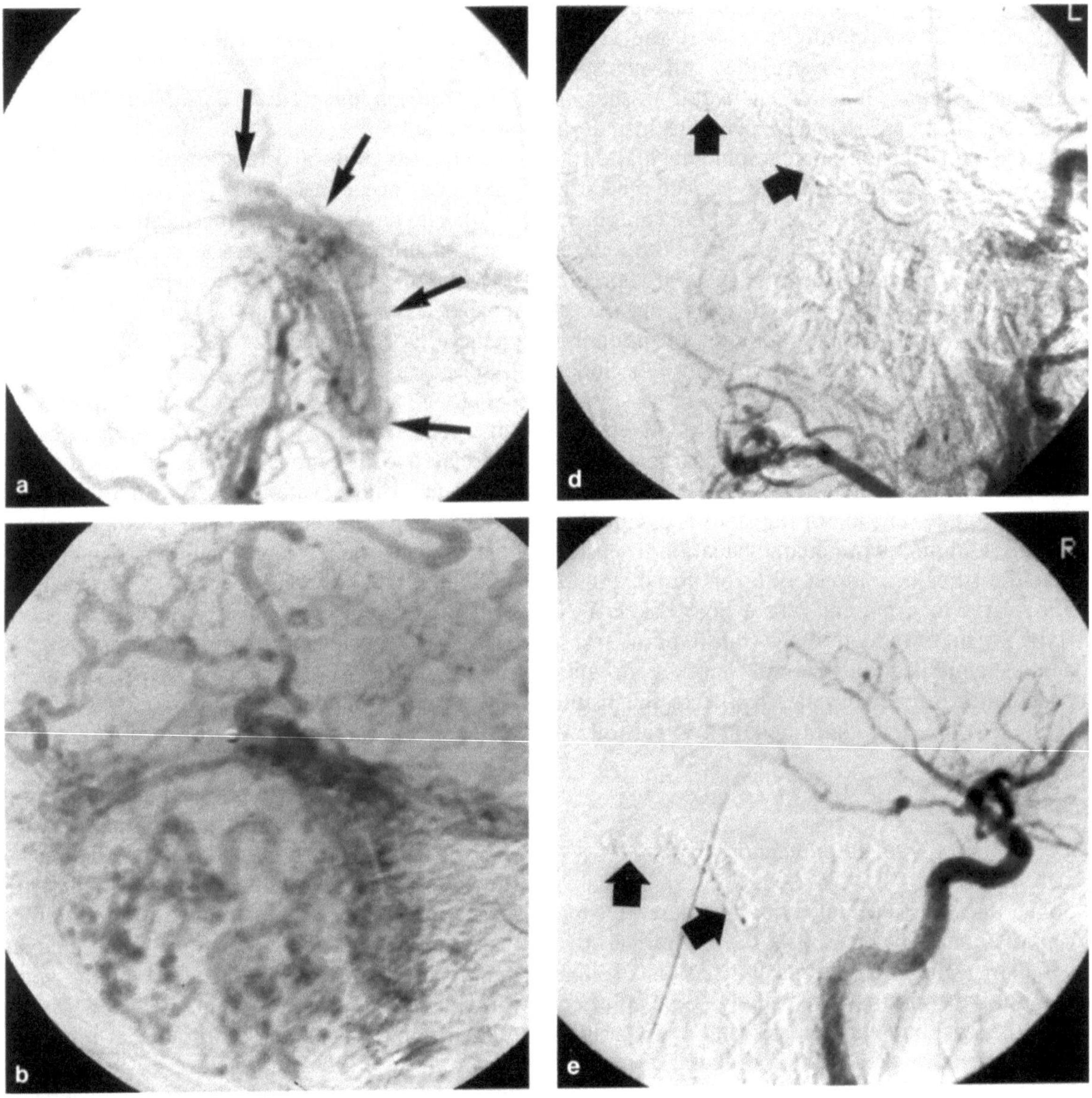

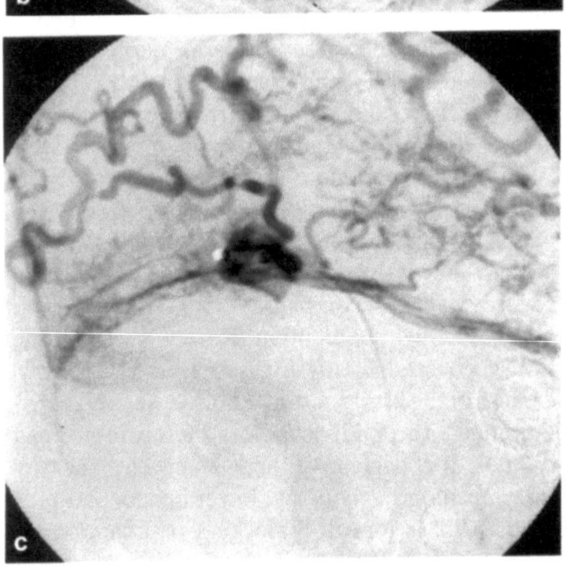

Fig. 3.3. a,b Left occipital artery injection, lateral view, early arterial (**a**) and late arterial (**b**) phases, demonstrates a dural fistula involving the sigmoid sinus (**a**) with venous drainage to cortical veins. The sigmoid sinus involved with the DAVF is illustrated by *arrows*. **c** Sigmoid sinus venogram, lateral projection. A small catheter has been navigated from a femoral venous access to the proximal (superior) end of the fistula site. Contrast injection demonstrates filling of the supratentorial veins draining the fistula. **d,e** Left internal (**d**) and external (**e**) carotid injections, lateral projections, demonstrate complete occlusion of the fistula site. The coils are outlined by *short arrows*

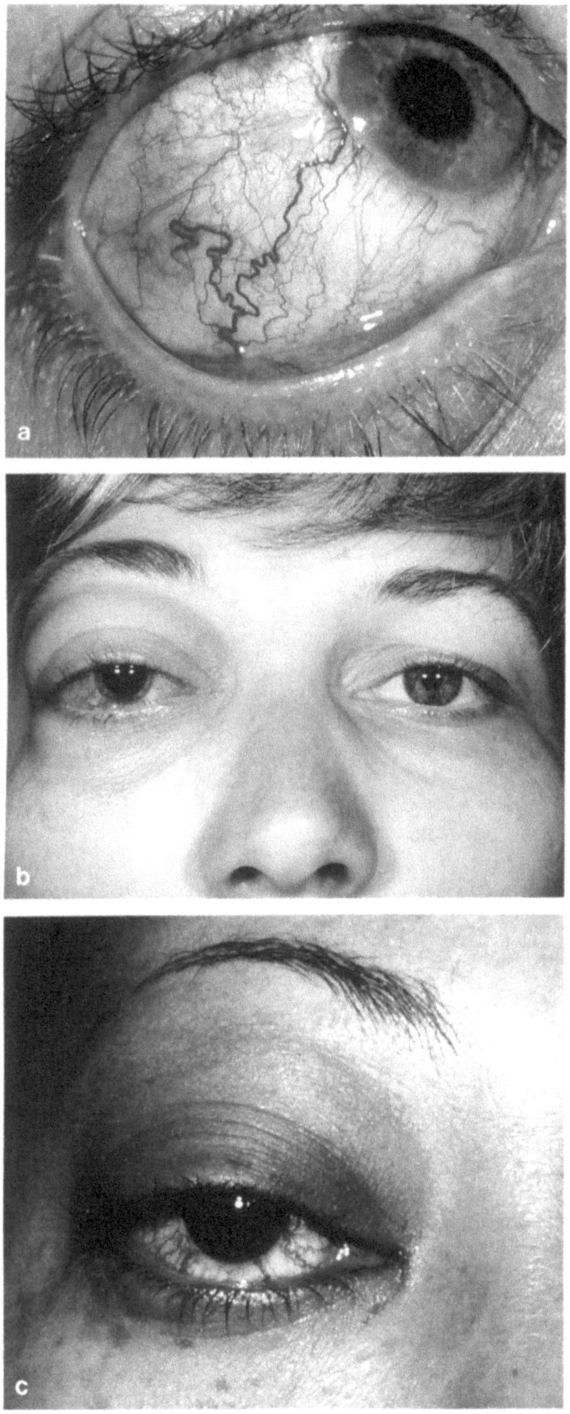

Fig. 3.4 a–c. Young woman with typical proptosis and conjunctival injection secondary to a dural fistula

be a useful adjunct in these instances but are no substitute for definitive fistula closure. Lateral canthotomy additionally can diminish retro-orbital pressure and improve ocular perfusion but only serves as a temporary measure until definitive fistula closure can be achieved. The severity of symptoms from cavernous dural fistulas rarely relates to the amount of arteriovenous shunting, but rather to the adequacy of venous drainage pathways. Occlusion of the anterior (proximal) superior ophthalmic vein produces diversion of the remaining arterialized blood to the vortex veins draining the retina. Diminished reabsorbtion of the aqueous humor results from markedly elevated venous pressure and produces severe clinical sequelae (Dowd et al. 1991). Similarly, occlusion of the inferior petrosal sinus, which can occur spontaneously or as the result of a therapeutic or diagnostic procedure, can divert the remaining fistula drainage toward the eye, producing acute aggravation of ocular symptoms. A small percentage of patients may have thrombosis of the distal (posterior) superior ophthalmic vein which can result in improvement of the ipsilateral eye but diverts flow to the contralateral eye. This anatomy occurred in 11% of our patients (Halbach et al. 1987b).

Thrombosis of the distal (posterior) superior ophthalmic vein and inferior petrosal sinus can divert flow to cortical veins through the sphenoparietal sinus and pontine veins and result in neurologic deficits, headaches, and, in rare instances, hemorrhage.

Of the 100 patients treated by our endovascular team with cavernous DAVFs, three had documented subarachnoid hemorrhage, all with occlusion of the primary venous drainage pathways and diversion of flow into cortical veins. Figure 3.5 pertains to a patient with a documented subarachnoid hemorrhage with only cortical drainage from a cavernous DAVF.

Headaches are produced by cavernous dural fistulas and are presumably related to mechanical stretch of the sensitive, highly innervated dura, or the result of thrombosis in a draining venous pathway or fistula site.

Diplopia is a common presenting symptom, usually resulting from sixth nerve and, less commonly, third nerve dysfunction. Approximately one-half of patients report a pulse-synchronous bruit (Halbach et al. 1987b). The turbulence created by the arteriovenous shunt is transmitted to the middle ear, producing the bruit. It occurs

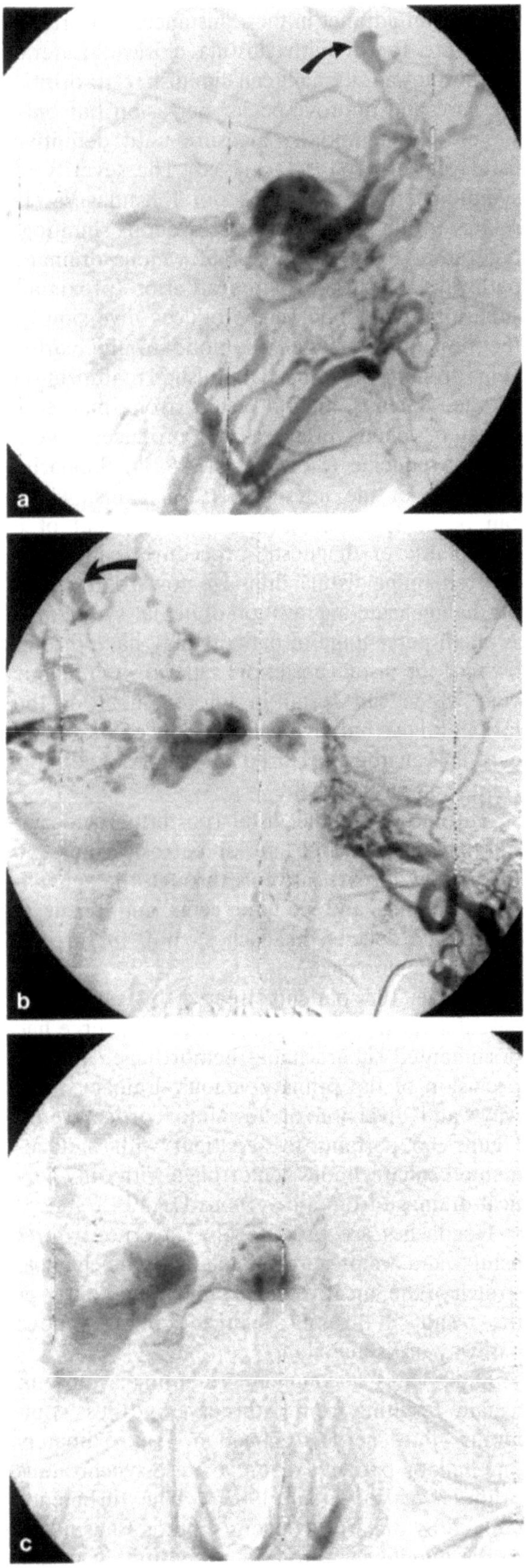

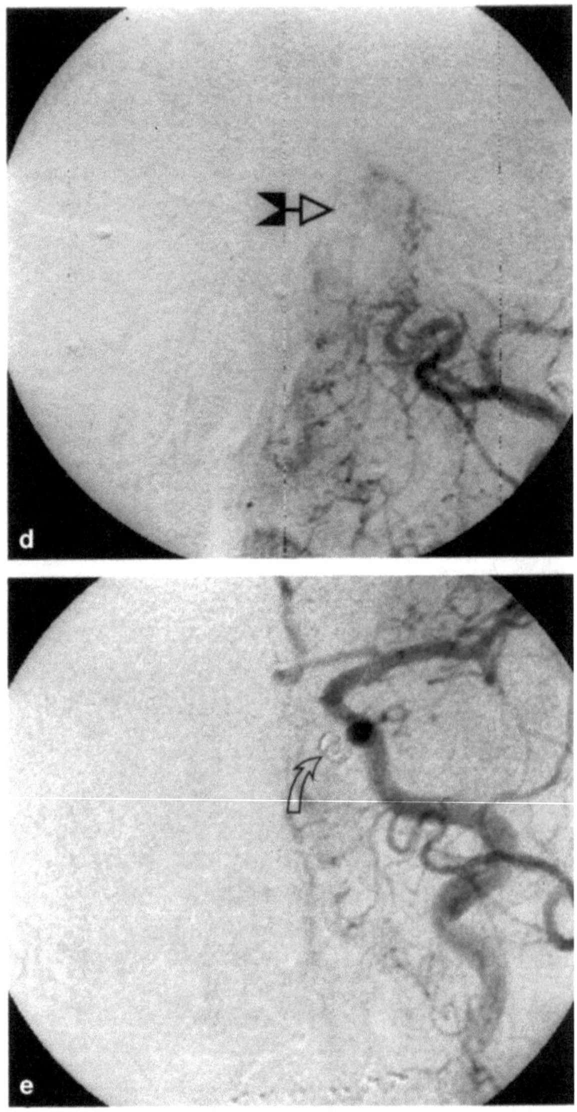

Fig. 3.5 a–e. A 77-year-old woman presented with subarachnoid hemorrhage localized to the right sylvian fissure. **a**, **b** Left external carotid injection, (**a**) lateral and (**b**) AP projections, demonstrates a dural arteriovenous fistula located in the left cavernous sinus. The venous drainage of this fistula is entirely to the contralateral cavernous sinus and eventually through the sphenoparietal sinus to cortical veins. A venous aneurysm (varix) is noted in the right sylvian region (*curved arrow*), which corresponds exactly to the location of hemorrhage on CT scan. **c** Left cavernous sinus injection, AP projection, demonstrates the same venous anatomy. A small microcatheter has been guided from a transfemoral venous access through the internal jugular vein up the inferior petrosal sinus to the fistulous site. Multiple platinum coils and silk suture were deposited at the fistula site. **d** External carotid injection, AP projection, post-embolization, demonstrates complete obliteration of the fistula with preservation of all normal branches. The multiple platinum coils are indicated by a *short horizontal arrow*.

often in patients with drainage posteriorly down the inferior or superior petrosal sinuses.

3.3.2 Radiographic Evaluation

Both CT and MRI can fail to elicit the diagnosis of a cavernous dural fistula if the fistula is small, is of relatively recent onset, or has an unusual venous drainage pathway. Commonly, the fistula itself is not imaged by CT or MRI but indirect evidence of the fistula, usually a dilated superior ophthalmic vein, can be detected. The gold standard for evaluation of a cavernous dural fistula is selective arteriography. Common carotid injections with filming of the carotid bifurcation should be obtained if compression therapy is to be entertained. Selective internal carotid arteriography commonly demonstrates dural supply arising from the meningohypophyseal trunk, inferolateral trunk, and occasionally ophthalmic branches. The distal internal maxillary artery usually supplies the cavernous DAVF through the artery of foramen rotundum. The middle meningeal and accessory meningeal arteries commonly have petrosal branches coursing towards the cavernous sinus. The ascending pharyngeal artery can supply the dural fistula through jugular and hypoglossal divisions of the neuromeningeal trunk. Arterial supply can arise from the internal and external carotid arteries bilaterally. Rapid arterial filming is essential to delineate whether a unilateral fistula site is present or if there is truly an unusual bilateral cavernous dural fistula. As with all dural fistulas, specific attention to the venous drainage pathways is important. BARROW et al. (1985) proposed a subclassification of cavernous connections into four major categories. Group B are cavernous DAVFs that are only supplied by dural branches of the internal carotid artery. Group C are cavernous DAVFs supplied by branches of the external carotid artery and group D are fistulas supplied by both internal and external carotid arteries. In our experience, group D are the most common. We have encountered an increasing number of group B fistulas as well as patients with group D fistulas who had initial embolization of the external carotid supply and converted to group B fistulas.

◁ **Fig. 3.5** (*continued*). **e** Common carotid injection, AP projection, 9-month follow-up arteriogram, demonstrates persistent closure of the fistula. The platinum coils are delineated by an *open curved arrow*. The patient has had complete resolution of symptoms and no further episodes of hemorrhage

3.3.3 Therapeutic Options

It is important to remember that spontaneous closure of cavernous dural fistulas can occur (BRISMAR and BRISMAR 1976; MAGIDSON and WEINBERG 1976). Other reports have documented closure following arteriography.

3.3.3.1 Carotid–Jugular Compression

Our primary therapy for compliant, motivated patients who demonstrate no contraindications is carotid–jugular compression (HALBACH et al. 1987b). Patients are excluded from this therapy if they have atherosclerotic or vascular disease involving the common carotid or carotid bifurcation since compressing this structure could result in dislodging plaque or thrombus. Additionally, patients with a hypercoagulable state should be excluded. Patients with cortical venous drainage should not further compromise their venous drainage by compressing their jugular vein, which could theoretically increase the risk of stroke and hemorrhage, and are therefore excluded. Patients who have an abrupt visual decline, intradural hemorrhage, or severe pain deserve more aggressive forms of therapy. Therapy is performed initially 10 s per compression four to six times an hour while awake. Gradually the duration of compression is increased to a maximum of 30 s. The compressions are continued for 4–6 weeks. The initial compressions are observed by a physician to ensure that cerebral ischemia or a vasovagal event does not occur. Patients are instructed to compress their involved carotid artery and jugular vein using the contralateral hand so that if the patient develops weakness from cerebral ischemia unrecognized by the patient, the hand will fall away and discontinue the therapy. The compressions are performed with the patient lying or sitting to reduce the risk of injury should a vagal event occur. The compression transiently decreases the arterial inflow while simultaneously increasing the venous pressure, promoting thrombosis in the fistula. We have instructed 45 patients with cavernous DAVFs to perform compression therapy with no deleterious effects and the treatment has resulted in complete cure in 15 patients (33%).

3.3.3.2 *Transarterial External Carotid Embolization*

Subselective catheterization and embolization of the feeding external carotid arteries has emerged as a highly successful therapy. PICARD et al. (1987) reported a series of 25 patients of whom 72% were completely cured and a further 24% had improvement in symptoms. Another series of nine cavernous DAVFs treated by external carotid embolization had excellent results (VINUELA et al. 1984). Both series had complications related to the use of liquid adhesives. Reflux of liquid embolic material through an anastomosis from the external to the internal carotid artery resulted in two strokes one of which was fatal. Our own results with external carotid embolization in 39 patients showed a complete cure in 80%, improvement in 18%, and a 5% complication rate (HALBACH et al. 1987b). Both particulate embolization and liquid adhesives have been shown to be effective in producing cure of a symptomatic cavernous DAVF (PICARD et al. 1987; HALBACH et al. 1987b). The use of Gelfoam powder should be discouraged as it can produce cranial nerve palsies and also result in late recanalization. The risk of cranial nerve injury can be reduced significantly with knowledge of the arterial supply to these structures, the avoidance of smaller particles or liquid adhesives as an embolic agent, and the use of provocative agents such as lidocaine as a functional test (HORTON and KERBER 1986). Dangerous anastomoses exist between the internal carotid artery, the vertebral artery, and nearly all of the external carotid branches involved in a dural fistula. These dangerous anastomoses as well as the critical arterial supply to the cranial nerves are beyond the scope of this chapter but are discussed in other texts (LASJAUNIAS and BERENSTEIN 1987). Transient aggravation of symptoms following complete closure of the fistula is uncommon and may be the result of thrombosis of the superior ophthalmic vein (SERGOTT et al. 1987).

3.3.3.3 *Transvenous Embolization*

Thrombosis of symptomatic cavernous dural fistulas was first described by a surgical exposure and placement of thrombogenic coils into the fistulous site (MULLAN 1979; HOSOBUCHI 1975). Subsequent endovascular occlusion of symptomatic cavernous DAVFs has been described (COURTHEOUX et al. 1987; TENG et al. 1988; HALBACH et al. 1989b; TAKAHASHI et al. 1989). Access to the cavernous sinus was described by surgical cutdown of the angular or superior ophthalmic vein (HOSOBUCHI 1975; COURTHEOUX et al. 1987; TENG et al. 1988; TAKAHASHI 1989). Transfemoral catheterization of the cavernous sinus through the inferior petrosal sinus or superior ophthalmic vein has also been reported (HALBACH et al. 1989b). The transvenous embolization of cavernous dural fistulas has emerged as our method of choice in symptomatic DAVFs that fail to respond to or are excluded from carotid–jugular compression. We have treated 42 patients by this technique, 31 patients through access via the inferior petrosal sinus and the remaining 11 through a superior ophthalmic vein approach. Our preferred approach is through the inferior petrosal sinus and commonly a microcatheter can be navigated through this structure even if it is not demonstrable on the initial arteriogram. Figures 3.5 and 3.6 both illustrate cases treated by transvenous embolization of the cavernous sinus accessed through the inferior petrosal sinus, even though it was not angiographically demonstrable. Figure 3.7 is an example of a DAVF treated by transvenous embolization through the superior ophthalmic venous approach. Roadmapping is often essential to localize the draining venous pathways and allow safe transvenous catheterization. Our preferred embolic material is thrombogenic platinum coils, usually containing Dacron or silk fibers, delivered through a small 3F microcatheter. Silk suture can be entangled with the coils to promote thrombosis. Rarely, liquid adhesives are utilized

Fig. 3.6a–f. A 32-year-old woman presented with ophthalmoplegia, left proptosis, and severe headaches. **a** Left external carotid arteriogram, lateral projection, demonstrates supply from distal internal maxillary and middle meningeal branches with drainage to cortical veins (*straight arrow*) and the superior ophthalmic vein (*curved arrow*). **b** Left internal carotid injection, lateral projection, demonstrates recruitment of supply to the fistula from internal carotid branches with drainage to the superior ophthalmic vein. **c**, **d** Left cavernous sinus injection, lateral (**c**) and AP (**d**) projections, demonstrates anterior compartment drainage to the superior ophthalmic vein. A total of 45 platinum coils and silk sutures were deposited in the fistula site and proximal superior ophthalmic vein. **e**, **f** Left internal carotid injection, lateral projection, (**e**) and left external carotid injection, lateral projection (**f**); status postembolization. Complete occlusion of the fistula site is demonstrated. A follow-up arteriogram at 3 months confirmed complete closure. The patient has had subsequent complete resolution of her presenting symptoms ▷

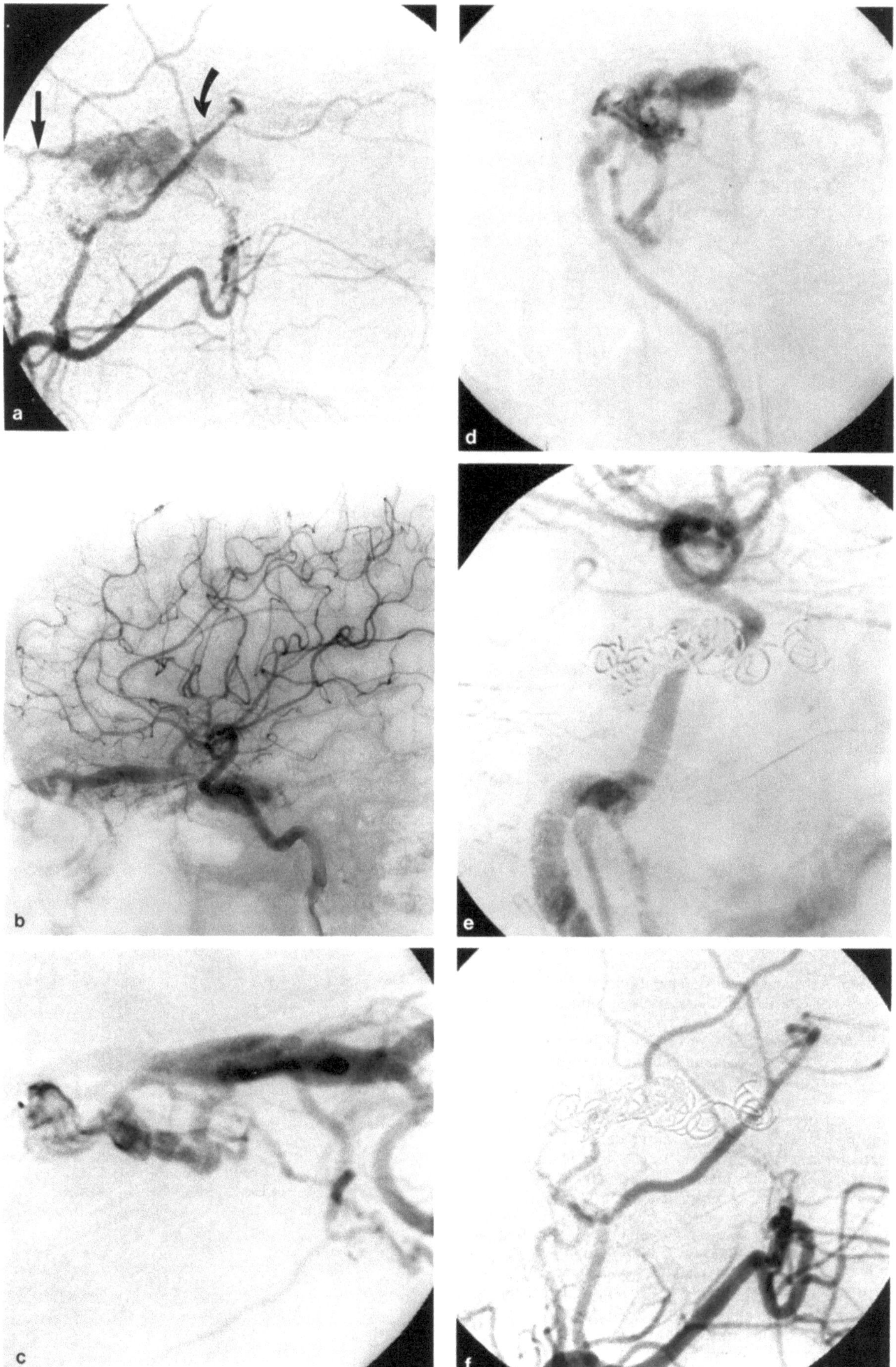
a
d
b
e
c
f

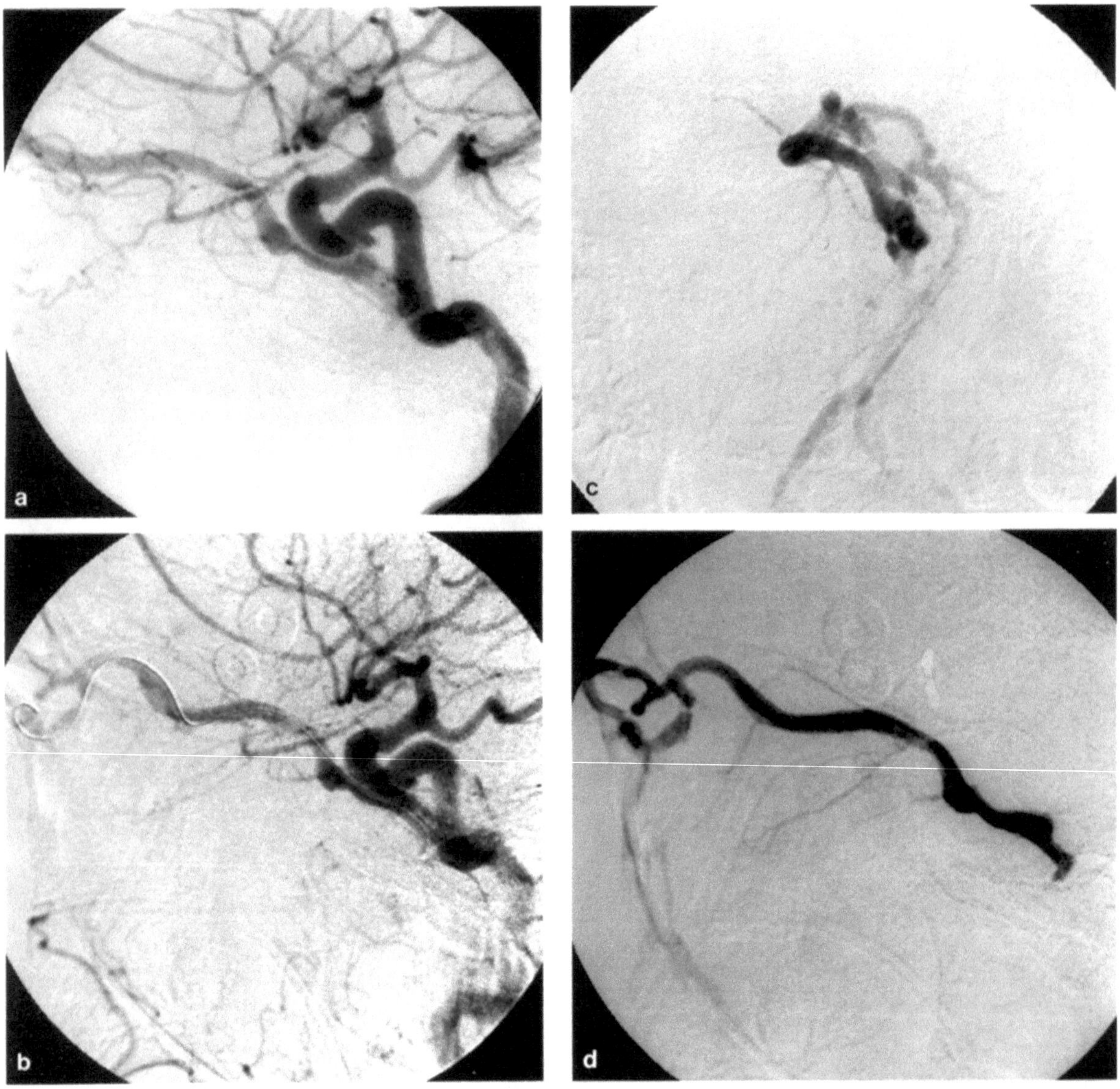

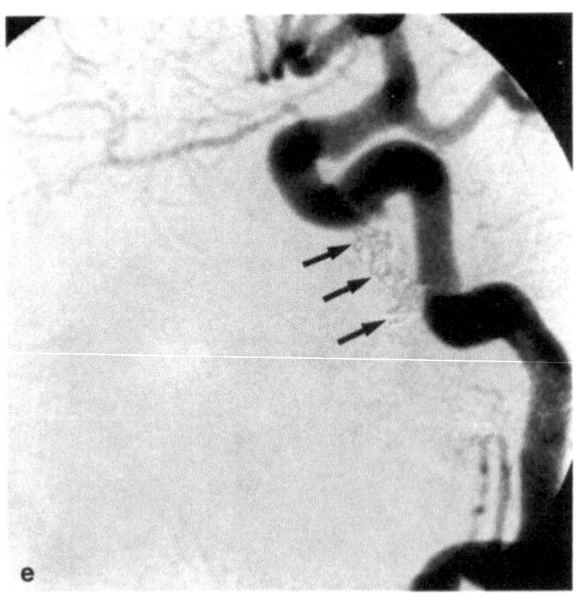

Fig. 3.7a–e. A 57-year-old woman presented with proptosis and chemosis secondary to a right cavernous dural fistula. At an outside hospital multiple coils were placed in the distal internal maxillary artery, producing only transient improvement in her symptoms. **a** Right internal carotid injection, lateral projection, demonstrates a cavernous dural fistula draining entirely to the superior ophthalmic vein supplied by the inferolateral trunk. The entire supply fistula arose from the internal carotid artery. **b** Right internal carotid injection, lateral projections, during retrograde catheterization of the fistula site. A catheter has been navigated from a transfemoral venous access through the internal jugular vein to the external jugular and angular vein and a small microcatheter has been navigated retrograde through the superior ophthalmic vein to the fistula site. **c**, **d** Injection of the microcatheter at the fistula site, in the AP (**c**) and the lateral projection (**d**), demonstrates the draining superior ophthalmic vein. **e** Right common carotid injection, status following embolization with 12 platinum coils. Complete closure of the fistula site is demonstrated. The platinum coils are outlined by *short straight arrows*. The patient has had complete resolution of her symptoms following closure of the fistula

when other agents fail. Complete angiographic obliteration was achieved in 33 of the 42 patients and clinical improvement was noted in the remaining nine. Two complications occurred, one with the use of a temporary balloon in the internal carotid artery, a technique no longer utilized. A second patient developed a cerebellar hematoma secondary to diversion of arterialized venous drainage in a high risk cavernous dural fistula without other venous drainage pathways. The development of more thrombogenic coils and softer delivery catheters and guide wires should make this an even more effective therapy in the future.

3.3.3.4 *Internal Carotid Embolization*

Rarely, severe symptomic cavernous DAVFs will fail both transvenous and arterial embolization of the external carotid supply. If the patient has rapidly declining vision or intradural hemorrhage, careful selective embolization of the dural supply arising from the internal carotid artery can be performed. We performed this technique in four patients using small microcatheters with the special curves near the distal tip to engage the origin of the inferolateral and meningohypophyseal trunk supply to a dural fistula (HALBACH et al. 1989). Figure 3.8 is an example of a highly symptomatic DAVF treated by embolization of the dural supply arising from the internal carotid artery. The potential risks of cerebral emboli make this the least attractive therapeutic option and therefore it is only recommended when all other avenues of therapy have failed.

Table 3.1 summarizes our experience with 123 patients with cavernous DAVF treated by our group. Our primary therapy for patients whose symptoms and angiographic features demand therapy and are not candidates or fail to respond to compression therapy is transvernous embo-

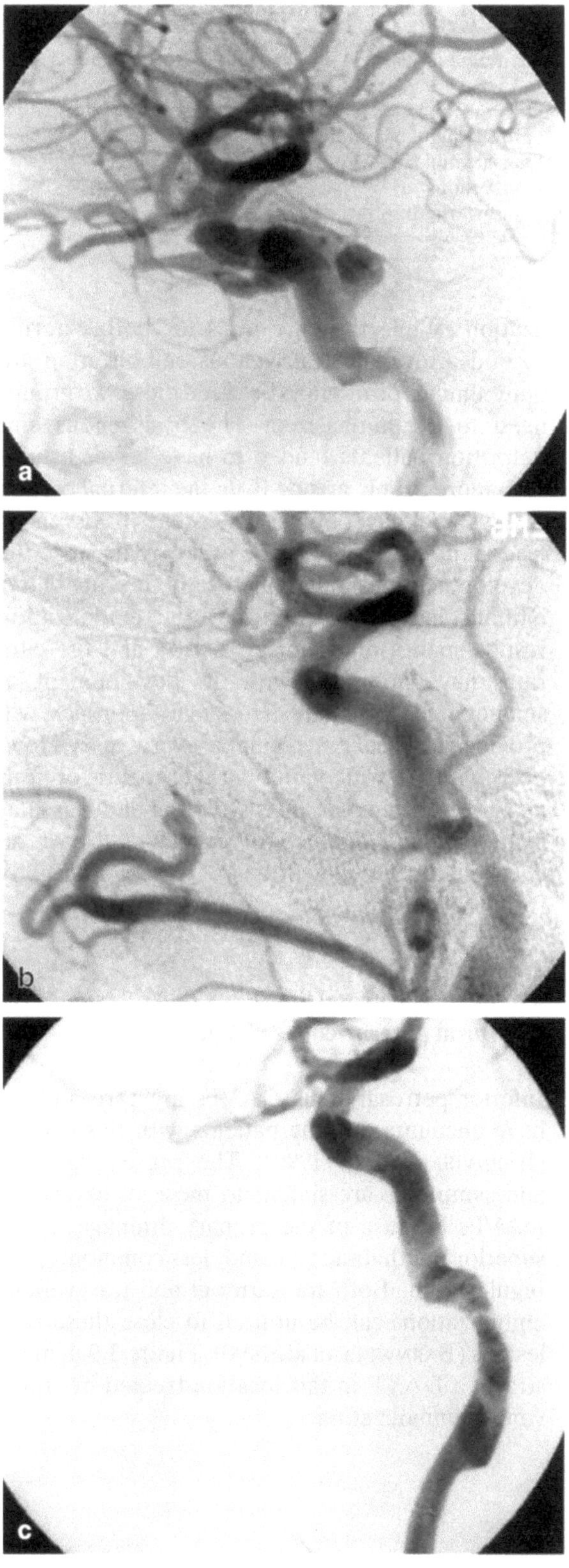

▷

Fig. 3.8a–c. A 66-year-old man presented with severe proptosis, chemosis, and abrupt visual decline. **a** Right internal carotid arteriogram, lateral projection, demonstrates a dural fistula supplied by the meningohypophyseal and inferolateral trunks. There was no external supply and attempts at transvenous embolization were unsuccessful. **b** Postembolization, carotid injection, lateral projection, demonstrates marked reduced filling of the fistula site. **c** Right internal carotid injection, lateral projection, 2 days following embolization, demonstrates complete closure of the fistula. The patient had complete recovery of vision

Table 3.1. Summary of cavernous dural treatments

Treatment modality	No. of patients treated	Cure (%)	Improved (%)	Permanent complications (%)
Carotid-jugular compression	47	17 (36%)		0 (0)
Transarterial ECA branches	45	34 (75%)	9 (20%)	2 (4%)
Transvenous	59	48 (81%)	11 (19%)	2 (3%)
Transarterial ICA branches	4	4 (100%)		1 (25%)

lization. While the cure rates for both external carotid artery and transvenous embolization are quite similar, differences between these two groups need to be emphasized. The transvenous embolization patients tended to have larger fistulas with more supply arising from the internal carotid artery. We have only utilized the transvenous treatment commonly in the past 6 years since the development of smaller microcatheters and better embolic agents. Our transarterial embolization results span a much longer period and the cure rates have improved with the development of smaller microcatheters. No single approach will provide an excellent result in every case. However, with the wide variety of therapeutic options available to treat this disease by the endovascular route, the vast majority of patients will have an excellent outcome with a low risk of morbidity from therapy.

3.4 Inferior Petrosal Sinus Dural Arteriovenous Fistulas

Inferior petrosal sinus DAVFs are rare and we have encountered nine patients with this disease (Barnwell et al. 1990). The presenting signs and symptoms are similar to those of cavernous DAVFs because of the primary drainage to the superior ophthalmic vein and, less commonly, the jugular bulb. Both transarterial and transvenous embolizations can be utilized to close these rare lesions (Barnwell et al. 1990). Figure 3.9 demonstrates a DAVF in this location treated by transvenous embolization.

3.5 Superior Sagittal Sinus Dural Arteriovenous Fistulas

3.5.1 *Clinical Presentation*

Superior sagittal sinus DAVFs are rare. We have only encountered 12 in this location. Because of the distance to the auditory apparatus, bruit audible to the patient is unusual but can sometimes be auscultated by an examiner listening over the vertex. The most common presenting symptom was headaches, present in one-half of our patients, followed by hemorrhage in 40% and stroke in 20%. The hemorrhage can be subdural, subarachnoid, or intraparenchymal. One patient presented with a dementia-like picture with cortical blindness. In the majority of our patients, the fistula was located in the middle third of the superior sagittal sinus. The remaining fistulas were seen in the posterior third.

3.5.2 *Radiographic Evaluation*

Plain skull radiography often reveals prominent dural grooves caused by enlarged middle meningeal arteries and veins. Longstanding fistulas can promote thickening of the overlying bone due to hyperemia. The arterial supply arises primarily from the middle meningeal and transosseous perforating branches from the occipital and superficial temporal artery. The arterial supply is usually bilaterally symmetric. We have seen one case where the entire supply to the fistula arose from external carotid feeders in a patient who presented with subarachnoid hemorrhage. This rare cause of subarachnoid hemorrhage must be considered in a patient with selective internal carotid and vertebral arteriograms in which a hemorrhage site has not been disclosed. Secondary arterial supply can arise from the ophthalmic artery, usually the anterior falx branch or posterior meningeal branches of the vertebral artery. As

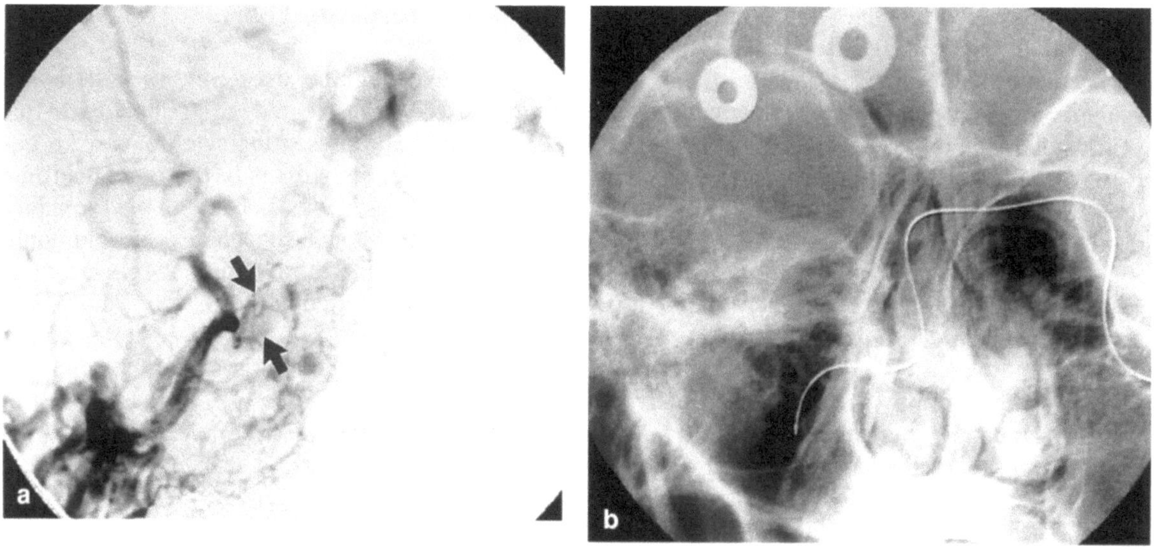

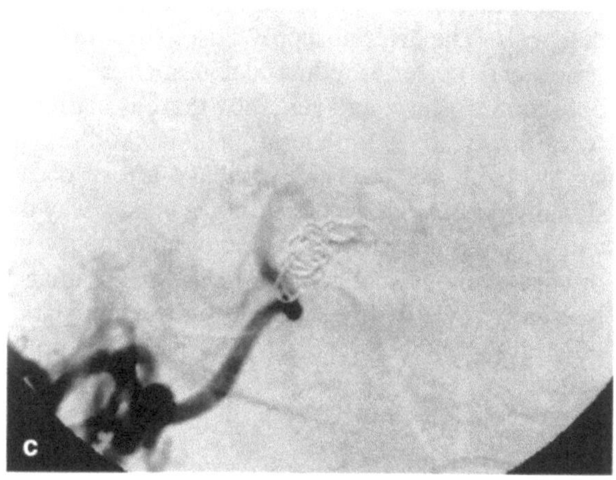

Fig. 3.9a–c. A 68-year-old man presents with bilateral proptosis, chemosis, and a right sixth nerve palsy. **a** Right external carotid injection, AP projection, demonstrates a dural fistula (*arrows*) located in the inferior petrosal sinus on the right side. The connection between the inferior petrosal sinus and the jugular bulb is occluded. The venous drainage is by way of the inferior petrosal sinus retrograde to the cavernous sinus to the contralateral inferior petrosal sinus and superior ophthalmic veins. **b** A plain skull film, AP projection, demonstrates a microcatheter coursing from a transfemoral access through the left inferior petrosal sinus across the circular sinus to the fistula site. **c** Postembolization right internal carotid injection, AP projection, demonstrates closure of the fistula by multiple platinum coils

with all dural fistulas, cortical venous drainage has a high affinity for producing hemorrhage. CT can be useful for detecting enlargement of the dural grooves in the inner table of the skull as well as bony thickening. The proximity of the draining veins to the inner surface of the skull can make detection by MRI and CT somewhat difficult.

3.5.3 Therapeutic Options

Excessive tortuosity can make placement of a catheter close to the fistula site difficult from a transfemoral access. Direct puncture of the distal superficial temporal artery in the scalp can permit embolization with liquid adhesives. Transvascular embolization alone was effective in 50% of the patients treated in our series. Thirty percent were treated by intraoprative exposure of the feeding arteries and embolization and 20% were treated by surgical excision of the fistulous site (HALBACH et al. 1988). All patients had complete cure of their fistulas and one complication occurred related to surgery.

Because of their unique midline location, multiplicity of arterial feeders, and critical venous drainage, dural fistulas involving the superior sagittal sinus often require unusual and aggressive forms of therapy.

3.6 Ethmoidal Dural Arteriovenous Fistulas

Dural fistulas located on the floor of the anterior cranial fossa are rare, with only 33 reported cases. The majority are solitary case reports (KOBAYASHI et al. 1988; HALBACH et al. 1990).

Unlike dural fistulas in other locations, there is a strong male predominance (87%). The presenting symptoms of dural fistulas located at the floor of the anterior cranial fossa are remarkably similar, with 91% presenting with hemorrhage, usually intercerebrally into the frontal lobe or subarachnoid hemorrhage. Because of the location on the anterior cranial fossa floor, the venous drainage is by way of olfactory veins or parasagittal veins, often with an associated venous aneurysm. Rarely, patients present with visual loss, with drainage posteriorly towards the cavernous sinus (HALBACH et al. 1990).

3.6.1 Radiographic Evaluation

Computed tomography and MRI are usually the primary modalities that disclose the intraparenchymal or subarachnoid hemorrhage resulting from the fistula. We have found that coronal MRI may disclose a dilated olfactory draining vein below the frontal lobe, thereby suggesting the diagnosis. The arterial supply arises from the anterior and posterior ethmoidal branches of the ophthalmic artery, and generally there is bilateral recruitment to a unilateral fistula. Additional supply from the internal maxillary artery occasionally occurs. The venous drainage is by way of a pial vein, often with associated pseudoaneurysm or varix (venous aneurysm). The venous drainage is usually towards the superior sagittal sinus and only rarely to the cavernous sinus or deep venous system.

3.6.2 Treatment

Surgical coagulation of the draining vein with or without resection of the fistulous site is a highly successful therapy for this disease. The procedure is associated with a high cure rate and low morbidity, usually with only diminished olfactory sensation resulting from elevation of the frontal lobe. Only a few cases of embolization in this disease have been reported (LASJAUNIAS et al. 1983; ABUMIYA et al. 1987). The primary arterial supply to these fistulas always arises from ethmoidal branches of the ophthalmic artery. While subselective catheterization of the ophthalmic artery is technically possible, the risk of retinal infarction with embolization remains high. We therefore reserve embolization for patients who cannot undergo a surgical procedure.

3.7 Deep Venous Dural Fistulas

Fistulas involving the deep venous system are unusual. We have treated 12 patients with this localization. The presenting symptoms were hemorrhage in seven, strokes in three, and chronic severe headaches in two. Because of the proximity to the aqueduct, hydrocephalus is commonly associated with the dural fistula at this location. The fistula was located in the straight sinus in six, the vein of Galen in five, and the posterior falx in one. The arterial supply arises from both middle meningeal arteries.

In addition there is recruitment of dural supply from the vertebral artery (posterior meningeal branch), posterior cerebral dural supply (artery of Davidoff and Schecter), internal carotid dural supply (marginal tentorial arteries), and rarely supply from the superficial temporal artery and anterior cerebral arteries. All patients were treated by preoperative embolization followed by a surgical procedure. Seven patients had intraoperative occlusion of the draining vein, direct puncture of the fistulous site, and embolization with liquid adhesives; all were cured by the procedure. Patients who had undergone ligation of the feeding arteries at surgery had subtotal occlusion of their fistula and required additional procedures of intraoperative embolization to achieve fistula cure. Coagulation of the fistula site was effective in the remaining cases in achieving complete cure. Three patients required ventricular shunting for hydrocephalus that was aggravated as a result of the treatment. Dural fistulas in this region have a high risk of hemorrhage and stroke and often require complex combined treatment strategies for definitive closure (HALBACH et al. 1989d).

3.8 Unusual Dural Fistulas

Intracranial dural fistulas that drain inferiorly towards the spinal cord can present with progressive radiculopathy and myelopathy similar to their radicular artery–medullary vein fistula counterparts (PICARD 1987). We have encountered two such fistulas in the craniocervical junction in patients who presented with slowly progressive lower extremity weakness (GAENSLER et al. 1990). Others have reported similar intracranial fistulas producing venous hypertension in the spinal cord and an ascending myelopathy (PICARD 1989).

Dural fistulas in children tend to have larger and more numerous connections than their adult counterparts. They can present with heart murmurs, macrocephaly, cardiac failure, elevated intracranial pressure, and hemorrhage (ALBRIGHT et al. 1983). Many of these larger fistulas require combined surgical and endovascular therapy. It is important to remember that congenital fistulas producing loud bruits are rarely reported by the child, who assumes the noise to be a normal part of its environment.

Multiple dural fistulas at separate locations can occur. We have encountered nine such patients (BARNWELL et al. 1991b). The etiology of these multiple dural fistulas is as yet unknown. Theoretically, a single dural fistula can produce elevated venous pressure, venous stagnation, and thrombosis at a distant site, yielding an additional dural fistula. In addition, hypercoagulable states (protein S, protein C, antithrombin 3 deficiency, elevated platelets, hyperviscosity syndrome) may also produce multiple venous thromboses, a known cause of dural fistulas.

Dural fistulas involving the torcula are rare, usually producing hemorrhage or dementia. Combined surgical and embolization techniques are usually effective in achieving complete cure.

We have encountered several DAVFs located in the tentorium. These fistulas usually recruit both internal and external dural supply. The cortical drainage associated with this location places the patients at high risk for stroke and hemorrhage, the most common presenting symptoms. Preoperative embolization followed by surgical exposure and embolization or excision is often required for complete cure. Figure 9.2 depicts an example of a tentorial DAVF cured by preoperative embolization and subsequent excision.

In conclusion, DAVFs are a complex disease that can present with a wide spectrum of clinical signs and symptoms. Abnormal venous drainage suggests a higher risk of hemorrhage and stroke, as do certain locations such as the deep venous system, superior sagittal sinus, tentorium, and ethmoidal dural region. The decision to treat an individual fistula must take into account the natural history of the disease, the patient's symptoms, the neurologic condition, and the risks and benefits of the treatment modalities. Endovascular treatment offers an excellent treatment option for the vast majority of dural fistulas that require therapy.

References

Abumiya T, Kamiyama H, Murata J et al. (1987) Dural arteriovenous malformation with uncommon draining veins in the anterior fossa. Case report. Neurol Med Chir (Tokyo) 27:1195–1200

Albright AL, Latchaw RE, Price RA (1983) Posterior dural arteriovenous malformations in infancy. Neurosurgery 13:129–135

Aminoff MJ, Kendall BE (1973) Asymptomatic dural vascular anomalies. Br J Radiol 46:662–667

Barnwell SL, Halbach VV, Higashida RT, Hieshima GB, Wilson CB (1989) Complex dural arteriovenous fistulas: results of a new combined neurosurgical and interventional neuroradiology treatment in 16 patients. J Neurosurg 7:352–358

Barnwell SL, Halbach VV, Dowd CF, Higashida RT, Hieshima GB (1990) Dural fistulas including the inferior petrosal sinus. AJNR 11:511–517

Barnwell SL, Halbach VV, Dowd CF, Higashida RT, Hieshima GB, Wilson CB (1991a) A variant of arteriovenous fistulas within the wall of dural sinuses: results of combined surgical and endovascular therapy. J Neurosurgery 24:199–204

Barnwell SL, Halbach VV, Dowd CF, Higashida RT, Hieshima GB, Wilson CB (1991b) Multiple dural arteriovenous fistulas of the spine and cranium. AJNR 12:441–446

Barrow DL, Spector RH, Braun IF, Landman JA, Tindall SC, Tindall GT (1985) Classification and treatment of carotid-cavernous sinus fistulas. J Neurosurg 62:248–256

Brismar G, Brismar J (1976) Spontaneous carotid cavernous fistulae: phlebographic appearance and relation to thrombosis. Acta Radiol [Diagn] 17:180–192

Castaigne P, Bories J, Brunet P, Cassan JL, Meninger V, Merland JJ (1975) Fistules arterio-veineuses de la duremere. Ann Med Interne (Paris) 126:813–817

Chaudhary M, Sachdev VP, Cho SH, Weitzner I Jr, Puljic S, Huang YP (1982) Dural arteriovenous malformation of the major venous sinuses: an acquired lesion. AJNR 3:13–19

Courtheoux P, Labbe D, Hamel C, Lecog PJ, Jahara M, Theron J (1987) Treatment of bilateral spontaneous dural carotid cavernous fistulas by coil and sclerotherapy. J Neurosurg 66:468–470

DeMarco JK, Dillon W, Halbach VV, Tsuruda JS (1990) Dural arteriovenous fistulas: evaluation with MR imaging. Radiology 175:193–199

Djindjian R, Cophignon J, Theron J (1973) Embolization by superselective arteriography from the femoral route; review of 60 cases: technique, indications, complications. Neuroradiology 6:20–26

Dowd CF, Halbach VV, Barnwell SL, Higashida RT, Hieshima GB (1991) Occlusion at the anterior superior ophthalmic vein in carotid cavernous fistulae acutely aggravating visual symptoms. Neuroradiology 33:142–143

Doyon D, Metzger J (1973) Malformations vasculaires duremeriennes sustentorielles. Acta Radiol 13:792–800

Gaensler EHL, Jackson P, Halbach VV (1990) Intracranial dural arteriovenous fistulas as a case of myelopathy. AJNR 11:513–523

Halbach VV, Higashida RT, Hieshima GB (1987a) Diagnosis and treatment of dural arteriovenous fistulae. In: Margulis AR, Gooding CA (eds) Diagnostic radiology. University of California Press, Berkeley, pp 303–308

Halbach VV, Higashida RT, Hieshima GB, Reicher M, Norman D, Newton TH (1987b) Dural fistulas involving the cavernous sinus: results of treatment in 30 patients. Radiology 163:437–442
Halbach VV, Higashida RT, Hieshima GB, Goto K, Norman D, Newton TH (1987c) Dural fistulas involving the transverse and sigmoid sinuses: results of treatment in 28 patients. Radiology 163:443–447
Halbach VV, Hieshima GB, Higashida RT, Reicher M (1987d) Carotid cavernous fistula: indications for urgent therapy. AJNR 8:627–633 and AJR 149:587–593
Halbach VV, Higashida RT, Hieshima GB, Cahan L, Rosenblum M (1988) Treatment of dural arterial venous malformations involving the superior sagittal sinus. AJNR 9:337–343
Halbach VV, Higashida RT, Hieshima GB, Hardin CW (1989a) Embolization of the dural branches arising from the cavernous internal carotid artery. AJNR 10:143–150
Halbach VV, Higashida RT, Hieshima GB, Hardin CW, Pribram H (1989b) Transvenous embolization of dural fistulas involving the cavernous sinus. AJNR 10:377–384
Halbach VV, Higashida RT, Hieshima GB, Mehringer CM, Hardin CW (1989c) Transvenous embolization of dural fistulas involving the transverse and sigmoid sinuses. AJNR 10:385–392
Halbach VV, Higashida RT, Hieshima GB, Wilson CW (1989d) Treatment of dural fistulas involving the deep cerebral venous system. AJNR 10:393–399
Halbach VV, Higashida RT, Hieshima GB, Wilson CW, Barnwell SL, Dowd CF (1990) Dural arteriovenous fistulas supplied by ethmoidal arteries. Neurosurgery 25:816–823
Hieshima GB, Reicher MA, Higashida RT et al. (1987) Intraoperative digital subtraction neuroangiography: a diagnostic and therapeutic tool. AJNR 8:759–767
Higashida RT, Hieshima GB, Halbach VV, Bentson JR, Goto K (1986) Closure of carotid cavernous sinus fistulae by external compression of the carotid artery and jugular vein. Acta Radiol [Suppl] (Stockh) 369: 580–583
Horton JA, Kerber CW (1986) Lidocaine injection into the external carotid branches: provocative test to preserve cranial nerve function therapeutic embolization. AJNR 7:105–108
Hosobuchi Y (1975) Electrothrombosis of carotid-cavernous fistula. J Neurosurg 42:76–85
Houser OW, Campbell JK, Campbell RJ, Sundt TM (1979) Arteriovenous malformations affecting the transverse dural sinus – an acquired lesion. Mayo Clin Proc 54:651–661
Ishii K, Goto K, Ihoico K et al. (1988) High risk dural arteriovenous fistulae at the transverse and sigmoid sinuses. AJNR 8:1113–1121
Jrgensen JS, Guthoff R (1988) Ophthalmoscopic findings in spontaneous carotid cavernous fistula: an analysis of 20 patients. *Graefes Arch Clin Exp Ophthalmol* 226:34–36
Kobayashi H, Hayashi M, Noguchi Y, Tsuji T, Handa Y, Caner HH (1988) Dural arteriovenous malformations in the anterior cranial fossa. Surg Neurol 30:396–401
Lasjaunias P, Ming C, Brugge KT, Atul T (1986) Neurological manifestations of intracranial dural arteriovenous malformations. J Neurosurg 64:724–730
Lasjaunias P, Berenstein A (1987) Surgical neuroangiography. Functional anatomy of craniofacial arteries, 1st edn. Springer, Berlin Heidelberg New York
Lasjaunias P, Halimi P, Lepez-Ibor L, Sichez JP, Hurth M, Tribolet ND (1983) Traitement endovasculaire des malformation vasculares durales (MVD) pures spontanees. *Neurochirurgie* 30:207–223
Magidson MA, Weinberg DE (1976) Spontaneous closure of a dural arteriovenous malformation. Surg Neurol 6:107–110
Mullan S (1979) Treatment of carotid cavernous fistulas by cavernous sinus thrombosis. J Neurosurg 50:131–144
Newton TH, Hoyt WF (1970) Dural arteriovenous shunts in the region of the cavernous sinus. Neuroradiology 1:71–78
Picard L, Bracard S, Mallet J, Per A, Glacobbe HL, Roland J (1987) Spontaneous dural arteriovenous fistulas. *Semin Intervent Radiol* 4:219–240
Sanders MD, Hoyt WF (1969) Hypoxic ocular sequelae of carotid cavernous fistulae. Br J Ophthalmol 53:82–97
Sergott RC, Grossman RI, Savino PJ, Bosley TM, Schatz NJ (1987) The syndrome of paradoxical worsening of dural cavernous sinus arteriovenous malformations. Ophthalmology 94:205–212
Sundt TM, Piepgras DG (1983) The surgical approach to arteriovenous malformations of the lateral and sigmoid dural sinuses. J Neurosurg 59:32–39
Takahashi A, Yoshimoto T, Kawakami K, Sugawara T, Suzuki J (1989) Transvenous copper wire insertion for dural arteriovenous malformations of cavernous sinus. J Neurosurg 70:751–754
Teng MM, Guo WY, Huang CI, Wu CC, Chang T (1988) Occlusion of arteriovenous malformations of the cavernous sinus via the superior ophthalmic vein. AJNR 539–546
Toya S, Shiobara R, Izumi J, Shinomiya Y, Shiga H, Kimura C (1981) Spontaneous carotid-cavernous fistula during pregnancy or in the postpartum stage. J Neurosurg 54:252–256
Vinuela F, Fox AJ, Debrun GM, Peerless SJ, Drake CG (1984) Spontaneous carotid-cavernous fistulas; clinical, radiological, and therapeutic considerations. Experience with 20 cases. J Neurosurg 60:976–984
Vinuela F, Fox AJ, Pelz DM, Drake CG (1986) Unusual clinical manifestations of dural arteriovenous malformations. Neurosurg 64:554–558

4 Embolization of Epistaxis

ANTON VALAVANIS and AVI SETTON

CONTENTS

4.1 Introduction

Epistaxis is a rather common, usually benign and self-limiting disease. Up to 60% of the adult population experiences an episode of nasal bleeding, but only 6% of these require medical attention (SMALL et al. 1982). Based on the bleeding site as revealed by nasal endoscopy, two topographically distinct types of epistaxis are distinguished, i.e., anterior and posterior epistaxis.

Anterior epistaxis is the most common type, being less severe than posterior epistaxis and usually self-limiting. The bleeding site is located in the anterior septum (Kisselbach's plexus), which is a readily accessible area to the ENT surgeon. When treatment is needed, simple measures such as anterior packing or cautery usually stop the bleeding effectively.

Posterior nasal hemorrhage occurs in a relatively inaccessible region and often requires active treatment. Advanced age and concurrent medical problems may further complicate the management of these patients. Different methods are utilized which vary in complexity, effectiveness, and stress to the patient. An ascending scale of treatment modalities for posterior epistaxis comprises cautery, injection of hemostatic agents to the pterygomaxillary space, anterior nasal packing, endoscopically guided electrocoagulation, posterior nasal packing, and surgical ligations, i.e., transantral internal maxillary artery ligation, sometimes in combination with ethmoidal artery ligation (CHANDLER and SERRINS 1965; WANG and VOGEL 1981; SCHAITKIN et al. 1987; METSON and LANE 1988).

In recent years endovascular embolization has evolved as an adjuvant or primary modality in epistaxis treatment (STRUTZ and SCHUMACHER 1990; VITEK 1991). A thorough clinical and endoscopic evaluation is essential to localize the bleeding source and to direct further treatment like packing, embolization, or surgical ligations. Posterior nasal packing is the immediate tool to control bleeding, even temporarily, in order to achieve hemodynamic and medical stabilization (e.g., blood transfusion if needed) and enable basic medical workup (i.e., coagulation profile, medical background). The packing is painful and stressful for the patient and prolonged packing may be complicated by aspiration, sinus infection, and alar necrosis by catheter pressure. Later sequelae include respiratory compromise, arterial hypoxia with secondary cardiac arrhythmias or cerebral ischemia, episodic nocturnal oxygen desaturation, and worsening of sleep disorders by overfilling of the nasopharynx and depression of the soft palate. A failure rate of up to 25%–50% and a complication rate of 20%–60% have been reported in the literature (WANG and VOGEL 1981; SCHAITKIN et al. 1987). Early removal of the posterior nasal packing after control of the bleeding is mandatory to prevent complications (STRUTZ and SCHUMACHER 1990).

When posterior nasal packing fails to stop the bleeding, the epistaxis is defined as intractable or uncontrollable, and further measures are needed. Internal maxillary artery ligation has been utilized since the early 1960s (CHANDLER and SERRINS

ANTON VALAVANIS, M.D., Professor and Head, Abteilung für Neuroradiologie, Departement Medizinische Radiologie, Röntgendiagnostisches Zentralinstitut, Universitätsspital Zürich, Frauenklinikstrasse 10, 8091 Zürich, Switzerland
AVI SETTON, M.D., Department of Radiology, Division of Interventional Neuroradiology, New York University Medical Center, 550 First Avenue, New York, NY 10016, USA

1965). A clinical failure rate of 10%–15% and a complication rate of up to 40%–47% have been reported (SCHAITKIN et al. 1987; METSON and LANE 1988). Furthermore, in approximately 6% of cases this approach is contraindicated because of the presence of a hypoplastic maxillary antrum (PEARSON et al. 1969). Investigation of surgical ligation failures revealed incomplete or inadequate ligation, incorrect vessel selection, anatomic variations, alternate dominance of blood supply, and reconstitution of flow to the nasal mucosa through collateral circulation to be the main underlying causes (BREDA et al. 1989; ROSNAGLE et al. 1980). The ethmoidal arteries, internal carotid artery (ICA) branches (i.e., inferolateral trunk, vidian artery), and nasopharyngeal vessels (ascending pharyngeal, descending palatine, ascending palatine, accessory meningeal artery) may reconstitute flow beyond the proximal occlusion to explain early recurrent hemorrhage (BREDA et al. 1989).

Endovascular embolization emerged as an attractive alternative in the treatment of epistaxis. Mapping the vascular system by superselective angiography and the ability to embolize the distal arteriolar bed in the bleeding territory may effectively control postsurgical failures (BREDA et al. 1989). Alternatively, embolization following superselective, distal catheterization of the bleeding nasal arterial territory may be employed as the primary modality of treatment and thus enable early removal of posterior nasal packing.

4.2 Etiology and Management Strategies

Multiple causes of epistaxis have been reported in different pathologic entities. Two major groups can be identified, i.e., a group with organic lesions as the source of bleeding and a second idiopathic group without identifiable underlying vascular or other pathology (LASJAUNIAS and BERENSTEIN 1987b).

In most cases the cause of bleeding is not determined. Inconsistent association with hypertension, heavy smoking, alcohol consumption, and hypercholesteremia can be found. In angiography and other imaging modalities no discrete lesions can be identified. Most of the patients are healthy with a sudden onset of severe epistaxis.

In the second group different pathologic entities should be considered: traumatic epistaxis in cases of facial trauma, and as a postsurgical or postbiopsy complication for vascular lesions. Tumoral epistaxis is a large group – juvenile angiofibromas, angiomatous polyp, capillary hemangioma, and primary or metastatic malignant tumors are some of the common hypervascular neoplastic lesions. Vascular pathology in the ICA or external carotid artery (ECA) territory may be an unusual source of severe hemorrhage. Aneurysms, arteriovenous fistulas, pseudoaneurysms, arteriovenous malformations (AVMs), and venous malformations should be considered. Systemic coagulopathy can present as severe intractable epistaxis.

In hemorrhagic hereditary telangiectasia of Osler-Weber-Rendu, recurrent epistaxis is the rule. The mucosal surfaces are the usual source of bleeding and in up to 85% of hemorrhagic events the nasal mucosa is the bleeding site. Multiple angiectasias are demonstrated angiographically in the early and late arterial phases (LASJAUNIAS and BERENSTEIN 1987b). The treatment of epistaxis in vascular lesions requires a multidisciplinary tailored approach to achieve palliation or cure. In idiopathic epistaxis the goal is to control and stop the bleeding, as no underlying pathology can be found.

4.3 Arterial Embolization

In 1974 SOKOLOFF et al. reported two cases in which selective arterial embolization with Gelfoam resolved intractable epistaxis and in 1976 DJINDJIAN et al. reported on the application of embolization in a larger series of patients with severe epistaxis. In 1979 WILLS and RUSSELL described a similar technique in bleeding diathesis. Although proven to be successful, embolization was utilized only secondarily, in patients who failed surgical ligation, in intractable bleeding in trauma or tumors, in coagulopathy, or in medically compromised patients when the risk of general anesthesia for surgical procedures was considered very high.

Following reports of arterial embolization (ROBERTSON and REARDON 1979; RICHE et al. 1979; WILLS and RUSSEL 1979), MERLAND et al. (1980) published a larger series of 54 patients with epistaxis managed by embolization. The effectiveness of the procedure, its low risk, and the minor yield of identifying the bleeding site by angiography were emphasized. Several further reports emphasizing the role of embolization in the treatment of severe and intractable epistaxis appeared in the 1980s (ROSNAGLE et al. 1980; VAN

WYCK et al. 1982; DAVIES 1986; PARNES et al. 1987; DEFILIPP et al. 1988; WEHRLI et al. 1988; HICKS and VITEK 1989). STRUTZ and SCHUMACHER, in 1990, documented a 90% success rate in controlling epistaxis. VITEK, in 1991, summarized his experience with microcatheter superselective embolization in 30 patients with idiopathic epistaxis. He reported a success rate of 87%–97% and one transient hemiparesis as the only complication in this group. The effectiveness and safety of the procedure in appropriately trained and experienced hands led the author to recommend endovascular embolization as the primary modality of treatment. In cases of idiopathic epistaxis the source of bleeding is not demonstrated clinically or angiographically.

The posterior septum is probably the territory where the bleeding most commonly originates. The possibility of occluding the small arteriolar bed in the septal area and nasal mucosa explains the high success rate in controlling the bleeding. The fact that proximal arterial clipping is quite successful suggests that decrease in the perfusion pressure in the nasal mucosa plays a role and that the physiologic hemostatic mechanisms can take over.

In failed cases of surgical arterial ligation, angiography reveals collateral blood supply to the nasal mucosa (BREDA et al. 1989). The contralateral internal maxillary artery plays a role mainly in the midline, i.e., in the septal territory. The ascending pharyngeal artery, the facial artery through the ascending palatine artery, the jugal and infraorbital arteries, and the accessory meningeal artery may reconstitute flow to the mucosa beyond a proximal ligation of the internal maxillary artery (PEARSON et al. 1969; BREDA et al. 1989). The vessels are usually amenable to arterial embolization with a high rate of bleeding control. When the ethmoidal arteries are prominent and reconstitute flow to the septal area, ethmoidal surgical ligation is necessary.

In Osler-Weber-Rendu disease, angiographic demonstration of the telangiectatic lesions and embolization with particles provide satisfactory immediate hemostasis for months to years. Recurrent events of epistaxis are almost the rule in this disease and repeated procedures are needed (LASJAUNIAS and BERENSTEIN 1987b). Arterial ligation should be avoided, except in cases of dominant supply from the ethmoidal arteries, in order to leave patent the arterial axis for repeated distal embolizations. Arterial changes in the form of irregularities and small aneurysms can be seen angiographically after several procedures and recurrent hemorrhages.

4.4 Vascular Anatomy of the Nasal Cavity

The blood supply to the nasal cavity is complex, originating from dual circulations, i.e., the ICA and ECA territories (LASJAUNIAS et al. 1979). In the ECA territory, the sphenopalatine artery is the dominant vessel, originating from the pterygopalatine segment of the internal maxillary artery. It exits the pterygopalatine fossa via the sphenopalatine foramen to enter the nasal cavity behind and above the middle choncha. This vessel ramifies into two major groups – the posterior lateral nasal branches or conchal arteries supplying the turbinates and parts of the maxillary, ethmoidal, and sphenoidal sinuses, and posterior medial nasal branches or septal arteries which supply the nasal septum. The anterior and posterior ethmoidal arteries originate from the ophthalmic artery beyond its second intraorbital segment. They mainly supply the superior parts of the septum at the level of the anterior and posterior ethmoidal cells and anastomose with the septal branches of the sphenopalatine artery – an anastomosis between the ECA and the ophthalmic artery.

The terminal branches of the descending palatine (greater palatine) artery may anastomose through the distal hard palate and the incisival foramen with the nasopalatine artery, the distal segment of the septal branch of the sphenopalatine artery, supplying the lower anterior portion of the nasal cavity.

The distal anterior septal branches of the superior labial artery, a branch of the facial artery, supply the anterior portion of the septum and occasionally the lateral nasal wall through alar branches. This anterior inferior portion of the septum – Kisselbach's plexus – is an arterial junction area between the facial, nasopalatine, and descending palatine arteries.

Additional possible supply to the nasal cavity territory is by collateral circulation through the accessory meningeal and ascending pharyngeal arteries. This will be seen in vascular lesions or after proximal ligations reconstituting blood supply to the mucoperiosteum (BREDA et al. 1989).

Transmedian anastomoses are common and are mainly encountered in vascular pathology.

They supply mainly the paramedian territory of the contralateral sphenopalatine artery.

4.5 Technique of Embolization

Angiography and embolization are performed in the neuroangiographic/interventional neuroradiology suite. The procedure is performed with the nasal packing in place (posterior and/or anterior nasal packings) and after thorough clinical examination of the patient by the ENT surgeon.

Preferably, general anesthesia is utilized, providing the advantages of a quite patient, controlled respiration (important with nasal packing), and less induced vascular spasm with catheter manipulation. Neuroleptic analgesia is considered for cooperative patients and in patients in whom general anesthesia entails a high degree of risk. A femoral approach using a conventional, preformed, neurodiagnostic 5-French (5F) catheter (Cook), catheter manipulation with or without a guidewire for selective catheterization, and hand injections using high quality digital subtraction angiography equipment are routine.

The diagnostic angiogram and superselective embolization are performed according to a protocol and depending on the clinically identified bleeding site and the type of epistaxis present (idiopathic, organic).

The detailed angiographic protocol described here is used by the senior author and applies to the idiopathic type of epistaxis. The ipsilateral common carotid artery is catheterized and injected first in frontal projection, to assess the ICA and ECA branches for pathologic processes, anatomic variations, and potentially dangerous anastomoses (Fig. 4.1a). Leaving the 5F catheter as a guiding catheter in the common carotid artery (CCA) below the bifurcation, a variable stiffness microcatheter (Tracker 18 or 10, Target Therapeutics) is inserted coaxially and advanced to the pterygopalatine portion of the internal maxillary artery using a microguidewire (Target Therapeutics). Verification of flow, possible descending palatine artery supply, and patent anastomoses to the ICA (artery of foramen rotundum) or ophthalmic artery is achieved by superselective angiography, preferably in frontal projection (Fig. 4.1b). If possible, the microcatheter will be advanced to the septal branch of the sphenopalatine artery and "septography" obtained (Fig. 4.1c). Careful manipulation is imperative to prevent arterial spasm. Embolization is then performed with low pressure injections of microparticles of polyvinyl alcohol foam (PVA) with size ranges of 40–150 or 150–250 μm ("Contour", Interventional Therapeutics) under careful fluoroscopic control, in order to detect any ophthalmic anastomoses through the ethmoidal arteries. It is essential to avoid filling of the ethmoidal artery to prevent potential embolization of the ophthalmic artery. With this catheter position a small volume of microparticles will usually suffice to block the arteriolar bed of the septum, which represents the origin of most cases of idiopathic intractable epistaxis.

Superselective catheterization of the ipsilateral facial artery is the next step, and angiography in the frontal projection is obtained, verifying or excluding supply to the anterior portion of the septum or alar area (superior labial artery branches). In the presence of supply, flow-guided embolization with microparticles is performed from a distal catheter position in the facial artery. In the absence of angiographically demonstrable supply, no embolization is performed.

A CCA injection in frontal projection is carried out for postembolization control, to confirm devascularization of the embolized territories and to detect any persisting residual ethmoidal supply via the ophthalmic artery to the septum (Fig. 4.1d).

The contralateral CCA is injected next. Ethmoidal and sphenopalatine arterial supply to the septum and potential vascular pathology are assessed. When there is angiographically demonstrable supply, coaxial superselective catheterization and embolization are performed as described above. When no arterial contribution is appreciated, the procedure is terminated without further embolization.

In cases with bilateral hemorrhage or lack of precise clinical determination of the bleeding source, bilateral embolization is performed. In certain pathologic conditions such as Osler-Weber-Rendu disease or nasopharyngeal tumors with epistaxis, bilateral embolization is performed, including vessels to the lateral wall (lateral branches of the sphenopalatine artery) and the inferior wall (descending palatine artery) of the nasal cavity and the nasopharynx (ascending pharyngeal, descending palatine, and ascending palatine arteries). A detailed description of the endovascular embolization of these entities is beyond the scope of this chapter and needs a tailored approach (Valavanis 1990).

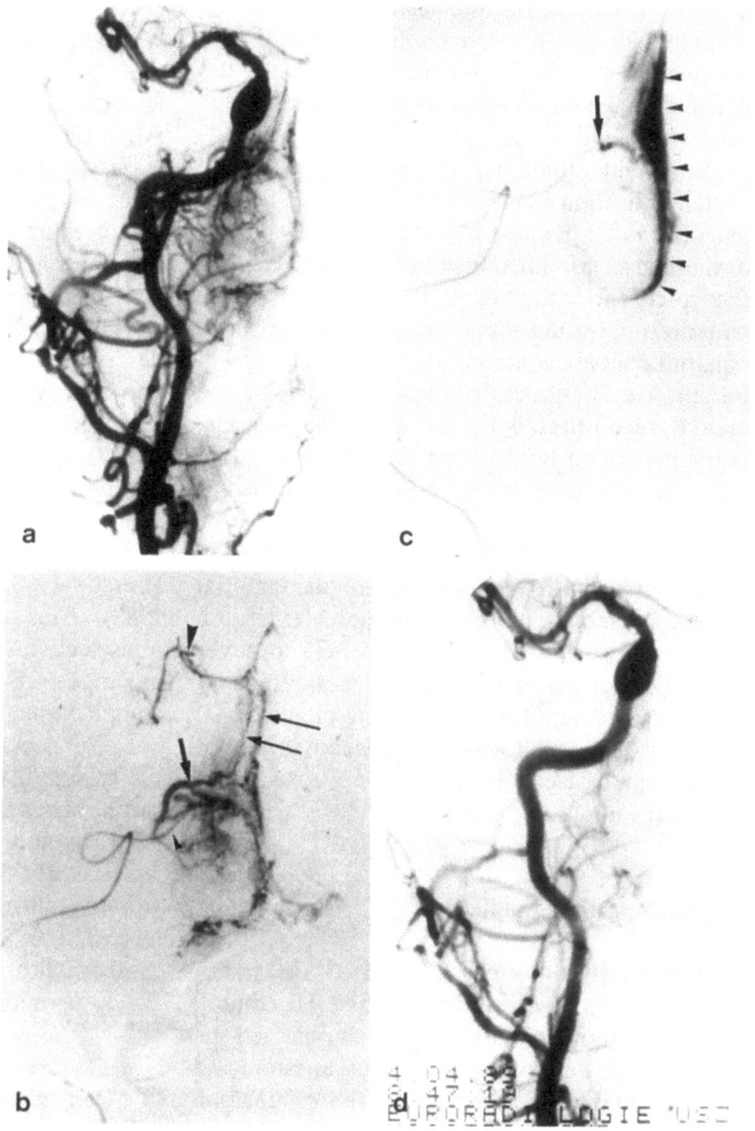

Fig. 4.1a–d. Angiographic evaluation and embolization, in frontal projection in a patient with idiopathic intractable epistaxis. **a** Right CCA angiography reveals unspecific hypervascularity of the septum and provides an overview of the arterial anatomy of the ICA and the ECA. **b** Right sphenopalatine artery angiography in frontal projection after superselective catheterization of the distal sphenopalatine artery with a Tracker microcatheter. There is clear visualization of the superior conchal branch (*small arrowhead*) with opacification of the superior turbinate, the septal branch (*thick arrow*), and the septum. Note dangerous anastomosis of the septal branch with the ophthalmic artery (*large arrowhead*) via anterior and posterior ethmoidal arteries (*thin arrows*). **c** Septography in frontal projection following distal superselective catheterization of the septal branch of the sphenopalatine artery distal to the origin of the ethmoidal arteries (*arrow*). Note intense and complete opacification of the septum (*arrowheads*) and absence of anastomoses with the ophthalmic artery. From this catheter position embolization with microparticles of PVA (45–150 μm) was performed. **d** Right CCA angiography following embolization confirms selective devascularization of the septum, absence of the collateral supply, and preservation of all ECA branches

In selected cases, septography and superselective embolization are achieved by using a bilateral approach. Using bifemoral punctures, simultaneous bilateral catheterization of both CCAs and concomitant bilateral coaxial catheterization of the septal branches of both sphenopalatine arteries is accomplished with Tracker microcatheters. Bilateral embolization or unilateral embolization with complete flow control by the contralateral microcatheter may facilitate distal embolization of the septal vascular bed.

On a routine basis the nasal packing is left in place for 6–8 h postembolization and then removed by the ENT surgeon. Alternatively, the packing can be removed in the neuroangiographic suite at the end of the procedure.

Prominent ethmoidal arteries in the control postembolization angiogram may predict further bleeding and a possible need for surgical clipping of these arteries. Since the ethmoidal arteries are the collateral pathways to the septal territory, embolization of the septal branch of the sphenopalatine artery beyond the site of anastomosis will be curative. If, in the control study, the septal area is reconstituted by the ethmoidal vessels, immediate or early recurrent bleeding will not be properly managed by additional endovascular therapy.

In Osler-Weber-Rendu disease, as embolization is a purely palliative procedure, embolic material injection is more extensive, and more vessels are superselectively catheterized bilaterally to cover the collateral circulation to the nasal mucosa territory. The importance of leaving the proximal arterial axis patent for future procedures cannot be overemphasized, as recurrent epistaxis is the rule in this disease.

4.6 Dangers and Complications

In 1979 Lasjaunias et al. reported the radioanatomic basis and protocol for arterial embolization for epistaxis. Further work emphasized the important evaluation of dangerous anastomoses between branches of the ECA, the ophthalmic artery, the ICA, and the vertebral artery (Lasjaunias and Berenstein 1987a). The potential damage to the ICA territory or ophthalmic artery territory through unrecognized anastomoses or reflux of embolic material explains the risk of stroke or blindness. Proper anatomic evaluation and distal superselective catheterization using variable stiffness microcatheters can minimize the danger of stroke.

Special attention is necessary to reduce the risk of blindness while embolizing the septal territory. Septography involves distal superselective catheterization. The importance of (a) gentle manipulation to prevent arterial spasm and (b) low injection pressures cannot be overemphasized; in this way potential filling of the ethmoidal arteries and inadvertent embolization of the ophthalmic artery are avoided.

Visualization of patent functional connections between septal branches and the ophthalmic artery via anterior and/or posterior ethmoidal arteries is a relative contraindication to embolization. Alteration of the catheter position and the embolic material size will permit safe embolization in these cases. Careful fluoroscopic monitoring and low pressure injection of the embolic material are mandatory, even when superselective angiography has not demonstrated dangerous anastomoses.

Ischemic changes and skin necrosis have been described as postembolization complications of epistaxis (Wehrli et al. 1988). Prevention can be achieved by anatomic recognition of cutaneous branches, superselective distal catheterization, and properly chosen particle size.

Rare case reports have discussed facial paralysis as a postembolization complication (Metson and Hanson 1983; Devries et al. 1986; Wehrli et al. 1988). This was possibly caused by proximal nonselective embolization of a dominant middle meningeal artery supply to the VIIth nerve. This complication is probably not applicable today, because superselective catheterization distal to the middle meningeal artery origin is routine. In recent series a complication rate of 3%–7% has been quoted (Strutz and Schumacher 1990; Vitek 1991). It seems that in the era of modern variable stiffness microcatheters and with the level of training and experience available today, the complication rate is significantly lower than the 50% reported earlier (Wehrli et al. 1988).

4.7 Conclusion

Distal embolization achieving blockage at the arteriolar bed level is essential for successful interventional management of intractable epistaxis. Proximal vessel occlusion, like proximal surgical clipping, reduces perfusion pressure to the nasal mucosa, but the rich collateral circulation can reconstitute flow to the bleeding territory with early recurrence of epistaxis.

The effectiveness, simplicity, and safety of the embolization procedure, in trained hands, make it the preferred primary modality of treatment in intractable epistaxis. In idiopathic epistaxis the importance of distal embolization of the posterior septal area is emphasized, as this is the usual source of bleeding which is inaccessible to clinical examination and cautery. In hereditary hemorrhagic telangiectasia (Osler-Weber-Rendu disease), more extensive embolization with preservation of the proximal vessels for future procedures is the rule. In organic lesions, angiography according to a specific protocol with tailored embolization and further surgical procedures will offer cure or palliation.

We recommend managing the patient with epistaxis by means of a multidisciplinary approach. Clinical endoscopic examination by an ENT surgeon and possible cautery are the first modes of treatment. Nasal packing is useful for immediate control of the bleeding and medical stabilization. Angiography and arterial embolization should be the next step, before any surgical procedure is attempted. Angiography according to a protocol, superselective catheterization using variable stiffness microcatheters, and microparticulate embolization offer a high success rate in controlling epistaxis and early removal of nasal packing. Only in the face of prominent ethmoidal vessels reconstituting flow to the nasal territory should surgical ligation be pursued. An escalating cascade of treatment modalities offers patients with epistaxis a tailored approach which is expected to yield a high success rate with minimal recurrence of bleeding and a low complication rate.

References

Breda SC, Choi IS, Persky NS, Weiss M (1989) Embolization in the treatment of epistaxis after failure of internal maxillary artery ligation. Laryngoscope 99:809–815

Chandler JR, Serrins AJ (1965) Transantral ligation of the internal maxillary artery for epistaxis. Laryngoscope 75:1151–1160

Davies KR (1986) Embolization of epistaxis and juvenile nasopharyngeal angiofibromas. AJNR 7:953–962

DeFilipp GJ, Steffey D, Rubinstein M, Drake A, Koopmann CH (1988) The role of angiography and embolization in the management of recurrent epistaxis. Otolaryngol Head Neck Surg 99:597–600

DeVries N, Vershuis RJ, Valk J, Snow GB (1986) Facial nerve paralysis following embolization for severe epistaxis. J Laryngol Otol 100:207–210

Djindjian R, Merland JJ, Theron J (1976) L'arteriographie superselective (A.S.S.) et l'embolisation dans les epistaxis graves. Ann Otol Laryngol (Paris) 93:23–33

Hicks JN, Vitek JJ (1989) Transarterial embolization to control posterior epistaxis. Laryngoscope 99:1027–1029

Lasjaunias P, Berenstein A (1987a) Surgical neuroangiography, vol 1: Functional anatomy of craniofacial arteries. Springer, Berlin Heidelberg New York

Lasjaunias P, Berenstein A (1987b) Surgical neuroangiography, vol 2: Endovascular treatment of craniofacial lesions. Springer, Berlin Heidelberg New York

Lasjaunias P, Marsot-Dupuch J, Doyon D (1979) The radio-anatomical basis of arterial embolization for epistaxis. J Neuroradiol 6:45–52

Merland JJ, Melki JP, Chiras J, Riche MC, Hadjean E (1980) Place of embolization in treatment of severe epistaxis. Laryngoscope 90:1694–1704

Metson R, Hanson DG (1983) Bilateral facial nerve paralysis following embolization for severe epistaxis. Otolaryngol Head Neck Surg 91:299–303

Metson R, Lane R (1988) Internal maxillary artery ligation for epistaxis: an analysis of failures. Laryngoscope 98:760–764

Parnes LS, Heenemann H, Vinuela F (1987) Percutaneous embolization for control of nasal blood circulation. Laryngoscope 97:1312–1315

Pearson BW, MacKensie RG, Goodman WS (1969) The anatomical basis of transantral ligation of the maxillary artery in severe epistaxis. Laryngoscope 79:969–984

Riche MC, Chiras J, Melki JP, Merland JJ (1979) The role of embolization in the treatment of severe epistaxis. J Neuroradiol 6:207–220

Robertson GH, Reardon EJ (1979) Angiography and embolization of the internal maxillary artery for posterior epistaxis. Arch Otolaryngol 105:333–337

Rosnagle RS, Allen WE III, Kier EL, Rochman LG (1980) Use of selective arteriography in the treatment of epistaxis. Arch Otolaryngol 106:137–142

Schaitkin B, Strauss M, Houck JK, Hershey PA (1987) Epistaxis: medical surgical therapy – a comparison of efficacy, complications and economic considerations. Laryngoscope 97:1392–1397

Small M, Murray J, Maran A (1982) A study of patients with epistaxis requiring admission to hospital. Health Bull (Edinb) 40:24–29

Sokoloff J, Wickbom T, McDonald D, Brahme F, Goergen TG, Goldberger LE (1974) Therapeutic percutaneous embolization in intractable epistaxis. Radiology 111: 285–287

Strutz J, Schumacher M (1990) Uncontrollable epistaxis. Arch Otolaryngol Head Neck Surg 116:697–699

Valavanis A (1990) Interventional neuroradiology for head and neck surgery. In: Cummings CW, Fredrickson JM, Harker LA, Krause CJ, Schuller DE (eds) Otolaryngology – head and neck surgery, update II. Mosby Year Book, St. Louis, pp 206–223

Van Wyck LG, Vinuela F, Heenemann H (1982) Therapeutic embolization for severe epistaxis. J Otolaryngol 11:271–274

Vitek JJ (1991) Idiopathic intractable epistaxis: endovascular therapy. Radiology 181:113–116

Wang L, Vogel DM (1981) Posterior epistaxis: comparison of treatment. Otolaryngol Heak Neck Surg 89:1001–1006

Wehrli M, Lieberherr U, Valavanis A (1988) Superselective embolization for intractable epistaxis: experience with 19 patients. Clin Otolaryngol 13:415–420

Wills PI, Russell RD (1979) Percutaneus embolization to control intractable epistaxis. Laryngoscope 89:1385–1388

5 Embolization of Intracranial and Skull Base Tumors

ANTON VALAVANIS

CONTENTS

5.1 Introduction

Embolization is now recognized as an established endovascular interventional neuroradiologic technique for the preoperative devascularization of vascular neoplasms of the intracranial space and of the skull base (LASJAUNIAS and BERENSTEIN 1987b; VALAVANIS 1990; HALBACH et al. 1992). The goal of embolization in cases of intracranial and skull base tumors is selective obliteration of the pathologic intratumoral vasculature while preserving the normal supply to surrounding tissues. In the majority of cases, selective obliteration of the intratumoral vasculature by appropriate embolic materials facilitates subsequent surgical tumor removal by improving the intraoperative conditions in terms of blood loss, almost bloodless tumor exposure, and easy identification of surgically important structures such as cranial nerves (VALAVANIS 1990). In conjunction with these advantages, embolization of intracranial and skull base tumors contributes to shortening of the operation time, increasing the rate of radical tumor removal, reducing the surgical complication rate, and possibly reducing the incidence of recurrence. In addition to embolization, the technique of permanent balloon occlusion of the internal carotid artery (ICA) in extensive tumors of the skull base with an intimate relationship to the ICA allows identification and resection of pericarotid tumor extensions without the fear of uncontrollable hemorrhage from the ICA and has thus contributed to safe and radical removal of skull base tumors previously regarded as inoperable (FISCH and MATTOX 1988).

As a general rule, embolization of tumors should be regarded as a purely preoperative measure and not as an alternative to surgery. Embolization acting only upon the vascular component of the tumor cannot cure neoplasms, but if properly performed, it can assist the neurosurgeon and the head and neck surgeon in treating their patients harboring hypervascular and challenging neoplasms. Only exceptionally (especially in elderly patients in a poor general clinical condition not allowing prolonged general anesthesia and in patients refusing surgery) can embolization be performed as a palliative measure in order to reduce temporarily the size and thus the mass effect of the tumor as well as related subjective or neurologic symptoms in certain, extensive intracranial and skull base tumors (VALAVANIS 1990).

ANTON VALAVANIS, M.D., Professor and Head, Abteilung für Neuroradiologie, Departement Medizinische Radiologie, Röntgendiagnostisches Zentralinstitut, Universitätsspital Zürich, Frauenklinikstrasse 10, 8091 Zürich, Switzerland

This chapter summarizes the indications, general principles, currently used interventional techniques, and potential complications of preoperative embolization of hypervascular tumors of the intracranial space and of the skull base.

5.2 Indications

The main indications for preoperative embolization of intracranial and skull base tumors are neoplasms which are characterized by a high degree of vascularity, by surgically inaccessible or less easily accessible supplying arteries, and/or by an intimate relationship to major arteries of the skull base, especially the ICA.

The histologic spectrum of tumors fullfilling the above-mentioned requirements for embolization is wide. As a general rule, embolization is mainly indicated in vascular tumors supplied by arterial branches of the external carotid artery (ECA), ICA, and vertebrobasilar system, which are amenable to superselective catheterization by flow-independent, variable stiffness microcatheters. These microcatheters have expanded the indications for tumor embolization because they allow distal catheterization of feeding arteries, selective catheterization of hitherto inaccessible small arterial pedicles (such as branches of the cavernous segment of the ICA, of the ophthalmic artery, and of the vertebral arteries), and the delivery of different embolic materials, such as microparticles, polymerizing fluids, and microcoils. Despite this technical progress, preoperative embolization of tumors is still mainly restricted to extra-axial intracranial and skull base tumors. Its role in the preoperative devascularization of intra-axial intracranial hypervascular neoplasms is currently limited to a very few types of tumors, such as solid, large hemangioblastomas, some exceptional types of glioblastoma multiforme with extensive intratumoral arteriovenous shunting, and intradural extensions of large and hypervascular skull base tumors.

The following is a list of tumors, classified by location and histology, which may represent an indication for preoperative embolization:

A. Intracranial tumors
1. Extra-axial tumors of bony origin
   a) Osteogenic tumors (osteoblastoma, osteosarcoma, osteochondroma)
   b) Hemangioma
   c) Plasmocytoma
   d) Metastasis
2. Extra-axial tumors of dural origin
   a) Meningioma (convexial, parasagittal, falcine)
   b) Fibrosarcoma
   c) Hemagiopericytoma
   d) Lymphoma
3. Intra-axial tumors (limited indication)
   a) Hemangioblastoma, solid
   b) Glioblastoma multiforme, solid with extensive arteriovenous shunts

B. Skull base tumors
1. Endocranial origin
   a) Meningiomas
   b) Neurinomas
2. Intrinsic to the skull base
   a) Glomus temporale tumor (tympanic, jugular)
   b) Chordoma
3. Exocranial origin
   a) Juvenile nasopharyngeal angiofibroma
   b) Glomus vagale and caroticum tumor
   c) Esthesioneuroblastoma
   d) Carcinoma
   e) Other (rare)

5.3 General Principles and Techniques

The goal of preoperative tumor embolization is selective obliteration of the intratumoral abnormal arteriocapillary bed, leading to tumor devascularization with preservation of the normal arterial supply to surrounding tissues. To achieve this goal a thorough pretherapeutic tumor evaluation by imaging techniques, a detailed angiographic workup, and the application of appropriate embolization techniques are necessary.

5.3.1 Pretherapeutic Evaluation by Imaging Techniques

Computed tomography (CT) and especially magnetic resonance imaging (MRI) are the basic imaging techniques for the primary evaluation of intracranial and skull base tumors. With regard to preoperative embolization, these techniques should provide information which is necessary for planning the angiographic workup and the embolization in each individual case. Specifically, this information should include (a) the specific location and site of origin of the tumor; (b) the topography of the tumor as it relates to surrounding bone, nerves, major vessels, brain, and dura; (c) the pattern of extension of the tumor (along fascial planes, soft tissue invasion, intraosseous, perineural, perivascular, transcranial, transdural); (d) the degree of vascularity based on the pattern of contrast enhancement as assessed by CT and/or MRI and on the presence of intratumoral vessels as assessed by MRI; (e) the vascular territory or territories involved by the tumor.

As a general rule, multiplanar, contrast-enhanced, T1-weighted, high-field MR is superior to high-resolution CT in reliably providing most of this information. High-resolution CT is, however, still needed as a complementary modality in order to assess subtle bony erosion and the pattern of intraosseous extension of certain skull base tumors.

5.3.2 Angiographic Workup

In the majority of cases both the angiographic workup of the tumor and its subsequent embolization are performed in one session, even in the case of extensive tumors with a complex vascular supply, provided that both procedures have been well planned according to the information provided by preceding CT/MRI investigations (Valavanis 1990).

Preferably, the procedures should be performed under general anesthesia. General anesthesia guarantees optimal working conditions for the interventional neuroadiologist and also minimizes the risk of spasm of the sensitive branches of the ECA. However, since the introduction of highly flexible microcatheters, the incidence of spasm in the ECA territory has significantly decreased, so that some procedures of tumor embolization can now be performed under local anesthesia. In cases where a permanent balloon occlusion of the ICA is planned, the procedure should be performed under local anesthesia because continuous control of the neurologic condition of the patient during the procedure is essential.

Irrespective of the type and the location of the tumor to be embolized, the optimal approach for both angiographic workup and embolization is through the femoral artery because this allows catheterization of both ICAs, ECAs, and vertebral arteries from a single puncture site.

Digital subtraction angiography (DSA) is today the preferred method when performing embolization procedures in the head and neck area. Besides providing instantaneously subtracted images, DSA has a higher contrast resolution than conventional film angiography without significant loss of spatial resolution and it allows the use of reduced amounts of diluted iodinated contrast material. Therefore, DSA provides excellent image quality and contributes to shortening of the procedure time.

The angiographic workup should follow a specific protocol developed for the individual tumor to be embolized. This protocol should be based on the vascular territory in which the tumor is located and should incorporate all functional vascular aspects known to be associated with the specific vascular territory. The angiographic workup, including selective and superselective functional neuroangiography, should provide information on the following:

1. Arterial supply
   a) Type, number, and geometry of feeding arteries (extracranial, dural, pial, abnormal origins)
   b) Collateral circulation
   c) Dangerous arterio-arterial anastomoses
   d) Cranial nerve supply
   e) Skin supply
2. Vascular composition and angioarchitecture of the tumor
   a) Mono- or multicompartmental
   b) Flow characteristics
   c) Arteriovenous shunts
3. Venous drainage
   a) Cortical/dural
   b) Dural sinuses
   c) Venous plexuses
   d) Obstruction of sinuses by intraluminal extension or external compression

For selective angiography, usually polyethylene, medium-sized catheters of a diameter of 4.5–5.5 French are used. Such catheters are flexible enough and have sufficient torque control to allow catheterization of individual feeding arteries in the head and neck. In addition, their relatively thin wall permits coaxial insertion of microcatheters for superselective angiography and embolization (Dion 1992).

The newly developed variable stiffness microcatheters such as the Tracker microcatheter (Target Therapeutics, Los Angeles) can be advanced over tortuous or angulated vascular segments and allow catheterization of the distal portion of feeding arteries as well as of arteries previously regarded as inaccessible to catheterization (KIKUCHI et al. 1987; DION 1992). This represents a major step forward in the superselective angiographic workup and embolization of head and neck and especially skull base tumors. Specifically, the following arteries can be frequently catheterized and embolized with the use of such microcatheters:

1. Ophthalmic artery branches, including the ophthalmic artery origin of the middle miningeal artery, in:
   a) Orbital, periorbital, frontobasal, and cavernous sinus meningiomas
   b) Intraorbital extension of juvenile nasopharyngeal angiofibromas
   c) Esthesioneuroblastomas
2. Branches of the cavernous portion of the ICA, in:
   a) Vascular tumors of the cavernous sinus (meningiomas, certain neurinomas)
   b) Sphenopetroclival meningiomas
   c) Tentorial and cerebello-pontine-angle (CPA) meningiomas
   d) CPA vascular neurinomas
   e) Intracavernous extension of juvenile nasopharyngeal angiofibromas and extensive glomus tumors of the temporal bone
3. Caroticotympanic branch of the ICA, in:
   a) Glomus tumors of the temporal bone
4. Dural branches of the vertebral artery, in:
   a) Intracranial extradural extensions of glomus tumors of the temporal bone
   b) Neurinomas of the jugular foramen
   c) Basal posterior fossa meningiomas and other tumors of this area
5. Temporal branches of middle cerebral artery, in:
   a) Intracranial intradural extensions of juvenile nasopharyngeal angiofibroma
6. Hemispheric branches of the posterior (PICA) and anterior inferior cerebellar arteries (AICA), in:
   a) Intracranial intradural extensions of large glomus tumors of the temporal bone

In addition, the angiographic workup should include determination of the intracranial collateral circulation at the level of the circle of Willis in every tumor of the skull base exhibiting a topographic relationship to any segment of the ICA (i.e., cervical, petrous, cavernous).

This combined angiographic–clinical tolerance test is essential in appraising the indication for permanent balloon occlusion of the ICA. It also provides the interventional neuroradiologist with useful information regarding the necessity to perform a temporary balloon occlusion of the ICA during embolization (vide infra). The test is performed by temporary occlusion of the ipsilateral ICA by means of manual compression or preferably by temporary endoluminal inflation of a nondetachable balloon and injection of contrast material into the contralateral ICA as well as into the dominant vertebral artery. Sufficient collaterals at the level of the circle of Willis are present if there is rapid and complete filling of the middle and anterior cerebral arteries on the side of the temporarily occluded ICA (VALAVANIS 1988).

5.3.3 Techniques of Tumor Embolization

As mentioned above, the main goal of tumor embolization is obliteration of the arteriocapillary bed of the tumor by intratumoral deposition of the embolic material. Additional, supplementary occlusion of the extratumoral supplying arteries may further augment the process of distal or intratumoral thrombosis (LASJAUNIAS and BERENSTEIN 1987b). Simple occlusion of the extratumoral segments of the supplying arteries without previous obliteration of the intratumoral microvasculature is in most cases not only ineffective regarding devascularization of the tumor but will stimulate the development of collateral supply. Collateral arteries supplying the tumor may then arise from unusual and surgically less easily accessible or even inaccessible sites, thus rendering the surgical removal of the tumor technically more difficult than it would have been without prior embolization.

From a technical point of view there are three principal factors that determine the success of intratumoral deposition of the embolic material: (a) the degree of catheterization selectivity, (b) the choice of the embolic material, and (c) the absence of spasm in the arteries to be embolized. Selective catheterization of the terminal supplying artery is an essential prerequisite to optimal tumor embolization. How distally such an artery can be catheterized is dependent on its inner diameter relative to the outer diameter of the catheter and on its geometry. Attempts at very distal catheterization of thin, very tortuous feeding arteries may induce spasm or cause flow cessation by blockage of the artery, thus preventing intratumoral deposition of the embolic agent. In these instances free flow embolization from a more proximal but still selective catheter position is preferable.

The recent introduction of special microcatheters and microguidewires not only allows very distal catheterization of the feeding branches of the ECA without causing spasm but also makes it possible to superselectively catheterize and embolize the supplying petrous, medial and lateral clival, and cavernous branches of the ICA, the ophthalmic artery, and dural branches of the vertebral arteries. Preshaping the microcatheters under steam so that their very distal segment assumes a slight curvature proved very useful for the superselective catheterization of these branches (DION 1992). If, however, superselective catheterization of these branches with a microcatheter is not possible, temporary balloon occlusion of the parent artery immediately distal to the origin of the supplying branch followed by microparticle embolization is an efficient alternative technique (VALAVANIS 1990). In order to avoid distal embolization of the microparticles into the cerebral vasculature after balloon deflation, multiple aspirations through the microcatheter and subsequent rinsing of the distal occluded segment of the parent artery with saline are essential prior to balloon deflation (THÉRON et al. 1986).

The fact that branches of the extradural portion of the ICA and of the vertebral artery are in hemodynamic balance with transcranial branches of the ECA can be used for "functional" embolization (LASJAUNIAS and BERENSTEIN 1987b). This can be accomplished by temporary balloon occlusion of the ICA or vertebral artery at the level of origin of the supplying branch and flow-controlled embolization of the tumor through that branch of the ECA which is in hemodynamic balance with the temporarily occluded branch arising from the ICA or vertebral artery (VALAVANIS 1990).

The embolic materials used in embolization of tumors of the intracranial space and the skull base include both particles and fluid materials. As a general rule, microparticles should be preferred to fluid materials in preoperative tumor embolization. They are easier and safer to use and, if properly sized, can reach the intratumoral microvasculature. Among the particulate materials the most commonly used are microparticles of polyvinyl alcohol foam (Ivalon), which are available in different sizes ranging from 45 to 500 µm (JACK et al. 1985; KERBER et al. 1988). In most cases the use of the smallest available size, in the range of 45–150 µm, is indicated. Gelfoam powder represents another alternative to microparticulate Ivalon embolization (BERENSTEIN and RUSSELL 1981). However, Gelfoam is more rapidly reabsorbable than Ivalon, a factor which should be taken into consideration when planning postembolization surgical removal of the tumor. With the use of Ivalon microparticles a delay of more than 4 weeks between embolization and operation should be avoided. Among the fluid materials used for tumor embolization, *N*-Butyl-2-cyanoacrylate (NBCA) has proved the most effective (BROTHERS et al. 1989). The polymerization time can be delayed if one adds oily iodinated contrast material (Pantopaque) (SPIEGEL et al. 1986). NBCA is made radiopaque and therefore visible fluoroscopically by the addition of a small amount of tantalum powder. If used for tumor embolization, the mixture of NBCA and tantalum should be such that the polymerization is significantly delayed in order for the NBCA to penetrate into the distal intratumoral vasculature. NBCA is considered a dangerous material because it can penetrate distally into vascular territories and thus cause ischemia of vital tissues, or it may polymerize rapidly, thus gluing the catheter tip within the arterial lumen (DION 1992).

5.3.4 Balloon Occlusion of the Internal Carotid Artery

Tumors of the skull base and of the upper neck may exhibit an intimate relationship to the wall of the ICA. Invasion of the adventitia of the ICA and/or significant arterial supply from extradural ICA branches represent major limiting factors for safe and radical removal of the tumor. Prior to the introduction of the technique of balloon occlusion of the ICA, the pericarotid tumor portion frequently had to be left in place in order to avoid laceration of the ICA wall and uncontrollable intraoperative hemorrhage.

These small pericarotid tumor residuals were a main cause of tumor recurrence. Attempts at excision of pericarotid tumor portions frequently caused laceration of the wall of the ICA with uncontrollable hemorrhage leading to significant morbidity and mortality. The introduction of preoperative permanent balloon occlusion of the ICA greatly contributed to safe and complete removal of extensive skull base tumors involving the adventitia, thus increasing the rate of radical tumor removal and decreasing both the recurrence rate and the intraoperative complication rate.

As a general rule, preoperative permanent balloon occlusion of the ICA should be considered in all skull base tumors and tumors of the upper neck which are shown by CT/MRI to encase or to invade the wall of the ICA and in tumors which are shown by angiography to receive significant supply from branches of the ICA. Specific indications for permanent preoperative balloon occlusion of the ICA include the following (VALAVANIS 1990):

1. Tumors originating within the cavernous sinus and involving the cavernous segment of the ICA, e.g., meningiomas and certain neurinomas
2. Skull base tumors secondarily extending into the cavernous sinus and involving the cavernous segment of the ICA, e.g., extensive glomus jugulare tumors, extensive juvenile nasopharyngeal angiofibromas, extensive nasopharyngeal and parapharyngeal carcinomas
3. Tumors involving the petrous segment of the ICA, e.g., glomus jugulare tumors
4. Tumors involving the extracranial portion of the ICA, e.g., glomus caroticum and vagale tumors

The procedure is preferably performed with the patient awake, so that the neurologic condition can be continuously controlled. As mentioned earlier (see Sect. 5.3.2), balloon occlusion of the ICA should be performed only after an angiographic tolerance test has demonstrated adequate collateral supply to the cerebral hemisphere ipsilateral to the ICA to be sacrificed and absence of any neurologic deficits during the test period (VALAVANIS 1988).

For permanent balloon occlusion of the ICA a nontapered, thin-walled guiding catheter is placed transfemorally into the proximal segment of the ICA. A latex microballoon attached to a microcatheter system is inserted coaxially through the guiding catheter into the ICA and advanced toward the cavernous segment of the ICA. The balloon is inflated with isotonic iodinated contrast material until the lumen of the ICA is occluded. Preferably the balloon is positioned between the origins of the inferolateral trunk of the cavernous segment of the ICA and of the ophthalmic artery. This will prevent anterograde thromboembolism from thrombus formed distal to the balloon and dislodged by inflow through the inferolateral trunk (VALAVANIS and FISCH 1989b).

Complete occlusion of the ICA is confirmed by a lateral carotid angiogram performed through the guiding catheter. The balloon is then detached by gently pulling on the microcatheter to which it is attached. After balloon detachment the pericarotid or intracavernous portions of the tumor may be embolized with microparticles injected through the guiding catheter into the ICA and flow-carried into the supplying branches. The procedure is terminated by detaching a second balloon within the proximal ICA. This will prevent distal migration of the first balloon in case it should deflate prematurely, and it also prevents extensive thrombus formation within the proximal ICA, which is known to carry the risk of ophthalmic artery embolism through the ECA system (LASJAUNIAS and BERENSTEIN 1987b).

Following the procedure the patient should be closely monitored for at least 12 h in an intensive care unit. During this time special care is taken to avoid a fall in blood pressure below the systolic level of 100 mm/Hg because this may cause ischemia in the cerebral hemisphere ipsilateral to the occluded ICA (VALAVANIS 1990).

5.4 Dangers and Complications

Several types of complications may occur during embolization of tumors of the intracranial space and of the skull base. The most serious complications associated with tumor embolization in the head and neck area include cerebral stroke, blindness, cranial nerve palsies, and skin necrosis (VALAVANIS 1986, 1990; LASJAUNIAS and BERENSTEIN 1987b). Cerebral stroke may occur when there is a reflux of embolic material from the ECA into the ICA or when embolic material refluxes from superselectively catheterized branches of the ICA or vertebral artery into the main stem of these vessels. Stroke may also occur when embolic material passes anterogradely through arterio-arterial anastomoses between the ECA and the ICA or vertebral artery. Blindness may occur when embolic material passes through anastomoses between the distal internal maxillary artery and the ophthalmic artery. Cranial nerve palsies may occur when branches of the ECA known to supply the transcranial course of the cranial nerves are occluded distally by certain embolic materials. Skin necrosis will occur when cutaneous branches of the ECA are intentionally or unintentionally occluded by embolic material. In addition to these complications which may occur during embolization, cerebral stroke and blindness are complications associated with the permanent balloon occlusion of the ICA. Since embolization of tumors is a preoperative measure to be followed by surgical removal of the tumor, every effort and caution should be undertaken to minimize the morbidity to nearly zero, because otherwise the patient has to face two management risks, i.e., an endovascular risk followed by a surgical risk.

5.4.1 Reflux of Embolic Material

Reflux of embolic material from the ECA into the ICA is a rare complication (LASJAUNIAS and BERENSTEIN 1987b) that may occur when embolization is being performed in the proximal branches of the main stem of the ECA and the injection pressure exceeds the systolic blood pressure. As mentioned earlier in this chapter, reflux of embolic material into the ICA can be avoided by injecting the embolic material synchronously with the heart beat and thereby during the systolic pulse wave of the arterial bloodstream.

Since the introduction of microcatheters allowing distal superselective catheterization and embolization of branches of the ECA, the risk of reflux of embolic material has been significantly reduced. However, embolization of small branches arising from the very proximal segment of the ECA, as is the case with glomus caroticum tumors, carries a relatively high risk for reflux of embolic material into the ICA. In these cases protection of the cerebral circulation with a temporarily inflated balloon in the proximal segment of the ICA is recommended.

Reflux of embolic material may also occur during embolization of branches of the ICA or the vertebral artery. Since these extradural branches are usually of small caliber and with relatively slow flow, the risk of reflux into the parent vessel is higher than when embolizing in the ECA territory. Embolization of these branches should be interrupted as soon as the blood flow is significantly decreased but before it ceases (VALAVANIS 1990).

5.4.2 Arterio-arterial Anastomoses

Since the routine performance of selective angiography and the widespread use of DSA, it has become evident that anastomoses between branches of the ECA and the ICA as well as the vertebral artery occur much more frequently than was previously assumed (LASJAUNIAS and BERENSTEIN 1987a). Such arterio-arterial anastomoses represent incomplete regressions of embryologic arterial connections. Embolic materials may pass through such anastomoses into the intracranial circulation and may cause cerebral stroke or, if they involve the ophthalmic artery system, blindness. The dangers associated with such anastomoses are higher in embolization of tumors than in vascular malformations because the flow in cases of tumors is slower than in cases of vascular malformations. Such anastomoses may be present but functionally inactive and therefore invisible on the preembolization angiogram. During embolization and with increasing pressure within the embolized vessel such an inactive anastomosis may become functionally active. Therefore special care is necessary in order to detect fluoroscopically the appearance of such anastomoses during embolization (VALAVANIS 1990).

Below is a list of the most frequently encountered anastomoses between branches of the ECA and the ICA, the ophthalmic artery, and the vertebral artery (LASJAUNIAS and BERENSTEIN 1987a).

Anastomoses between the internal maxillary artery and the cavernous segment of the ICA:
- Cavernous branch of middle meningeal artery
- Cavernous branch of the accessory meningeal artery
- Artery of the foramen rotundum

Anastomoses between the ascending pharyngeal artery and the cavernous segment of the ICA:
- Carotid branch of the superior pharyngeal artery
- Lateral clival branch of the jugular division of the ascending pharyngeal artery
- Medial clival branch of the hypoglossal division of the ascending pharyngeal artery

Anastomoses between the internal maxillary artery and the petrous segment of the ICA:
- Anterior tympanic artery
- Vidian artery

Anastomoses between the ascending pharyngeal artery and the petrous segment of the ICA:
- Mandibular anastomosis of the superior pharyngeal artery
- Inferior tympanic artery

Anastomoses between the posterior auricular artery or the occipital artery and the petrous segment of the ICA:
- Stylomastoid branch

Anastomoses between the occipital artery and the vertebral artery:
- C1 anastomotic branch
- C2 anastomotic branch

Anastomoses between the ascending pharyngeal artery and the vertebral artery:
- Hypoglossal branch of the odontoid arch system
- Musculospinal artery

Anastomoses between the ascending cervical artery and the vertebral artery:
- C3 anastomosis
- C4 anastomosis

Anastomoses between the posterior cervical artery and the vertebral artery:
- C2 anastomosis
- C3 anastomosis
- C4 anastomosis

Anastomoses between the ECA trunk and the vertebral artery:
- C4 collateral

Anastomoses between the internal maxillary artery and the ophthalmic artery:
- Orbital branch of the infraorbital artery
- Anterior ethmoidal branch of the sphenopalatine artery
- Meningo-ophthalmic branch of the middle meningeal artery
- Recurrent meningeal branch of the middle meningeal artery
- Orbital branch of the anterior deep temporal artery

The presence of such anastomoses does not represent an absolute contraindication to embolization. Several techniques can be applied in order to avoid the risks associated with the presence of such anastomoses (LASJAUNIAS and BERENSTEIN 1987b). These techniques are (VALAVANIS 1986, 1990):

1. The use of particles larger in size than the diameter of the anastomotic artery
2. Positioning of the catheter tip distal to the origin of the anastomotic artery
3. Temporary occlusion of the anastomotic artery by a large reabsorbable piece of embolic material such as Gelfoam
4. Temporary balloon occlusion of the vertebral artery or the ICA at the level of entry of the anastomotic artery

By applying one or more of these techniques, in the presence of an arterio-arterial anastomosis, it is usually possible to perform complete tumor embolization. As a general rule, fluid materials should not be used because their passage into the cerebral circulation cannot be reliably avoided by the techniques mentioned above.

5.4.3 Cranial Nerve Palsies

The transcranial and extracranial segments of the cranial nerves are supplied by terminal branches of the ECA system. Occlusion of such branches during embolization of tumors may result in a cranial nerve palsy (LASJAUNIAS and BERENSTEIN 1987a,b). Depending upon the type of embolic material and on the presence or absence of collateral supply, such cranial nerve palsies may be permanent or transient. With the use of microparticulate materials and with care to avoid occlusion of nerve supplying branches, the risk of inducing a permanent cranial nerve palsy during embolization of tumors is low.

The following branches of the ECA participate in the supply of the trans- and extracranial segments of the cranial nerves: The neuromeningeal trunk of the ascending pharyngeal artery supplies the lower cranial nerves (IX–XII). The petrosal branch of the middle meningeal artery and the stylomastoid branch of the occipital artery supply the intratemporal segments of the facial nerve. The accessory meningeal artery participates in the supply of the cavernous courses of the cranial nerves IV–VI (LASJAUNIAS and BERENSTEIN 1987a).

5.4.4 Occlusion of Cutaneous Branches of the External Cartoid Artery

Occlusion of cutaneous branches of the ECA may cause necrosis of the skin in the craniotomy area. This may lead to postoperative wound healing retardation and infection. Occlusion of cutaneous branches of the ECA should be avoided in preoperative embolization. Cutaneous branches of the ECA that supply the skin in the area of craniotomy include the superficial temporal artery and its branches, the posterior auricular artery, and the cutaneous branches of the occipital artery (VALAVANIS 1990; ADLER et al. 1986).

5.5 Embolization of Meningiomas

5.5.1 General Remarks

Meningiomas are usually benign, slowly growing tumors originating from the arachnoid cells of the dural coverings of the brain and accounting for approximately 15% of all primary intracranial tumors (HALBACH et al. 1992). Because of their frequency and their frequent hypervascularity, meningiomas represent an important indication for preoperative embolization (RICHTER and SCHACHENMAYR 1983; TEASDALE et al. 1984; MANELFE et al. 1986; RODESCH and LASJAUNIAS 1991). Because meningiomas arise from the meningeal sheaths, they obligatorily receive meningeal arterial supply. The meningeal arterial supply of meningiomas typically arises from the dural base of the tumor. The cerebral surface of meningiomas, however, frequently receives additional arterial supply from pial-cortical arteries. Depending on the contribution of the meningeal and pial arterial systems to the supply of meningiomas, these tumors can be classified by selective angiography into four types, i.e.:

1. Meningiomas with exclusive meningeal supply
2. Meningiomas with dominant meningeal supply
3. Meningiomas with balanced meningeal and pial supply
4. Meningiomas with dominant pial supply

The angiographic protocol for the evaluation of meningiomas will depend on the specific location of the tumor and on the vascular territory or territories occupied by the tumor as assessed by imaging techniques and preferably by multiplanar, contrast-enhanced MRI.

The angiographic evaluation should provide the following information:

1. Dural arteries supplying the tumor
2. Pial arteries supplying the tumor
3. Relationship of dural/pial arterial supply to the tumor
4. Detection of arterio-arterial anastomoses
5. Detection of abnormal origin of dural supplying arteries
6. Displacement of pial arteries
7. Transosseous supply of the tumor
8. Compression and/or encasement of the internal carotid, vertebral, or basilar arteries with skull base meningiomas
9. Collateral circulation to the brain
10. Intensity of tumor staining and flow characteristics of the tumor
11. Venous drainage of the tumor
12. Cortical venous changes
13. Status and patency of adjacent major dural venous sinuses

Meningiomas exhibit a characteristic angiographic appearance consisting of dilated meningeal feeding arteries converging towards the dural site of tumor attachment, radiating intratumoral dural arteries, and a more or less homogeneous blush of variable intensity, usually persisting into the late venous phase (LASJAUNIAS and BERENSTEIN 1987b).

The type of meningeal arteries supplying a meningioma depends primarily on the location, size, and extension of the tumor in respect of meningeal vascular territories. The introduction of microcatheters and steerable guidewires allows superselective catheterization and embolization not only of meningeal arteries arising from the ECA but also of dural branches participating in the supply of meningiomas and originating from the ICA and vertebral arteries. However, at the current state of development of interventional technology, superselective catheterization and embolization of the multiple, small pial supplying arteries originating from cortical arteries is technically not possible. Therefore, the most efficient embolization of meningiomas will be achieved in those types with exclusive or dominant meningeal supply. The effect of embolization will be moderate in meningiomas with balanced meningeal-pial supply and minimal in meningiomas with dominant pial supply. In this last group, embolization is indicated if the minimal dural supply to the tumor is in a surgically less easily accessible site. This applies especially to certain basal meningiomas, such as frontobasal meningiomas, tuberculum sellae meningiomas, and posterior fossa meningiomas, which receive their meningeal supply from dural arteries of the skull base. Embolization of purely intraventricular meningiomas does not represent an established indication.

5.5.2 *Vascular Supply and Embolization of Meningiomas According to Location*

5.5.2.1 *Meningiomas of the Convexity, the Parasagittal Area, and the Falx Cerebri*

Meningiomas of the convexity, the parasagittal area, and the falx cerebri receive their dural supply from the branches of the ipsilateral middle meningeal artery. Meningiomas located in the parasagittal area or in the falx and meningiomas extending into the contralateral side may receive additional supply from the corresponding branches of the contralateral middle meningeal artery. Depending on the specific location of the meningioma one or more of the following branches will participate in its supply (RODESCH and LASJAUNIAS 1991):

1. The branch of the frontal convexity supplies the dura over the frontopolar area. It may also arise from the anterior ethmoidal artery.
2. The frontal branch of the middle meningeal artery supplies the dura over the anterior parietal region. Occasionally, this branch may originate directly from the ophthalmic artery or from the intraorbital lacrimal artery.
3. The parieto-occipital trunk of the middle meningeal artery supplies the dura of the posterior parietal and occipital region of the convexity.
4. The petrosquamosal branch of the middle meningeal aratery supplies the petrosquamosal groove as well as the basal edge of the tentorium cerebelli.

Meningiomas of the anterior portion of the falx also receive supply from the artery of the falx cerebri, which arises from the anterior ethmoidal artery. Meningiomas involving the free margin of the falx and the wall of the inferior sagittal sinus may receive supply from dural branches of the pericallosal and callosomarginal arteries. Because of their size and distal origin, these meningeal branches of the ethmoidal and anterior cerebral arteries are usually not accessible to superselective catheterization and embolization.

The middle meningeal artery supplying a meningioma may not always originate from the internal maxillary artery. The most frequent variation in origin of the middle meningeal artery is the ophthalmic artery (LASJAUNIAS and BERENSTEIN 1987a). In these cases, the middle meningeal artery or one of its major branches arises from the second segment of the ophthalmic artery distal to the origin of the central retinal artery. In the author's experience, the use of microcatheters (Tracker, Target Therapeutics) allows, in the majority of these cases, superselective catheterization of the proximal trunk of the middle meningeal artery through the ophthalmic artery and thus safe embolization of the meningioma with appropriately sized microparticles. Navigation through the ophthalmic artery and catheterization of the proximal trunk of the middle meningeal artery are facilitated in cases of meningioma by the fact that both vessels are slightly or moderately dilated (Fig. 5.1).

Other rarer variations in the origin of the middle meningeal artery include an origin from the inferolateral trunk or from the petrous segment of the ICA, from the ascending pharyngeal artery, from the contralateral internal maxillary artery, and, extremely rarely, from the basilar artery. Catheterization of these origins of the middle meningeal artery is not always possible and

Fig. 5.1a–f. Lateral sphenoid wing meningioma. **a** Sagittal T1-weighted MRI after gadolinium-DTPA injection shows a homogeneously and intensively enhancing medium-sized meningioma with broad attachment to the dura of the lateral sphenoid wing. **b** Common carotid angiography in lateral projection shows a dilated ophthalmic artery in its proximal portion (*black arrow*), the origin of the middle meningeal artery from the ophthalmic artery (*white arrow*), and tumor opacification. **c** Selective ophthalmic artery angiography shows more clearly the origin of the middle meningeal artery (*white arrow*) and intense, homogeneous tumor opacification corresponding to tumor enhancement on MRI (**a**). There is dominant meningeal supply to the tumor. Note the central retinal artery (*black arrows*) and the retinal blush (*black arrowheads*). **d** Superselective catheterization of the origin of the middle meningeal artery (*arrow*) and intratumoral embolization with microparticles of PVA. **e** Internal carotid angiography in lateral projection after embolization shows devascularization of the tumor and preservation of the ophthalmic artery. **f** Sagittal T1-weighted MRI after gadolinium-DTPA injection 3 days after embolization shows extensive central necrosis of the tumor with only a peripheral thin rim of enhancement probably arising from persisting pial supply ▷

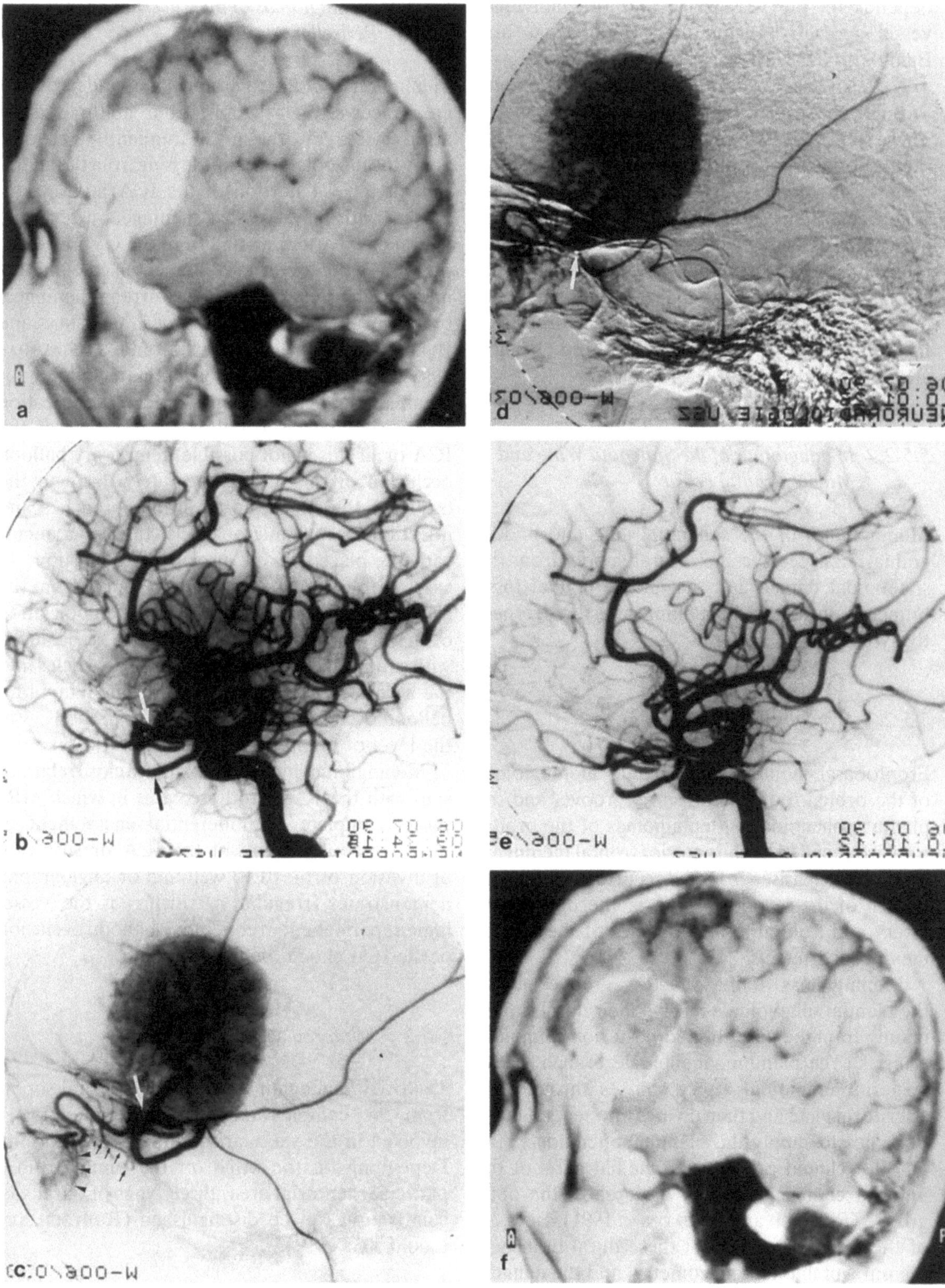
a
b
c
d
e
f
P

depends on the vessel size and the individual vessel geometry encountered (Lasjaunias and Berenstein 1987a).

Meningiomas of the convexity may extend through the calvaria into the subgaleal space. These transosseous extracranial extensions receive their supply from scalp arteries. Depending on their location, these extensions are supplied by branches of the superficial temporal, posterior auricular, or occipital arteries. Embolization of these cutaneous vessels should be targeted towards the distal supplying branches while avoiding occlusion of their proximal trunks in order not to compromise postoperative wound healing (Rodesch and Lasjaunias 1991).

5.5.2.2 *Meningiomas of the Sphenoid Wing and Middle Cranial Fossa*

Meningiomas of the sphenoid wing and middle cranial fossa receive their dural supply from the sphenoidal branch and the middle cranial fossa branches of the middle meningeal artery, respectively (Fig. 5.1).

5.5.2.3 *Frontobasal Meningiomas*

Frontobasal meningiomas include meningiomas of the orbital roof, the olfactory groove, and the planum sphenoidale. Meningiomas of the orbital roof are supplied by the anterior frontal meningeal artery, which arises from the recurrent meningeal branch of the second portion of the ophthalmic artery and from anterior branches of the middle meningeal artery.

Meningiomas of the olfactory groove and of the planum sphenoidale receive their dural supply mainly from the anterior and posterior ethmoidal arteries. The planum sphenoidale branch of the posterior ethmoidal artery courses through the cribriform plate and then divides into several dural branches to supply the planum sphenoidale, the anterior clinoid process, the medial parts of the anterior cranial fossa, and the area of the optic groove (Rodesch and Lasjaunias 1991). Because of the rather small size of these dural branches, the unfavorable vessel geometry, and the dangers associated with the ophthalmic artery territory, the role of embolization in frontobasal meningiomas is rather limited.

5.5.2.4 *Meningiomas of the Cavernous Sinus and Perisellar Area*

Meningiomas of the cavernous sinus and perisellar area receive their supply from multiple dural arterial sources, the most frequently observed being the inferolateral trunk arising from the lateral wall of the C4 portion of the ICA and anastomosing with the accessory meningeal artery, the lateral clival artery arising from the C5 portion of the ICA, the cavernous branch of the middle meningeal artery, and the recurrent meningeal branch of the ophthalmic artery (Lasjaunias and Berenstein 1987a; Rodesch and Lasjaunias 1991). An efficient embolization technique for meningiomas in this region is direct catheterization of the supplying C4 and/or C5 branches of the ICA or, if this is not possible, temporary balloon occlusion of the ICA immediately distal to the origin of the supplying cavernous branches and injection of small microparticles through a microcatheter placed in the proximal C5 portion. In cases with dominant or balanced supply from the accessory meningeal artery, efficient embolization of major portions of the tumor can be achieved with superselective injection of microparticles into the accessory meningeal artery during temporary balloon occlusion of the C4 portion of the ICA at the level of origin of the inferolateral trunk.

Meningiomas in this area exhibit a close relationship with the ICA. In those cases in which MRI shows complete circumferential encasement of the cavernous portion of the ICA or suspicion of invasion of the ICA wall and/or angiography demonstrates irregular narrowing of the vessel lumen, permanent preoperative balloon occlusion of the ICA should be considered.

5.5.2.5 *Tentorial Meningiomas*

Tentorial meningiomas receive their dural supply from the complex meningeal arterial network involved in the vascularization of the tentorium. Depending on the origin of the tumor from a particular tentorial area, three types of dural vascularization can be distinguished (Rodesch and Lasjaunias 1991):

1. Meningiomas arising from the medial tentorial edge or from the medial third of the tentorium are mainly supplied by the marginal tentorial artery. This artery has a highly variable origin

including the C5 portion of the ICA (formerly called Bernasconi's artery), the superior branch of the inferolateral trunk, the ophthalmic artery, the lacrimal artery, and the accessory meningeal artery.

2. Meningiomas arising from the anterior lateral two-thirds of the tentorium are mainly supplied by the lateral branch of the lateral clival artery, which usually arises from the C5 portion of the ICA, by the basal tentorial branch of the petrous branch of the middle meningeal artery, and by the basal tentorial branch of the petrosquamosal branch of the middle meningeal artery.
3. Meningiomas arising from the posterior portion of the tentorium, which is peripherally attached to the occipital bone, may receive their supply from supra- and/or infratentoral dural arteries. Supratentorially, the main supply is derived from tentorial branches of the parieto-occipital and petrosquamosal branches of the middle meningeal artery. Infratentorially, the supply is derived from three sources: The lateral parts are supplied by the meningeal branch of the mastoid artery, arising from the horizontal portion of the occipital artery. The central parts are supplied by the multiple superior branches of the artery of the cerebellar fossa, which is a branch of the posterior meningeal artery. The posterior meningeal artery has a variable origin and may arise from the extradural segment of the vertebral artery, the occipital artery, the neuromeningeal trunk of the ascending pharyngeal artery or the PICA. The medial parts around the confluens sinuum and the straight sinus are mainly supplied by the artery of the falx cerebelli, which may arise from the vertebral artery, the occipital artery, or the PICA.

5.5.2.6 *Meningiomas of the Posterior Fossa*

Meningiomas of the posterior fossa include clival, petroclival, cerebellopontine angle and posterior surface of petrous bone, jugular foramen, cerebellar convexity, and foramen magnum meningiomas. Several arterial trunks, including the ICA, the middle meningeal, the occipital, the ascending pharyngeal, the vertebral, and the cerebellar arteries, contribute to the dural supply of posterior fossa meningiomas. The specific supply of an individual tumor will depend on its location and site of attachment to a certain dural territory as well as on its secondary extension along the posterior fossa dura (Rodesch and Lasjaunias 1991).

Petroclival meningiomas and meningiomas of the posterior surface of the petrous bone and of the cerebellopontine angle are supplied by the clival branches of the ICA anteriorly, branches of the petrosal branch of the middle meningeal artery superiorly, the ascending branch of the mastoid artery posteriorly, and the jugular and hypoglossal branches of the ascending pharyngeal artery inferiorly and centrally. In addition, the AICA with its distal dural branch, i.e., the subarcuate artery, frequently contributes to the dural supply of meningiomas in this region (Fig. 5.2).

Meningiomas of the cerebellar convexity receive their dural supply from the branches of the artery of the cerebellar fossa, the posterior meningeal artery, and the artery of the falx cerebelli.

Depending on their location, size, and extension, posterior fossa meningiomas frequently receive additional pial supply arising from the superior cerebellar artery, the AICA, and/or the PICA.

5.5.3 *Results and Complications*

The success of embolization of meningiomas depends mainly on the amount of dural supply present, on the accessibility to selective catheterization of dural feeders arising from the ICA or vertebral artery, and on the ability to achieve intratumoral deposition of the embolic material. The best results in terms of degree of devascularization are achieved with supratentorial convexity, parasagittal, falcine, and sphenoid wing meningiomas with a dominant meningeal supply. Embolization is less effective in those basal meningiomas with partial supply from inaccessible dural arteries. In the author's experience this is especially the case with frontobasal meningiomas.

The effect of embolization on the vascularity of the meningioma is best assessed with postembolization CT or MRI (Rodesch and Lasjaunias 1991). Depending on the degree of devascularization achieved, focal or diffuse areas of absent contrast enhancement will be seen within the tumor, indicating areas of intratumoral necrosis (Manelfe et al. 1986). However, radiologic-pathologic correlations disclosed a discrepancy between the CT appearance of embolized men-

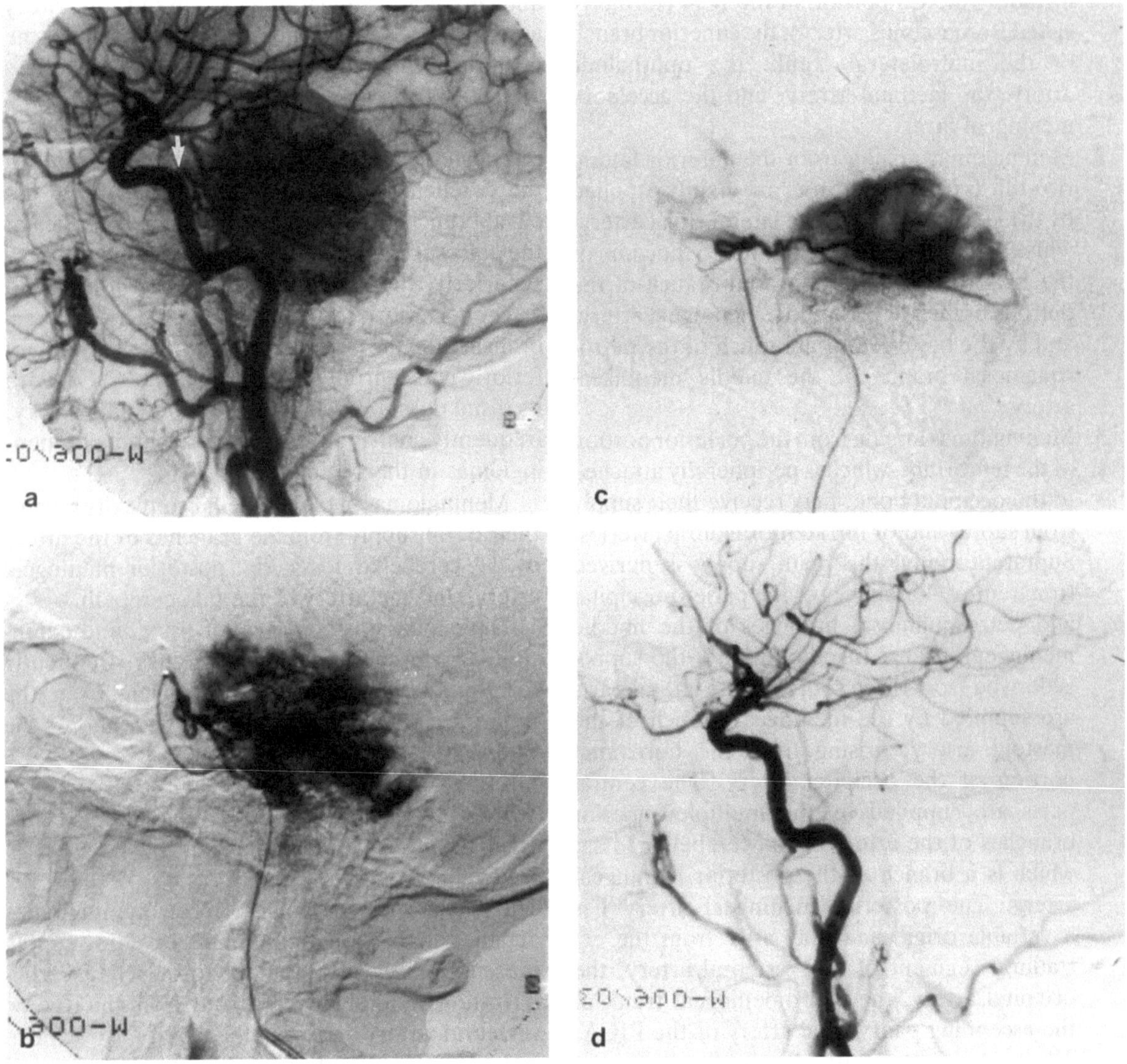

Fig. 5.2a–d. Cerebellopontine angle meningioma. **a** Common carotid angiography in lateral projection shows dominant meningeal supply to the tumor from the lateral and medial clival branches of the C5 portion of the ICA (*arrow*). Note intense and homogeneous opacification of the tumor, typical for a hypervascular meningioma. Additional supply to the tumor was from the neuromeningeal trunk of the ascending pharyngeal artery, the petrous branch of the middle meningeal artery, and the AICA (not shown). **b** Selective catheterization of the medial clival branch of the C5 portion of the ICA shows opacification of the medial tumor compartment. This was embolized with microparticles of PVA. **c** Selective catheterization of the lateral clival branch of the C5 portion of the ICA shows opacification of the lateral tumor compartment. This was embolized with microparticles of PVA. **d** Common carotid angiography in lateral projection after embolization of the clival branches of the ICA and of the middle meningeal and ascending pharyngeal arteries shows devascularization of the tumor

ingiomas and histologic findings in some cases, for reasons which are not understood (Manelfe et al. 1986).

Embolization of meningiomas should not be associated with mortality or morbidity because the disease is a benign one and the procedure is a preoperative and not a curative one. Theoretically, major complications such as cerebral stroke, blindness, or cranial nerve palsies may result from the application of inappropriate techniques or from ignoring relevant angiographic findings (cranial nerve supply arising from feeding arteries, dangerous anastomoses between feeding arteries and cerebral or ophthalmic arteries) and should be avoided in the majority of cases. Minor complications are related to inadvertent occlusion of cutaneous, muscular, or osseous branches of the ECA and include pain, skin necrosis, and trismus (MANELFE et al. 1986; LASJAUNIAS and BERENSTEIN 1987b). Intratumoral, peritumoral, or subarachnoid hemorrhage occurring during embolization has been reported in a few cases (WATANABE et al. 1986; SUYAMA et al. 1987; HAYASHI et al. 1987). Most probably, this is caused by high injection pressure of the embolic material or contrast agent with subsequent rupture of intratumoral vessels or vessels located at the surface of the tumor (RODESCH and LASJAUNIAS 1991). It is detected by extravasation of contrast agent during embolization or on postembolization CT. Depending on the location of the tumor and on the degree of hemorrhage, this complication may be clinically asymptomatic or may cause transient seizures, focal neurologic deficits, or headache (LASJAUNIAS and BERENSTEIN 1987b).

In a large series of cases of meningioma embolization the overall incidence of permanent neurologic deficits was reported to be 1.6%, the mortality, 0%, and the incidence of minor or transient complications, 2.7% (LASJAUNIAS and BERENSTEIN 1987b).

5.6 Embolization of Juvenile Nasopharyngeal Angiofibroma

5.6.1 General Remarks

Juvenile nasopharyngeal angiofibroma (JNA) is a histologically benign, fibrovascular tumor with the potential for locally aggressive behavior. The great majority occur in young males around puberty (LASJAUNIAS and BERENSTEIN 1987b).

Most commonly the tumor originates from the sphenopalatine foramen. In its early stage of development the tumor occupies the nasopharynx eccentrically and the ipsilateral posterior nasal fossa (VALAVANIS and FISCH 1989c). From here the tumor may secondarily extend into the paranasal sinuses, the infratemporal fossa, the central and paracentral middle cranial fossa, and finally intracranially and into the orbit. Presenting symptoms of JNA are nasal obstruction and variable degrees of epistaxis. Depending on the specific pattern of tumor extension, further symptoms may develop and include sinusitis, otitis, temporal swelling, exophthalmos, and cranial nerve palsies (LASJAUNIAS and BERENSTEIN 1987b). The modality of choice for management of JNAs is preoperative embolization followed by radical surgical tumor removal. High-resolution CT and multiplanar, T1-weighted, gadolinium-DTPA-enhanced MRI are essential imaging modalities for planning the angiographic workup and the embolization procedure and for selecting the surgical approach (VALAVANIS and FISCH 1989c).

In 1982 FISCH introduced a detailed topographic classification of JNA which has proved useful in planning the angiographic workup and in selecting the appropriate operative approach for a given case of JNA (FISCH et al. 1984; ANDREWS et al. 1989). This classification is derived from the evaluation of tumor extension and associated bone destruction as seen on CT and/or MRI. According to this classification JNAs are subdivided into the following classes:

- *Class I*: Tumors limited to the nasopharynx and nasal cavity and not causing significant bone destruction
- *Class II*: Tumors that invade the maxillary, ethmoid, and sphenoid sinuses and cause significant bone destruction
- *Class IIIa*: Tumors that invade the pterygopalatine fossa, the infratemporal fossa, and the orbit
- *Class IIIb*: Additional intracranial extradural extension lateral to the cavernous sinus
- *Class IVa*: Tumors with extension into the cavernous sinus
- *Class IVb*: Tumors with intracranial intradural extension or extension into the pituitary fossa or suprasellar area

Angiographically the tumor has a typical appearance and can be differentiated from other nasopharyngeal and nasal cavity hypervascular lesions such as angiomatous polyp, hemangioma, hemangiopericytoma, angiosarcoma, and extracranial meningioma. The supplying arteries arising from the ECA and ICA are only minimally dilated (Fig. 5.3). The tumor blush is intense but slightly inhomogeneous; it appears during the arterial phase but persists until the late venous phase of the angiogram. The draining veins appear during the later part of the venous phase. Only exceptionally may JNAs exhibit intratumoral arteriovenous shunting, and in these cases there is early appearance of the draining veins. As a general rule, angiographic exploration of a given case of angiofibroma should be performed according to an individual protocol derived from the CT and MRI appearance of the tumor. Besides a detailed

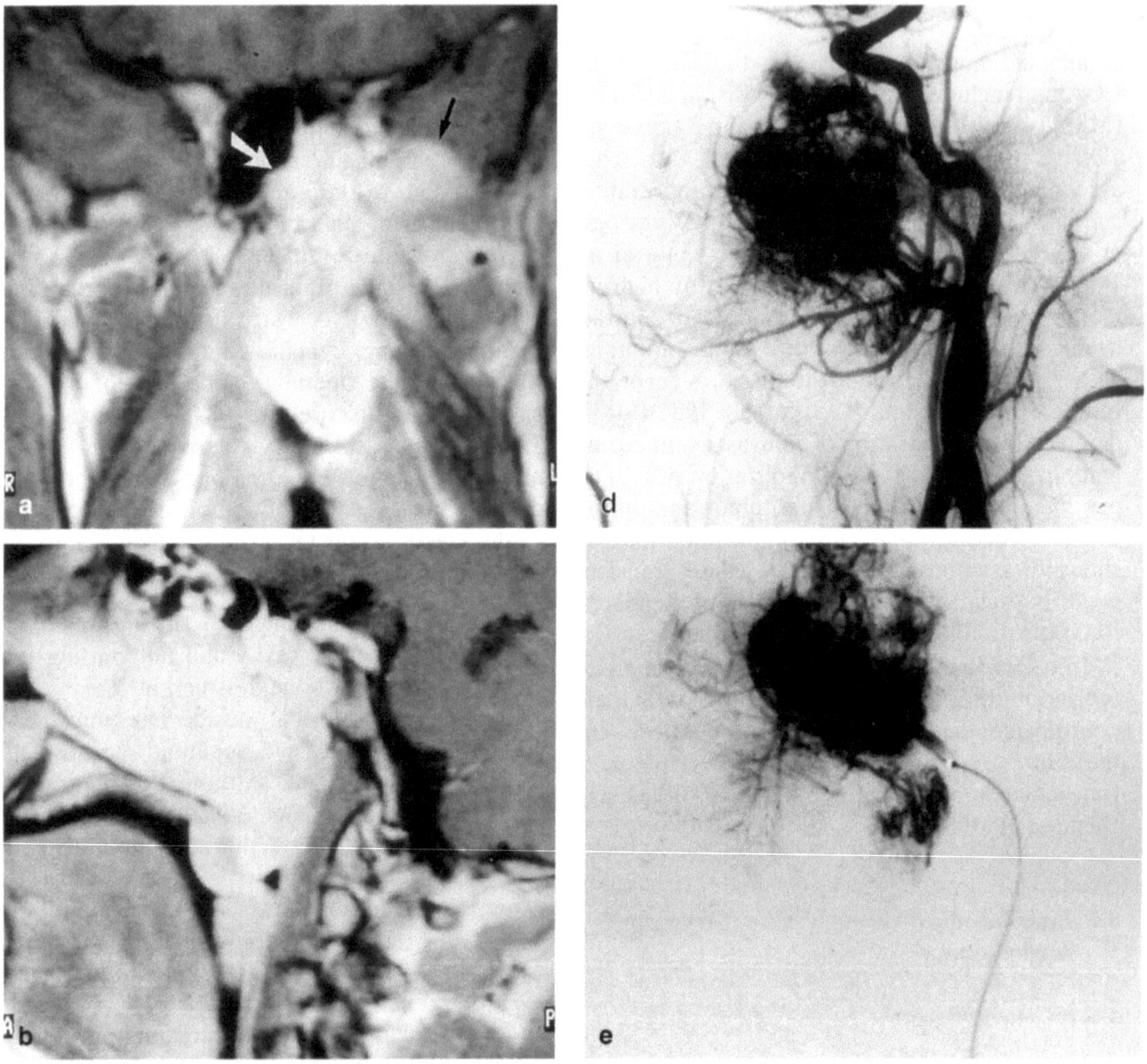

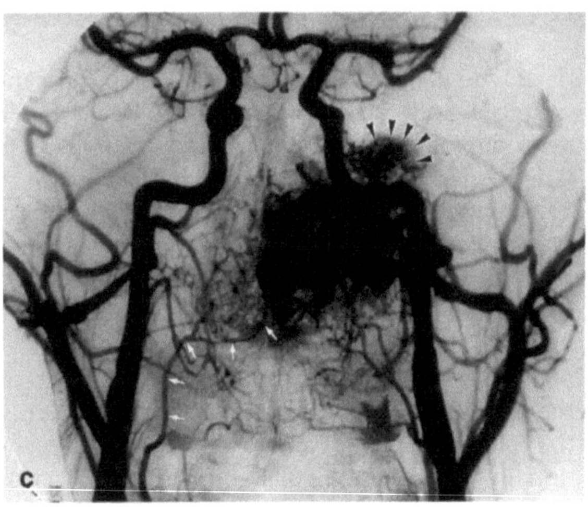

Fig. 5.3a–j. Juvenile nasopharyngeal angiofibroma (JNA) class IIIb. **a** Coronal T1-weighted MRI after gadolinium-DTPA injection shows a larger, strongly and homogeneously enhancing tumor mass obliterating the nasopharynx with its epicenter located eccentrically on the left side. The tumor extends through the floor of the sphenoid sinus into the left part of the sphenoid sinus (*white arrow*) and through the foramen ovale intracranially into the left extradural temporobasal space (*black arrow*). **b** Sagittal T1-weighted MRI after gadolinium-DTPA injection shows the anterior extension of the tumor into the nasal cavity, its superior extension into the sphenoid sinus, and its caudal extension towards the oropharynx. **c** Simultaneous, bilateral common carotid angiography in frontal projection shows the typical intense but inhomogeneous blush of JNA. The tumor is located on the left side but reaches the midline. The inferior midline parts of the tumor are supplied by the contralateral, slightly dilated ascending palatine artery (*white arrows*). The intracranial extradural extension of the tumor is located superolateral to the petrous ICA (*black arrow-heads*). **d** Left common carotid angiography in lateral projection shows the typical blush of JNA and its supply from the internal maxillary artery, the ascending pharyngeal artery, and the ascending palatine artery. The intracranial extradural extension is supplied by the inferolateral trunk.

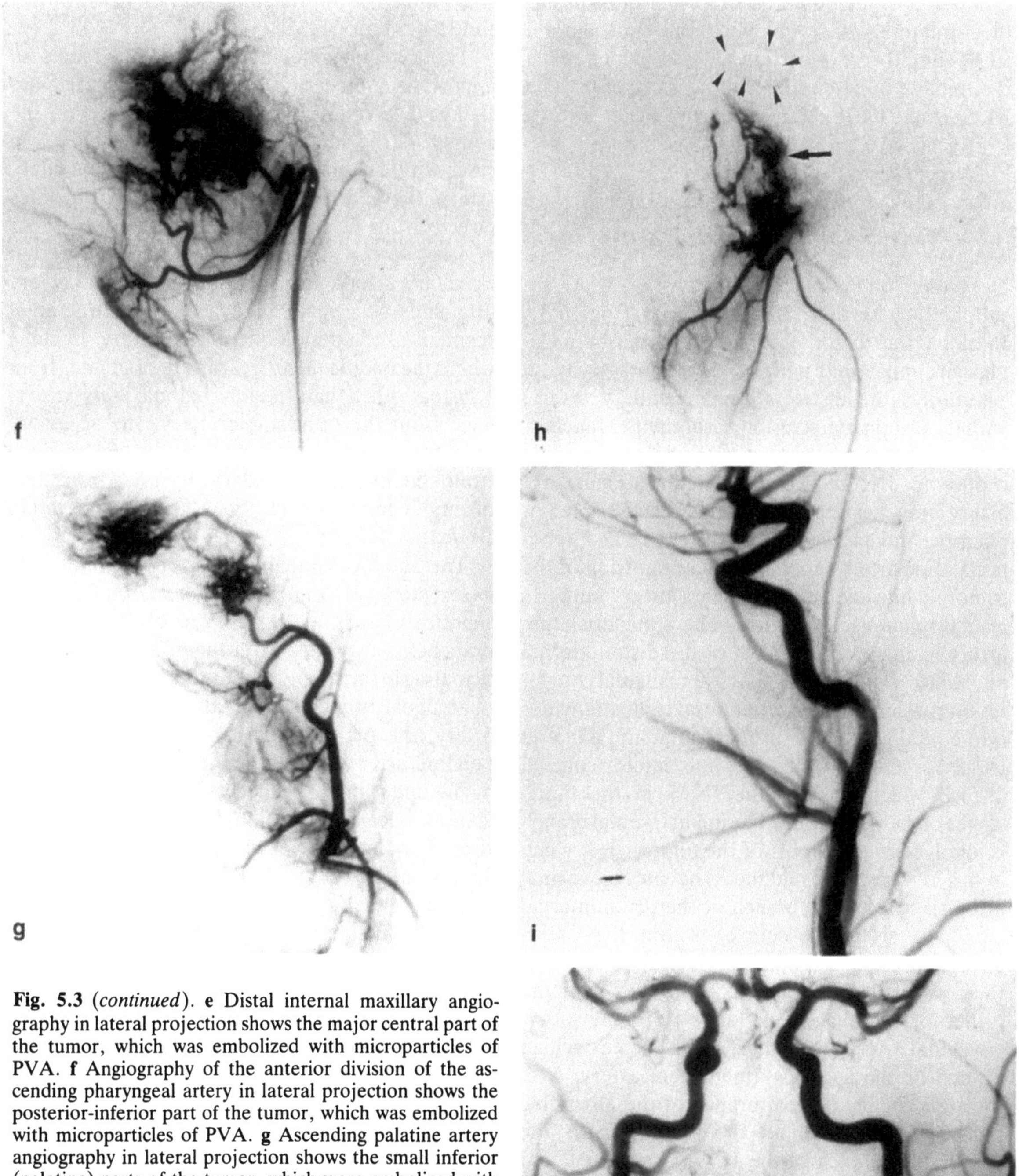

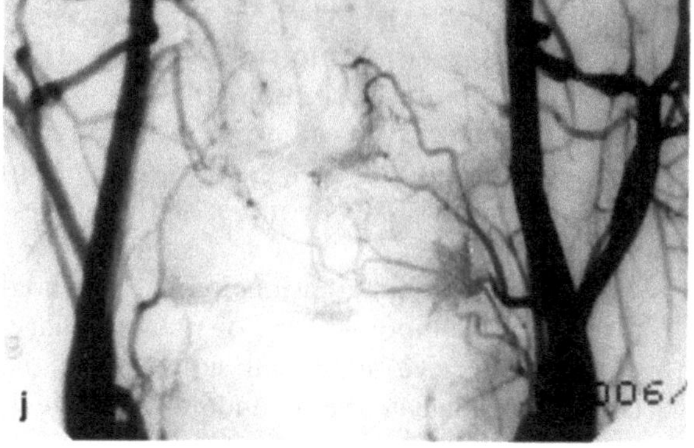

◁ **Fig. 5.3** (*continued*). **e** Distal internal maxillary angiography in lateral projection shows the major central part of the tumor, which was embolized with microparticles of PVA. **f** Angiography of the anterior division of the ascending pharyngeal artery in lateral projection shows the posterior-inferior part of the tumor, which was embolized with microparticles of PVA. **g** Ascending palatine artery angiography in lateral projection shows the small inferior (palatine) parts of the tumor, which were embolized with microparticles of PVA. **h** Angiography of the accessory meningeal artery in lateral projection during temporary balloon occlusion of the ICA (*arrowheads*) at the level of origin of the inferolateral trunk shows opacification of the intracranial extradural extension of the tumor (*arrow*), which was safely embolized with microparticles of PVA. **i** Left common carotid angiography in lateral projection after embolization shows complete devascularization of the tumor, including its intracranial extension (compare with **d**). **j** Simultaneous, bilateral common carotid angiography in frontal projection after embolization of all ipsilateral and contralateral supply to the tumor confirms its complete devascularization (compare with **c**)

evaluation of the potential supplying branches of the ipsilateral ECA and ICA, the contralateral ECA should be explored in all cases which reach the midline or extend beyond it (Lasjaunias and Berenstein 1987b; Valavanis and Fisch 1989c).

5.6.2 Vascular Supply and Embolization According to Size and Extension

Depending on their size and extension, JNAs are supplied by several specific arteries (Fig. 5.3). Initially, the tumor occupies the anterior nasopharynx unilaterally and the posterior nasal cavity. Therefore, the distal internal maxillary artery, with its nasopharyngeal and nasal cavity branches, is the first and constant arterial system providing supply to JNAs. The distal internal maxillary artery branches supplying JNAs are the sphenopalatine and pterygovaginal arteries. The sphenopalatine artery supplies the nasal portion of the tumor, while the pterygovaginal artery supplies its nasopharyngeal portion. The sphenopalatine artery is an anterior branch of the distal internal maxillary artery and has a lateral to medial course. Upon reaching the posterior nasal cavity it divides into a medial branch for the septum and a lateral trunk for the conchae. It is this lateral conchal branch which supplies the JNAs in the initial stages of their evolution. The medial, septal branch is involved in the supply of the tumor later, when it has reached the midline. The pterygovaginal artery is a recurrent branch of the distal internal maxillary artery. It courses within the pterygovaginal canal, supplies the lateral portions of the roof of the nasopharynx, and ends near the orifice of the eustachian tube. Here the pterygovaginal artery anastomoses with the eustachian branch of the accessory meningeal artery, with the superior pharyngeal branch of the ascending pharyngeal artery, and inconstantly with the mandibular branch of the ICA (Lasjaunias and Berenstein 1987a). Therefore, "proximal" occlusion of the distal internal maxillary artery without intratumoral deposition of microparticles through the pterygovaginal artery will invariably result in reconstitution of the arterial supply to the tumor through one or more of these anastomotic channels.

Larger tumors with extensions into the sphenoid sinus, the infratemporal fossa, or the parapharyngeal space receive additional supply from the accessory meningeal, the ascending pharyngeal, and the ascending palatine arteries (Lasjaunias and Berenstein 1987b).

The accessory meningeal artery represents an important source of supply to JNAs of classes II–IV. The origin of this vessel depends on the course of the internal maxillary artery, i.e., in cases with a deep course of the internal maxillary artery, the accessory meningeal artery originates directly from the internal maxillary artery, whereas in cases with a superficial course of the internal maxillary artery, the accessory meningeal artery originates as a main branch of the extracranial segment of the middle meningeal artery. In cases where the middle meningeal artery originates from a system other than the internal maxillary artery, e.g., from the ophthalmic artery, the accessory meningeal artery always originates directly from the internal maxillary artery, irrespective of its course (Lasjaunias and Berenstein 1987a).

The accessory meningeal artery supplies with its extracranial branches the posterolateral and superior extracranial extensions of JNAs. These branches anastomose with the other arteries participating in the supply of the area, i.e., the superior pharyngeal branch of the ascending pharyngeal artery, the pterygovaginal artery, the ascending palatine artery, and the mandibular artery. This again underlines the necessity of distal embolization, because occlusions proximal to the anastomotic points will result in reconstitution of the supply to the tumor. In addition to these extracranial branches and their anastomoses, the accessory meningeal artery also has a transcranial branch, which courses through either the foramen ovale or the foramen of Vesalius and anastomoses with the inferolateral trunk of the ICA. While the two systems are usually in a hemodynamic balance, in some cases one of them is dominant (Lasjaunias and Berenstein 1987a).

If the accessory meningeal artery is hypoplastic, the inferolateral trunk will be dominant and will supply with its posterior branch most of the tumor portion located in the territory of the accessory meningeal artery. In these cases angiography of the ICA will opacify through the dilated inferolateral trunk the extracranial tumor compartment, which – in a balanced situation – would be supplied by the extracranial branches of the accessory meningeal artery. This may provide the erroneous impression of intracranial tumor extension. Careful analysis of the angiogram and correlation with CT/MRI help in the correct identification of the position of the tumor blush (LASJAUNIAS and BERENSTEIN 1987b).

The ascending pharyngeal artery participates via its superior pharyngeal branch in the supply of the posterior and posteromedial portions of JNAs. This branch anastomoses with the accessory meningeal, the pterygovaginal, and the mandibular arteries. Furthermore, it gives off the carotid branch, which courses through the foramen lacerum and anastomoses with the inferolateral trunk as well as the recurrent artery of the foramen lacerum, arising from the C5 portion of the ICA (LASJAUNIAS and BERENSTEIN 1987a).

The inferior extension of JNAs towards the soft palate receives its supply from the terminal segment of the ascending palatine artery. The ascending palatine artery usually arises from the mandibular segment of the facial artery, but it may also arise directly from the external carotid trunk, the medial pharyngeal branch of the ascending pharyngeal artery, or even the accessory meningeal artery. The terminal segment of the ascending palatine artery anastomoses with the descending palatine artery, which, in cases of proximal embolization of the ascending palatine artery, may reconstitute the supply to the inferior portion of the tumor.

Extensions into the sphenoid sinus receive their supply from sphenoidal branches of the vidian–mandibular anastomotic system and should be distinguished from intracranial, extradural, parasellar extensions. Extensions into the ethmoid sinus receive their supply from anterior and posterior ethmoidal branches of the ophthalmic artery and should be distinguished from true intraorbital extensions (LASJAUNIAS and BERENSTEIN 1987b).

Intraorbital extensions occur mainly through the inferior orbital fissure and may receive their supply directly from the ophthalmic artery branches or the infraorbital artery. If the intraorbital extension occurs through the superior orbital fissure, then the anteromedial branch of the inferolateral trunk will also be involved in the supply of the tumor (LASJAUNIAS and BERENSTEIN 1987b).

Intracranial extradural tumor extensions into the middle cranial fossa and into the cavernous sinus occur through the basal foramina (ovale, rotundum, lacerum) or after destruction of the sphenoid sinus walls and/or the greater wing of the sphenoid bone. The arterial supply is mainly provided by the branches of the inferolateral trunk, which are in a hemodynamic balance with the transcranial branches of the internal maxillary artery and with the recurrent branches of the ophthalmic artery. If there is dominance of the internal maxillary system over the inferolateral trunk, the intracranial extradural tumor extension will be mainly opacified during internal maxillary angiography. This represents a favorable hemodynamic situation for embolization of the intracranial extradural extension through the accessory meningeal artery and/or the artery of the foramen rotundum and/or the carotid branch of the superior pharyngeal branch of the ascending pharyngeal artery. In cases with a balanced supply between the inferolateral trunk and the accessory meningeal artery, temporary occlusion of the inferolateral trunk with a balloon inflated within the C4 portion of the ICA will induce increased flow through the transcranial branch of the accessory meningeal artery towards the intracranial portion, thus enabling embolization of the intracranial extradural tumor extension. In cases with dominance of the ICA supply, selective catheterization of the inferolateral trunk with an appropriately preshaped microcatheter and embolization with NBCA or microparticles should be attempted. If this fails, embolization can be performed after temporary balloon occlusion of the ICA immediately distal to the origin of the inferolateral trunk followed by injection of microparticles through a microcatheter placed proximal to the origin of the inferolateral trunk. These techniques are also used for embolization of the mandibular artery supply or supply from other branches of the ICA (Fig. 5.3).

Intracranial intradural extensions are rare. They occur at the temporobasal area and are supplied by cortical branches of the temporopolar and/or anterior temporal arteries arising from the middle cerebral artery. Currently available microcatheters usually allow distal catheterization of these temporal branches of the middle cerebral artery and thus enable safe embolization of these rare intradural tumor extensions (VALAVANIS 1990).

Permanent preoperative balloon occlusion of the ICA should be considered in the rare class IVb and in some class IVa JNAs exhibiting extensive invasion of the cavernous sinus and encasement of the cavernous portion of the ICA (VALAVANIS and FISCH 1989b,c).

5.6.3 *Effect of Embolization; Endovascular Protocol*

Before the routine application of preoperative embolization, patients who underwent surgery for JNAs were at distinct risk of exsanguination (CUMMINGS 1980). The average blood replacement without previous embolization is reported in the literature to be approximately 2000 cc. Since the routine application of embolization the risk of exsanguination has almost disappeared and the blood loss during surgery has been reduced to less than 1000 cc (DAVIS and DEBRUN 1987; LASJAUNIAS and BERENSTEIN 1987b; VALAVANIS and FISCH 1989c). Embolization itself, if properly performed after precise evaluation of the superselective angiograms, today carries a very low risk (LASJAUNIAS 1980). Below a brief protocol is outlined for the endovascular exploration and embolization of JNAs of classes III, IVa, IVb.

1. Contralateral common carotid angiography in frontal projection with manual compression of the ipsilateral ICA.
   - Identification of contralateral supply
   - Preliminary evaluation of patency of circle of Willis
2. Ipsilateral common carotid angiography in frontal projection
   - Overall assessment of tumor extent (extracranial, intracranial, orbital, towards or beyond midline, lateral)
3. Ipsilateral common carotid angiography in lateral projection
   - Overall assessment of tumor extent (extracranial, intracranial, orbital, anterior/posterior)
   - Identification of external carotid supply and origin of feeders
4. Ipsilateral internal carotid angiography in lateral projection
   - Identification of internal carotid supply to:
     a) Extracranial tumor portions (mandibular artery, recurrent artery of foramen lacerum, inferolateral trunk)
     b) Ethmoidal extension (ethmoid branches of ophthalmic artery)
     c) Orbital extension (ophthalmic artery)
     d) Intracranial extradural extension (inferolateral trunk)
     e) Intracranial intradural extension (temporopolar and anterior temporal branches of middle cerebral artery)
   - Evaluation of the wall of the C5, C4, and C3 portions of the ICA
5. Ipsilateral distal internal maxillary angiography in lateral projection
   - Identification of supplying arteries (sphenopalatine, pterygovaginal, descending palatine arteries)
   - Identification of dangerous anastomoses with ICA (vidian artery, artery of foramen rotundum) or ophthalmic artery (ethmoidal arteries, infraorbital artery)
   - Embolization of tumor compartment through identified feeding arteries
6. Ipsilateral proximal internal maxillary angiography in lateral projection
   - Identification of supplying arteries (accessory meningeal and middle meningeal arteries)
7. Ipsilateral accessory meningeal angiography in lateral projection
   - Identification of extracranial supplying branches
   - Identification of dangerous anastomoses with ICA (transcranial branch, mandibular artery)
   - Identification of transcranial supply to intracranial extradural extension
   - Embolization of tumor compartment(s)
8. Ipsilateral ascending pharyngeal angiography in lateral projection
   - Identification of supplying arteries (superior pharyngeal branch)
   - Identification of dangerous anastomoses (carotid branch)
   - Embolization of tumor compartment
9. Ipsilateral ascending palatine angiography in lateral projection (variable origin: facial artery, external carotid trunk, middle pharyngeal artery)
   - Identification of supplying artery (soft palate branch)
   - Embolization of tumor compartment
10. Ipsilateral common carotid angiography in lateral projection
    - Confirmation of devascularization of entire external carotid supply to tumor
    - Identification of persisting ICA supply to tumor
11. Ipsilateral internal carotid angiography in lateral projection
    - Identification of ICA branches supplying tumor (mandibular artery, inferolateral trunk, other cavernous branches, ophthalmic artery)

- Embolization after direct catheterization or, if this is not possible, free-flow embolization during temporary balloon occlusion. (If the ICA has to be permanently occluded, embolization should be performed after detachment of the first (i.e., distal) balloon.

12. Ipsilateral common carotid angiography in lateral projection
    - Final ipsilateral postembolization control
13. Contralateral common carotid angiography in frontal projection
    - Identification of persisting contralateral supply
14. Depending on arteries participating in tumor supply, continue as with steps 5–9 described above
15. Contralateral common carotid angiography in frontal projection
    - Final contralateral postembolization control

5.7 Embolization of Glomus Tumors

5.7.1 General Remarks

Glomus tumors or paragangliomas are usually benign but locally invasive, highly vascular tumors which arise from glomus bodies distributed in the middle ear cavity, the jugular fossa, and the extracranial parasympathetic chain of the neck, as well as in other areas of the head and neck. The majority of glomus tumors (48%) arise within the temporal bone, i.e., glomus tympanicum and glomus jugulare tumors. The next most frequent localization of glomus tumors is the carotid body (35%) followed by glomus vagale tumors (11%). The remaining 6% arise from glomus bodies located in other sites of the head and neck such as the orbit, the larynx, the nasal cavity, and the naso- and oropharynx. In approximately 10% of cases multifocal glomus tumors are encountered. Familial cases with an autosomal dominant inheritance do occur and have a high incidence (30%) for multifocal tumors. Up to 5% of glomus tumors exhibit secretory activity (catecholamines and serotonin) causing hypertensive crises, palpitations, and headaches. Between 3% and 18% of glomus tumors may undergo malignant transformation with lymph node involvement or distant metastasis. The incidence of malignant transformation is higher in glomus vagale and caroticum tumors than in glomus tumors of the temporal bone (Zak and Lawson 1982; Lasjaunias and Berenstein 1987b).

The therapy of choice for glomus tumors is surgical removal. Because of their high degree of vascularity and their intimate relationship with cranial nerves and the wall of the ICA, in the past the rate of radical removal was low and the associated surgical morbidity and mortality high. The introduction of surgical microtechniques, the invention of new surgical approaches, and the routine application of preoperative embolization significantly improved the radicality of tumor removal, minimized morbidity, and almost totally eliminated the surgical mortality (Fisch and Mattox 1988).

The neuroradiologic evaluation of glomus tumors proceeds in sequential steps and includes CT, MRI, and superselective angiography in order to ascertain the precise localization and topographic delineation of the tumor, to assess its relationship with the wall of the ICA, to demonstrate its intrinsic vascular architecture, and finally to detect or exclude any further, coexisting, asymptomatic glomus tumor (Valavanis and Fisch 1989a).

High-resolution CT provides useful information concerning the relationship of the tumor to surrounding bony structures such as enlargement and erosion of the jugular foramen, infiltration of the petrous bone, erosion of the carotid canal, involvement of the facial nerve canal, labyrinthine destruction, erosion of the hypoglossal canal, and the relationship of extracranial glomus tumors to the exocranial aspect of the skull base (Valavanis et al. 1987). Gadolinium-enhanced T1-weighted MRI is primarily applied to assess the intrinsic soft tissue morphology of the tumor and the degree of its vascularity but also to detect invasion of the adventitia of the ICA and any intracranial extra- or intradural tumor extension (Valavanis and Fisch 1989a).

The angiographic workup of glomus tumors should be performed according to a specific protocol elaborated for each individual tumor and derived from the preceding CT/MRI evaluation of the lesion. Irrespective of their location, glomus tumors have a characteristic angiographic appearance consisting of enlarged feeding arteries, an early, intense, slightly inhomogeneous tumor blush, and early appearing draining veins. This angiographic appearance reflects the intrinsic vascular architecture of glomus tumors (Lasjaunias and Berenstein 1987b). As can be shown histologically, the intrinsic vascular architecture of glomus tumors consists of (a) centripetally oriented intratumoral arterioles with a diameter of approximately 90 μm at the tumor periphery and of 300–600 um in the central parts of the tumor, (b) intratumoral arteriolo-arteriolar anastomoses, and (c) direct communications between intratumoral arterioles and venules and sinusoids, i.e., arteriovenous shunting (WILLIS and BIRRELL 1955). These features, i.e., progressively increasing vessel diameter from the periphery towards the center of the tumor, presence of an anastomosing arteriolocapillary bed, and arteriovenous shunts, are the principal determinants of the embolic material to be used in embolization of glomus tumors. In order that the embolic microparticles reach the central parts of the intratumoral vasculature, their diameter must be less than the diameter of the peripheral tumor arterioles, i.e., less than 90 μm. Furthermore, the presence of intratumoral arteriovenous shunting justifies the use of NBCA in certain cases.

Based on the superselective angiography, two types of glomus tumors are distinguished, i.e., multi- and monocompartmental tumors. Approximately 85% of glomus tumors of any location have a multicompartmental vascular composition. Each compartment represents a hemodynamic but not a morphologic unit. It is supplied by the artery normally supplying the vascular territory in which this tumor compartment has evolved and it is drained by its own veins. Injection of each supplying artery will only opacify the tumor compartment supplied by this artery. In contrast, in monocompartmental tumors consisting of a single compartment, injection of each identified feeding artery will opacify the entire tumor. Therefore, in monocompartmental glomus tumors, intratumoral embolization through an easily accessible and safe supplying artery may result in complete devascularization of the entire tumor without the need for embolization of all feeding arteries. Complete devascularization of multicompartmental glomus tumors requires embolization of all compartments through all identified feeding arteries (VALAVANIS 1986).

5.7.2 Glomus Tumors of the Temporal Bone

Glomus tumors of the temporal bone include glomus tympanicum and glomus jugulare tumors as well as some intratemporal glomus tumors of unusual origin such as the infralabyrinthine compartment or the medial wall of the petrous ICA. Glomus temporale tumors represent by far the most common type of glomus tumor and one of the most important indications for preoperative embolization in the head and neck area (VALAVANIS 1990). Initial symptoms of glomus temporale tumors include pulsatile tinnitus and a reddish-bluish mass within the middle ear. The appearance of additional symptoms depends on the pathways of extension of the tumor and include facial nerve palsy, lower cranial nerve palsies, and symptoms simulating a cerebellopontine angle mass.

In 1982 Fisch introduced a detailed classification of glomus temporale tumors which has subsequently been further refined to incorporate the experience of the interventional neuroradiologic and otoneuromicrosurgical techniques (FISCH and MATTOX 1988). This classification has proved highly useful both for planning the embolization and for selection of the appropriate surgical approach. According to this classification, glomus temporale tumors are categorized into the following classes and subclasses:

Class A: Glomus tympanicum tumors confined to the tympanic cavity.

Class B: Glomus tympanicum tumors extending into the mastoid bone but leaving the cortical outline of the jugular bulb intact.

Class C: Glomus jugulare tumors with variable degrees of extension into the infralabyrinthine portion of the temporal bone and along the petrous carotid canal. Depending on the degree of involvement of the carotid canal, class C glomus tumors are further subdivided into subclasses C1–C4.

Class C1: Glomus tumors causing only minimal erosion of the vertical segment of the carotid canal.

Class C2: Glomus tumors causing extensive erosion of the vertical segment of the carotid canal.

Class C3: Glomus tumors characterized by additional erosion of the horizontal segment of the carotid canal.

Class C4: Glomus tumors that reach the foramen lacerum and may extend into the cavernous sinus.

Class D: Glomus jugulare tumors with intracranial extension. If the intracranial extension is extradural, the tumor is classified as class *De1 to De3*, depending on the size of the extradural extension. If there is additional intradural extension the tumor is classified as *Di1–Di3*, depending on the size of the intradural extension.

Correlation of the CT and MRI findings with superselective angiographic studies in individual cases of glomus temporale tumors led to the development of detailed protocols for the angiographic evaluation, embolization, and, if indicated, balloon occlusion of the ICA for each class of glomus temporale tumor (VALAVANIS 1990). The type and the number of arteries participating in the supply of glomus temporale tumors correlate well with the class of tumor present. However, branches of the ascending pharyngeal artery (inferior tympanic artery, neuromeningeal trunk) are always involved in the supply of glomus temporale tumors bacause the ascending pharyngeal artery normally supplies the glomus bodies of the tympanic cavity and jugular fossa, from which these tumors arise (LASJAUNIAS and BERENSTEIN 1987b).

The angiographic evaluation of glomus temporale tumors should include the identification of all supplying arteries, the presence of dangerous anastomoses between supplying arteries and the ICA or vertebral artery, identification of cranial nerve supply by feeding arteries, and identification of the vascular composition of the tumor (i.e., multicompartmental versus monocompartmental). Furthermore, delineation of the relationship of the tumor mass to the internal jugular vein and the adjacent dural sinuses as well as detection of extraluminal compression or intraluminal extension is of special importance for subsequent postembolization surgical removal of the tumor. This is best done by analysis of the venous phase of the ipsilateral vertebral artery angiography, performed in frontal projection, in conjunction with the information obtained previously by CT and MRI. Angiographically two-thirds of glomus temporale tumors exhibit a multicompartmental composition, while one-third are composed of a single compartment. A multicompartmental tumor can have maximally four compartments. These are the inferomedial, the posterolateral, the anterior, and the superior compartment (VALAVANIS 1986, 1990; LASJAUNIAS and BERENSTEIN 1987b).

The inferomedial compartment is located in the jugular fossa and in the hypotympanum. It is the first compartment to develop in the evolution of a multicompartmental glomus tumor. Its hypotympanic portion is supplied by the inferior tympanic branch of the ascending pharyngeal artery while its jugular fossa portion is supplied by the neuromeningeal trunk (Fig. 5.4). The jugular and hypoglossal branches of the neuromeningeal trunk also supply small medial extensions of this compartment into the intracranial extradural space at the level of the jugular foramen and hypoglossal canal. If the intracranial extension is large, the inferomedial compartment receives additional supply from the lateral clival branch of the ICA anteriorly and from dural branches of the vertebral artery posteriorly. If there is additional intradural extension of the inferomedial compartment, this intradural extension receives its supply from the PICA and the AICA.

The posterolateral compartment occupies the posterior tympanic cavity and the mastoid bone in close relationship to the mastoid segment of the facial nerve canal. This compartment is present in class B–D tumors. Its main supply is from the stylomastoid artery, which enters the temporal bone through the stylomastoid foramen and arises from either the occipital or, more rarely, the posterior auricular artery.

Intracranial extradural extensions of the posterolateral compartment are supplied by the meningeal branch of the occipital artery (i.e., mastoid artery), which enters the skull through a transmastoid foramen. Larger extradural extensions receive additional supply from meningeal branches of the vertebral artery.

The anterior compartment occupies the anterior tympanic cavity and exhibits a close topographic relationship with the carotid canal. The main supply of this compartment is from the anterior tympanic as well as the caroticotympanic arteries. The anterior tympanic artery arises from the proximal internal maxillary artery and enters the tympanic cavity through the chroda tympani canal. It supplies the lateral portion of this compartment. On the other hand, the caroticotympanic artery, which is an embryologic remnant of the hyoid artery, enters the tympanic cavity through the hyoid canal at the junction of the vertical and horizontal segments of the carotid canal. It supplies the pericarotid portion of this compartment. Extensions of this compartment along the horizontal segment of the carotid canal toward the foramen lacerum or even the cavernous sinus receive additional supply from the cavernous branches of the ICA as well as the carotid branch of the anterior ramus of the ascending pharyngeal artery.

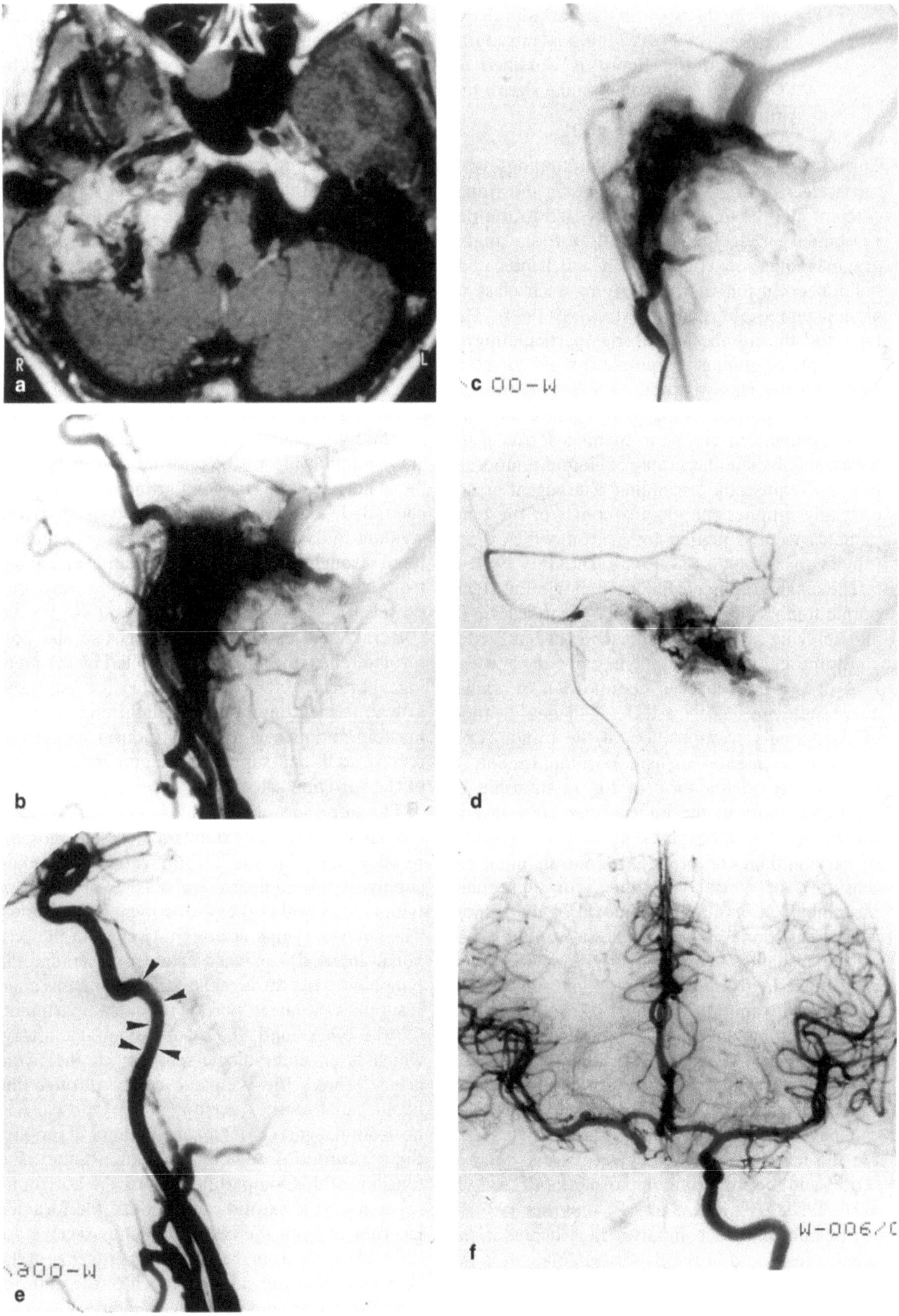
R
L
a
c
b
d
e
f

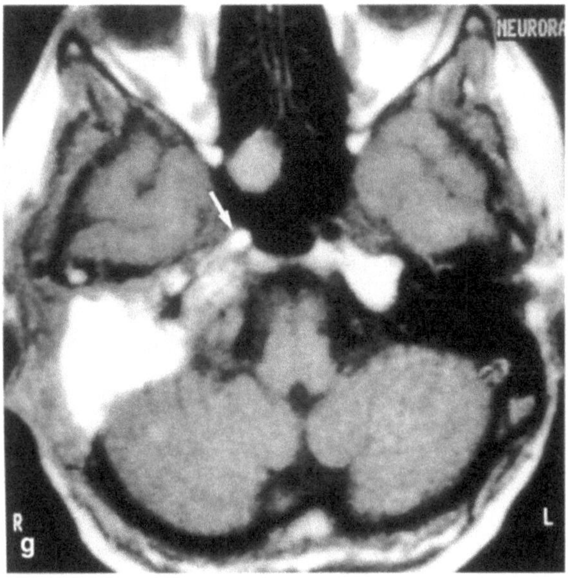

◁ **Fig. 5.4a–g.** Glomus tumor of temporal bone, class C3De2. **a** Axial, T1-weighted MRI after gadolinium-DTPA injection shows a glomus jugulare tumor with intense enhancement and typical intratumoral flow voids. Note tumor extension along the horizontal segment of the carotid canal and medium-sized intracranial extradural extension. **b** Common carotid angiography in lateral projection shows the typical early, intense blush of glomus tumor with early appearing draining veins. **c** Selective angiography of the ascending pharyngeal artery in lateral projection shows the inferomedial compartment of the tumor, which was embolized with microparticles of PVA. **d** Selective middle meningeal artery angiography shows the superior compartment of the tumor, which was embolized with microparticles of PVA. **e** Common carotid angiography in lateral projection after embolization confirms devascularization of the tumor. Note circumferential narrowing of the vertical and proximal horizontal segments of petrous ICA, indicating tumor encasement (*arrowheads*). **f** Contralateral ICA angiography in frontal projection during temporary balloon occlusion of the right ICA shows excellent collateral supply to the right hemisphere. The patient tolerated this test occlusion lasting for 20 min without any neurologic deficit. Because of extensive involvement of the carotid canal, the ICA was subsequently permanently occluded with two detachable balloons, one detached in the cavernous segment and the second in the proximal, cervical segment of the ICA (not shown). **g** Axial T1-weighted MRI after gadolinium-DTPA injection, performed 1 week postoperatively, confirms radical tumor removal. The operative cavity contains high signal intensity fatty tissue. Note also high signal intensity of the occluded ICA (*arrow*)

The superior compartment occupies the superior aspect of the tympanic cavity. It is supplied by the superior tympanic artery arising from the superficial temporal artery. Intracranial extradural extensions of this compartment into the middle temporal fossa are supplied by the petrosal branch of the middle meningeal artery as well as by the accessory meningeal artery.

Embolization of multicompartmental glomus tumors is carried out with microparticles of PVA with a size of less than 90–100 μm. For complete and effective devascularization of multicompartmental glomus tumors it is essential that supplying branches from the ICA and vertebral artery also be embolized. The use of the newer variable stifness microcatheters allows safe superselective catheterization and embolization of these branches (Fig. 5.5). If, however, this is technically not possible, temporary balloon occlusion of the parent artery distal to the origin of the supplying branch followed by microparticle embolization represents an efficient alternative technique. In exceptional cases with large intradural extensions, distal selective catheterization and embolization of the supplying branches of the AICA and the PICA is also possible (Valavanis 1990).

Monocompartmental tumors with geometrically easily accessible feeding arteries may be embolized with a fluid material such as NBCA provided that these feeders represent safe arteries (a safe feeder is an artery which is not involved in the supply of cranial nerves and not anastomosing with the ICA or the vertebral artery) (Valavanis 1986).

Large glomus tumors with intracranial extension may require permanent preoperative balloon occlusion of the ICA in order to reduce the risks of mobilization of the pericarotid tumor portion from the ICA wall and to achieve a radical tumor removal. Glomus tumors with the following features regarding the relationships with the ICA should undergo permanent balloon occlusion of the ICA:

1. Tumors with extensive destruction of the horizontal segment of the carotid canal
2. All class C4 tumors with extension into the cavernous sinus
3. Tumors with erosion of the carotid canal and extensive supply from the caroticotympanic and cavernous branches of the ICA

Embolization of glomus tumors of the temporal bone is associated with a high degree of efficiency and a low complication rate if properly performed (Lasjaunias and Berenstein 1987b; Valavanis 1990). The effectiveness of embolization of glomus temporale tumors is best appreciated on postembolization preoperative MRI showing extensive intratumoral areas of absence of contrast

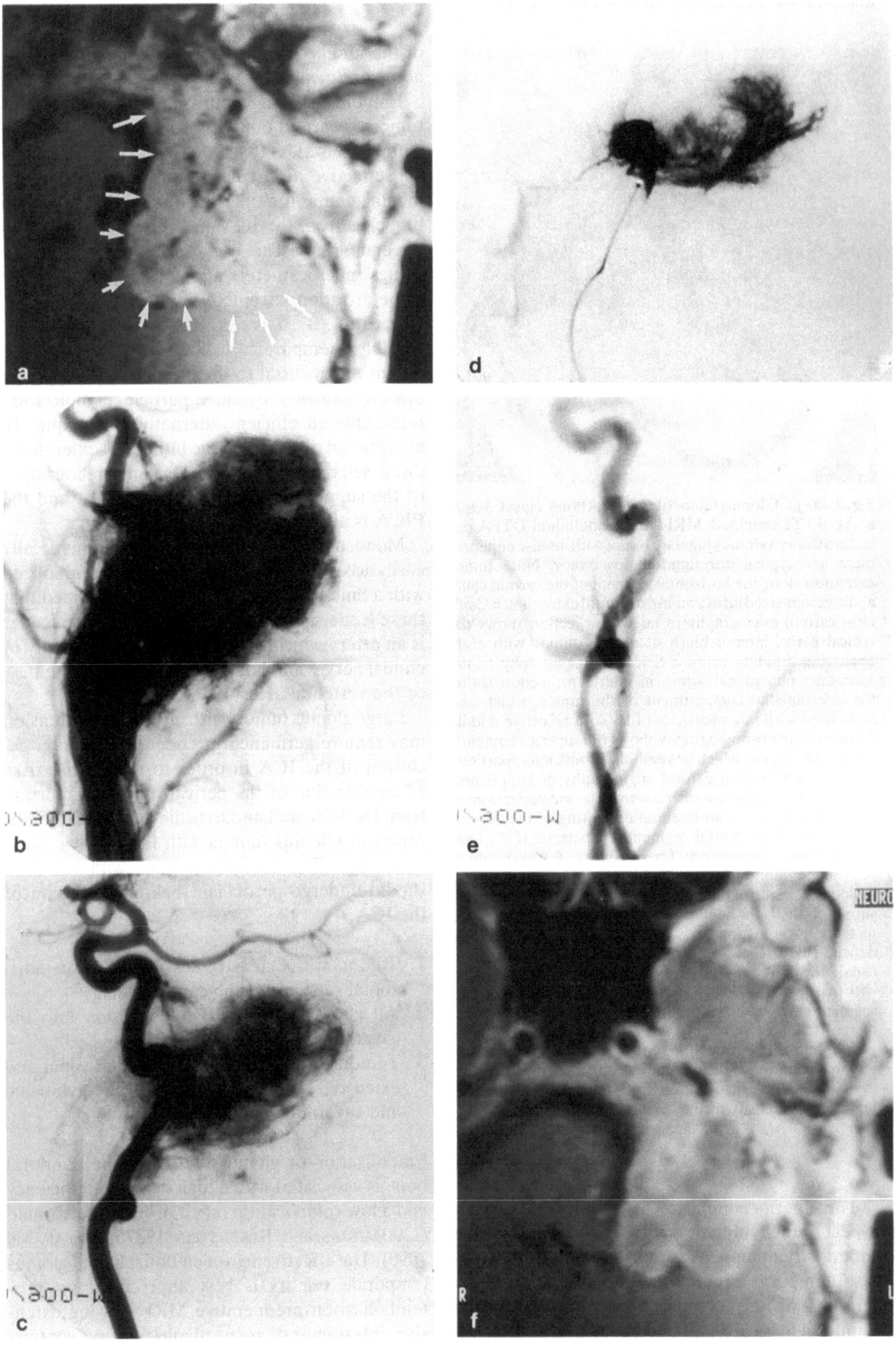

enhancement representing intratumoral ischemic necroses.

5.7.3 Glomus Caroticum Tumors

Glomus caroticum tumors originate from the carotid body itself. With further growth these tumors displace the ICA posterolaterally and the main trunk of the ECA anteromedially. They therefore occupy the soft tissue space enclosed by the carotid bifurcation. Multiplanar MRI is superior to CT in showing the craniocaudal extension of glomus caroticum tumors, their relationship to the exocranial aspect of the skull base, and their specific relation to the wall of the ICA. Glomus caroticum tumors exhibit on MRI an intrinsic appearance identical to that of glomus tumors of the temporal bone or the vagal body. Glomus caroticum tumors should be differentiated by MRI and angiography from other lesions of the carotid bifurcation which may mimic the presence of a glomus tumor clinically. These lesions include hypervascular metastases, neurinomas, and neurofibromas, aneurysms of the proximal ICA, and a dolichoectatic carotid sinus (LASJAUNIAS and BERENSTEIN 1987b).

The main supply to glomus caroticum tumors is provided by the musculospinal branch of the ascending pharyngeal artery (LASJAUNIAS and BERENSTEIN 1987a,b). The musculospinal branch arises from the posterior wall of the proximal ascending pharyngeal artery, courses posterosuperiorly, and then curves in an acute angle inferiorly to enter the carotid space. It supplies the larger superior compartment of the tumor. The musculospinal artery anastomoses with the extracranial high cervical ipsilateral vertebral artery. If such a patent anastomosis is present, embolization should be carried out only after catheterization of the musculospinal branch distal to the anastomotic vessel, or if particles are used which are larger than the anastomotic vessel itself. The small inferior compartment is supplied by the so-called artery of the carotid body (LASJAUNIAS and BERENSTEIN 1987b; VALAVANIS 1990). This artery arises directly from the carotid bifurcation. Newer variable stifness microcatheters usually allow selective catheterization of the artery of the carotid body. Embolization of the carotid body artery carries a significant risk of reflux of embolic material into the ICA. Embolization of this artery should be performed with a very low injection pressure. If catheterization of the carotid body artery is not technically possible, temporary ballon occlusion of the proximal ICA with free-flow embolization is an alternative technique. However, this technique carries a definite risk of blindness due to occlusion of the central retinal artery. Temporary proximal ICA occlusion may reverse the flow in the ophthalmic artery and particles may be carried from the main trunk of the ECA into the ophthalmic artery. Flow reversal within the ophthalmic artery must be excluded before embolization is carried out during temporary occlusion of the proximal ICA.

Large glomus caroticum tumors are also supplied by branches of the lingual artery and the superior laryngeal artery, as well as by the ascending and deep cervical arteries and the muscular branches of the occipital artery. Complete embolization of larger glomus tumors is usually possible after selective catheterization and embolization of the mentioned vessels (VALAVANIS 1990).

◁ **Fig. 5.5a–f.** Glomus tumor of the temporal bone, class C3De2Di1. **a** Axial T1-weighted MRI after gadolinium-DTPA injection shows a large glomus jugulare tumor with intense enhancement and typical intratumoral flow voids. The tumor extends along the petrous ICA within the infralabyrinthine compartment of the temporal bone and medially into the intracranial extradural (*long arrows*) and intradural space (*short arrows*). **b** Common carotid angiography in lateral projection shows this unusually large glomus tumor with its typical angiographic blush. **c** Following embolization with microparticles of PVA of the ECA-supplying branches (not shown), angiography of the ICA shows a large anterior compartment supplied by the caroticotympanic artery. **d** Selective angiography of the caroticotympanic artery with opacification of the anterior compartment. This was embolized with microparticles of PVA. **e** Common carotid angiography in lateral projection after embolization shows devascularization of the tumor. Note preservation of cutaneous branches (occipital, superficial temporal arteries) of the ECA. **f** Axial T1-weighted MRI after gadolinium-DTPA injection performed 4 days after embolization shows extensive intratumoral necroses including the intracranial intradural extension

5.7.4 Glomus Vagale Tumors

Glomus vagale tumors arise from the nodose ganglion or from extravagal paraganglions (LASJAUNIAS and BERENSTEIN 1987b). These tumors are located in the upper parapharyngeal space and displace the ICA anteromedially. Therefore, in contrast to carotid body tumors, vagal tumors displace both the main trunk of the ECA and the extracranial ICA in an anterior direction (VALAVANIS 1990).

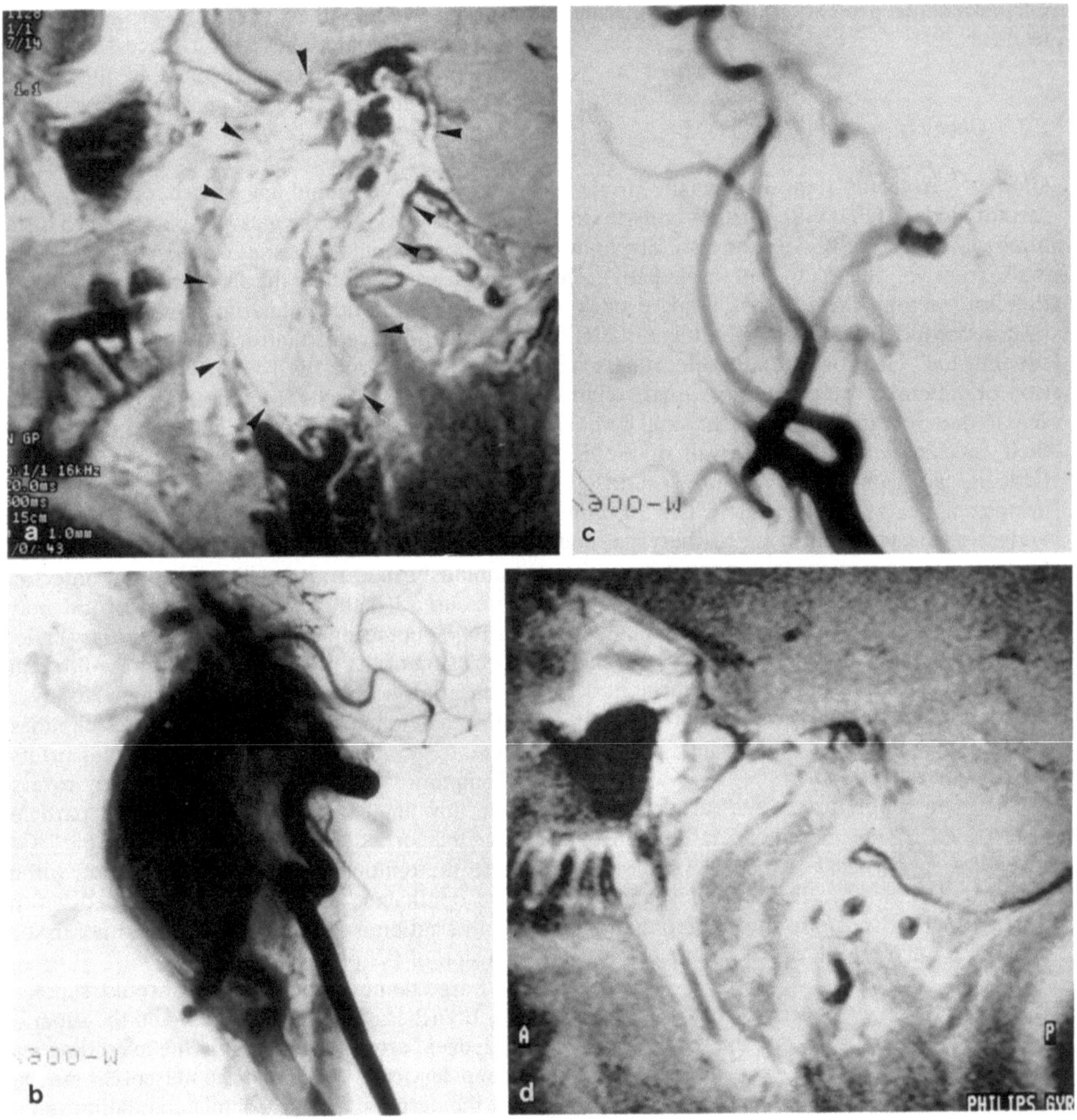

Fig. 5.6 a–d. Large glomus vagale tumor. **a** Sagittal T1-weighted MRI after gadolinium-DTPA injection shows a large glomus vagale tumor (*arrowheads*) with characteristic intratumoral flow voids. The tumor extends superiorly into the infralabyrinthine compartment of the temporal bone and inferiorly towards the level of the carotid bifurcation. **b** Simultaneous, left-sided common carotid and vertebral artery angiography in lateral projection shows the entire extent of the tumor. Note typical anterior displacement of both the ICA and the ECA. **c** Simultaneous, left-sided common carotid and vertebral artery angiography in lateral projection following embolization with microparticles of PVA of all identified feeding arteries (i.e., musculospinal and neuromeningeal branches of the ascending pharyngeal artery, muscular branches of the occipital artery, muscular branches of the vertebral artery) shows devascularization of the tumor. **d** Sagittal T1-weighted MRI after gadolinium-DTPA injection performed 6 days after embolization shows extensive necrosis of the tumor

Larger glomus vagale tumors may reach the skull base and extend into the jugular foramen. Multiplanar MRI is highly useful in depicting the relationship of the tumor to the wall of the ICA as well as its extention into the skull base and specifically into the jugular foramen. The main arterial supply is derived from the musculospinal branch of the ascending pharyngeal artery and from muscular branches of the occipital artery.

Larger tumors with extensions into the jugular foramen receive additional supply from the neuromeningeal trunk of the ascending pharyngeal artery but also from the ascending cervical and the ipsilateral vertebral artery.

For complete embolization of vagal body glomus tumors the same techniques are applied as for embolization of carotid body and temporal bone glomus tumors (Fig. 5.6).

Glomus vagale and caroticum tumors with invasion of the wall of the ICA represent a major limitation for safe and radical removal. In these cases permanent preoperative balloon occlusion of the ICA should be considered. This usually allows the complete resection of the tumor.

References

Adler JR, Upton J, Wellman J, Winston KR (1986) Management and prevention of necrosis of the scalp after embolization and surgery for meningioma. Surg Neurol 25:357–360

Andrews JC, Fisch U, Valavanis A (1989) The infratemporal fossa approach for extensive nasopharyngeal angiofibromas. In: Fisch U, Valavanis A, Yasargil MG (eds) Neurological surgery of the ear and skull base. Kugler and Ghedini, Amsterdam, pp 249–255

Berenstein A, Russell E (1981) Gelatin sponge in therapeutic neuroradiology: a subject review. Radiology 141:105–112

Brothers MF, Kaufmann JCE, Fox AJ, Deveikis JP (1989) *N*-Butyl-2-cyanoacrylate: substitute for IBCA in interventional neuroradiology-histopathologic and polymerization time studies. AJNR 10:777–786

Cummings BJ (1980) Relative risk factors in the treatment of juvenile nasopharyngeal angiofibroma. Head Neck Surg 3:21–26

Davis KR, Debrun GM (1987) Embolization of juvenile nasopharyngeal angiofibromas. Semin Intervent Radiol 4:309–320

Dion JE (1992) Principles and methodology. In: Vinuela F, Halbach VV, Dion JE (eds) Interventional neuroradiology: endovascular therapy of central nervous system. Raven, New York, pp 1–15

Fisch U, Mattox D (1988) Microsurgery of the skull base. Thieme, New York

Fisch U, Fagan P, Valavanis A (1984) The infratemporal fossa approach for the lateral skull base. Otolaryngol Clin North Am 17:513–522

Halbach VV, Hieshima GB, Higashida RT, David CF (1992) Endovascular therapy of head and neck tumors. In: Vinuela F, Halbach VV, Dion JE (eds) Interventional neuroradiology: endovascular therapy of central nervous system. Raven, New York, pp 17–28

Hayashi T, Shojima K, Utsunomiya H, Moritakea K, Honda E (1987) Subarachnoid hemorrhage after preoperative embolization of a cystic meningioma. Surg Neurol 27:295–300

Jack CR Jr, Forbes G, Dewanjee MK, Brown ML, Earnest FN (1985) Polyvinyl alcohol sponge for embolotherapy: particle size and morphology. AJNR 6:595–597

Kerber CW, Bank WP, Horton JA (1988) Polyvinyl alcohol foam: prepacking emboli for therapeutic embolization. Radiology 130:1993–1994

Kikuchi Y, Strother CM, Boyer M (1987) New catheter for endovascular and interventional procedures. Radiology 165:870–871

Lasjaunias P (1980) Nasopharyngeal angiofibromas. Hazards of embolization. Radiology 136:119–123

Lasjaunias P, Berenstein A (1987a) Surgical neuroangiography, vol I: Functional anatomy of craniofacial arteries. Springer, Berlin Heidelberg New York

Lasjaunias P, Berenstein A (1987b) Surgical neuroangiography, vol II: Endovascular treatment of craniofacial lesions. Springer, Berlin Heidelberg New York

Lasjaunias P, Ter Brugge K, Chin M, Lopez Ibor L (1987) Embolization and balloon-occlusion techniques in the management of cranial base tumors. In: Sekhar L, Schramm VL Jr (eds) Tumors of the cranial base: diagnosis and treatment. Futura Mount Kisco, New York, pp 95–104

Manelfe C, Lasjaunias P, Ruscalleda J (1986) Preoperative embolization of intracranial meningiomas. AJNR 7:963–972

Richter HP, Schachenmayr W (1983) Preoperative embolization of intracranial meningiomas. Neurosurgery 13:261–268

Rodesch G, Lasjaunias P (1991) Embolization and meningiomas. In: Al-Mefty O (ed) Meningiomas. Raven, New York, pp 285–297

Spiegel SM, Vinuela F, Glodwasser MJ, Fox AJ, Pelz DM (1986) Adjusting polymerization time of isobutyl-2-cyanoacrylate. AJNR 7:109–112

Suyama T, Tamaki N, Fujiwara K, Hamano S, Kimura M, Matsumoto S (1987) Peritumoral and intratumoral hemorrhage after gelatin sponge embolization of malignant meningioma: case report. Neurosurgery 21:944–946

Teasdale E, Patterson J, McLellan D, MacPherson P (1984) Subselective preoperative embolization for meningiomas. A radiological and pathological assessment. J Neurosurg 60:506–511

Théron J, Cosgrove R, Melanson D, Ethier R (1986) Embolization with temporary balloon occlusion of the internal carotid or vertebral arteries. Neuroradiology 28:246–253

Valavanis A (1986) Preoperative embolization of the head and neck: indications, patient selection, goals and precautions. AJNR 7:943–952

Valavanis A (1988) Interventional neuroradiology of skull base tumors. In: Fisch U, Mattox D (eds) Microsurgery of the skull base. Thieme Medical, New York, pp 634–655

Valavanis A (1990) Interventional neuroradiology for head and neck surgery. In: Cummings CW, Fredrickson JM, Harker LA, Krause CJ, Schuller DE (eds) Otolaryngology – head and neck surgery. Update II. Mosby Year Book, St. Louis, pp 206–223

Valavanis A, Fisch U (1989a) Glomus tumors of the temporal bone: imaging and classification. In: Fisch U, Valavanis A, Yasargil MG (eds) Neurological surgery of the ear and skull base. Kugler and Ghedini, Amsterdam, pp 63–68

Valavanis A, Fisch U (1989b) Balloon-occlusion of the internal carotid artery in extensive skull base tumors. In: Fisch U, Valavanis A, Yasargil MG (eds) Neurological surgery of the ear and skull base. Kugler and Ghedini, Amsterdam, pp 81–86

Valavanis A, Fisch U (1989c) Juvenile nasopharyngeal angiofibroma: imaging, classification and embolization. In: Fisch U, Valavanis A, Yasargil MG (eds) Neurological surgery of the ear and skull base. Kugler and Ghedini, Amsterdam, pp 235–244
Valavanis A, Schubiger O, Naidich TP (1987) Clinical imaging of the cerebellopontine angle. Springer, Berlin Heidelberg New York
Watanabe K, Matsumura K, Matsuda M, Handa J (1986) Meningioma with intratumoral and subdural hemorrhage as an immediate complication of therapeutic embolization. Case report. Neurol Med Chir 26:904–907
Willis AG, Birrell JH (1955) The structure of a carotid body tumor. Acta Anat (Basel) 25:220–265
Zak FG, Lawson W (1982) The paraganglionic chemoreceptor system. Physiology, pathology and clinical medicine, Springer, New York Berlin Heidelberg

6 Endovascular Treatment of Arteriovenous Malformations of the Brain

ALEX BERENSTEIN, PIERRE LASJAUNIAS, and IN SUP CHOI

CONTENTS

6.1 Introduction

The endovascular approach to arteriovenous malformations dates back to the original work by LUESSENHOP in the 1960s. LUESSENHOP employed free-floated particulate material introduced into the internal carotid artery after surgical exposure of the carotid artery. The original material was steel particles covered with methyl methacrylate. This approach was then refined by using barium-impregnated Silastic spheres. The technique was inspired by the original work of BROOKS, who injected muscle particles into the internal carotid artery in an attempt to occlude carotid cavernous fistulas. The rationale of silicone sphere embolization was to obliterate the feeding pedicles to large, surgically inaccessible malformations. Subsequently the percutaneous transcatheter technique was developed by KRICHEFF in the early 1970s; this permitting greater flexibility, enabling either the anterior or the posterior circulation to be approached. The major drawback of such an approach was the size of the embolic particles that could be injected. This nonselective technique was employed as a palliative measure in large malformations, or for presurgical embolization, or as part of a staged procedure (HILAL and MICHELSEN 1975; WOLPERT et al. 1981). The more modern era of endovascular embolization was pioneered by KERBER (1976), assisted by the possibility of employing flow-guided microballoon catheters with a calibrated leak microballoon system. This catheter assembly system consisted of very flexible and soft Silastic tubing to which a Silastic balloon with a calibrated "leak" was attached. Modifications of this technique included the use of a pressure chamber (PEVSNER 1977) and the use of calibrated leak latex balloons (BERENSTEIN 1981; DEBRUN et al. 1982). The latest generation of variable stiffness microcatheters has revolutionized the approach to cerebrovascular navigation in the endovascular treatment of arteriovenous malformations of the brain (BAVMs).

When deciding to treat or not to treat a BAVM, it is important to understand not only the anatomy and the technical possibilities but also the disease, its clinical manifestation, and its natural history. Such knowledge is crucial to the decision to introduce a catheter into the brain.

6.2 Natural History

Accurate determination of the natural history of a BAVM is a difficult task in the individual case,

---

ALEX BERENSTEIN, M.D., Professor of Radiology and Neurosurgery, Department of Radiology, New York University Medical Center, 560 First Avenue, New York, NY 10016, USA

PIERRE LASJAUNIAS, M.D., Ph.D., Professor of Radiology and Neurosurgery, Unité de Neuroradiologie Vasculaire Diagnostique et Thérapeutique, Hôpital Bicêtre, Université Paris Sud, 78, Rue du Général Leclerc, 94275 Kremlin-Bicêtre, France

IN SUP CHOI, M.D., Radiology, Massachusetts General Hospital, Fruit Street, Boston, MA 02114, USA and may not even be possible. Many studies, including CRAWFORD et al.'s (154 cases, 1988) and ONDRA et al.'s (160 cases, 1990), have suggested some clues as to the natural behavior of BAVMs in symptomatic patients.

6.2.1 Clinical Features

Presenting symptoms vary depending upon the size of the BAVM, its location, and the degree of AV shunt. Except for vein of Galen malformations and arteriovenous fistulas in the pediatric age group, the most common single presenting symptom of BAVMs is hemorrhage, followed by seizures and recurrent headaches.

6.2.1.1 Hemorrhage

According to various neurosurgical reports, intracranial hemorrhage is the initial presenting symptom in approximately 50% of BAVMs (PATERSON and MCKISSOCK 1956; PERRET and NISHIOKA 1966; SVIEN and MCRAE 1965; TROUPP et al. 1970; STEIN and WOLPERT 1980; WALTIMO 1973a,b). This figure is corroborated by our own experience: hemorrhage was the initial clinical sign of BAVM in 47.3% of our 279 patients. The rate of first hemorrhage in unruptured BAVM was estimated to be 2%–3% yearly by GRAF et al. (1983). The rate of recurrent hemorrhage was as high as 6% for the 1st year and 2% thereafter. ONDRA et al. (1990) recently reported a prospective study of untreated symptomatic BAVM in 160 patients. They reported a hemorrhage rate of 4% per year regardless of the initial presentation, and this rate was constant throughout the follow-up period of 23.7 years.

The true incidence of hemorrhage is probably higher than these figures since it has been postulated that sudden headaches with or without seizures and other acute symptoms may represent hemorrhages. Evidence of such minor hemorrhages has been documented in the neurosurgical literature (STEIN and WOLPERT 1980; YAMADA 1982). STEIN and WOLPERT found evidence of previous hemorrhage in one-third of BAVMs operated on.

It is generally accepted that spontaneous rupture of a BAVM occurs in the nidus or veins near the nidus or associated aneurysms (YASARGIL 1988; MCKENZIE 1953; MOODY and POPPEN 1970; STEIN and WOLPERT 1980). Various investigators (WILLINSKY 1988; MARKS et al. 1990) have analyzed the relationship between the angioarchitecture and the incidence of hemorrhage. They have found that intranidal aneurysms correlated strongly with hemorrhage, though it is not clear whether such aneurysms represent true aneurysms or pseudoaneurysms that occur after hemorrhage. Whichever is the case, we can postulate that these aneurysms represent weakness of the angioarchitecture and that treatment planning therefore should be aimed toward these parts of the BAVM when partial treatment is the only possibility (Fig. 6.1). WILLINSKY (1988) concluded that hemorrhage is more likely to occur with deep lesions and posterior fossa AVMs, and that arterial aneurysms and venous stenosis are more common features associated with hemorrhage (Fig. 6.2). Many recent reports suggest that there is no direct correlation between size of the lesion and hemorrhage (CRAWFORD et al. 1986; WILLINSKY 1988; MARKS et al. 1990; ONDRA et al. 1990).

Hemorrhage in patients with BAVMs is most frequently intracerebral (approximately 63% of cases) (PERRET and NISHIOKA 1966). Subarachnoid hemorrhage is seen in about one-third and intraventricular hemorrhage is the least frequent, occurring in 6% of cases. Intracranial hemorrhage due to BAVMs is considered relatively benign compared to other types, such as hemorrhage due

Fig. 6.1a–f. 43-year-old male with seizure disorder and migraine-type headache. Digital subtraction angiography (DSA) of the left vertebral artery, **a** frontal and **b** lateral view, demonstrates a large flow-related aneurysm (*curved arrow*) in the parieto-occipital artery. The aneurysm is proximal to the nidus. Note the partial opacification of a large venous ectasia. **c** DSA of the left internal carotid artery, lateral view. The anterior and lateral portions of the nidus are supplied by the angular and parietal branches of the middle cerebral artery. Note that the aneurysm of the posterior cerebral artery is not opacified. The presence of a large venous ectasia suggests that there is outflow restriction. **d** Superselective DSA of the left parieto-occipital artery, lateral view. This pedicle was given priority because of a flow-related aneurysm. The aneurysm and the feeding pedicle are included in the acrylic cast. Note that a larger portion of the nidus is filled than in vertebral artery injection since systemic hypotension is used. **e** Postembolization DSA of the left vertebral artery reveals complete occlusion of the parieto-occipital artery supply to the AVM and the aneurysm. There is increased collateral supply from the calcarine branch (*arrows*), as compared with the preembolization angiogram (**a**). **f** Postembolization control DSA of the left internal carotid artery. The nidus is occluded except for residual supply from a small network of arteries of the posterior parietal branch (*open arrow*) ▷

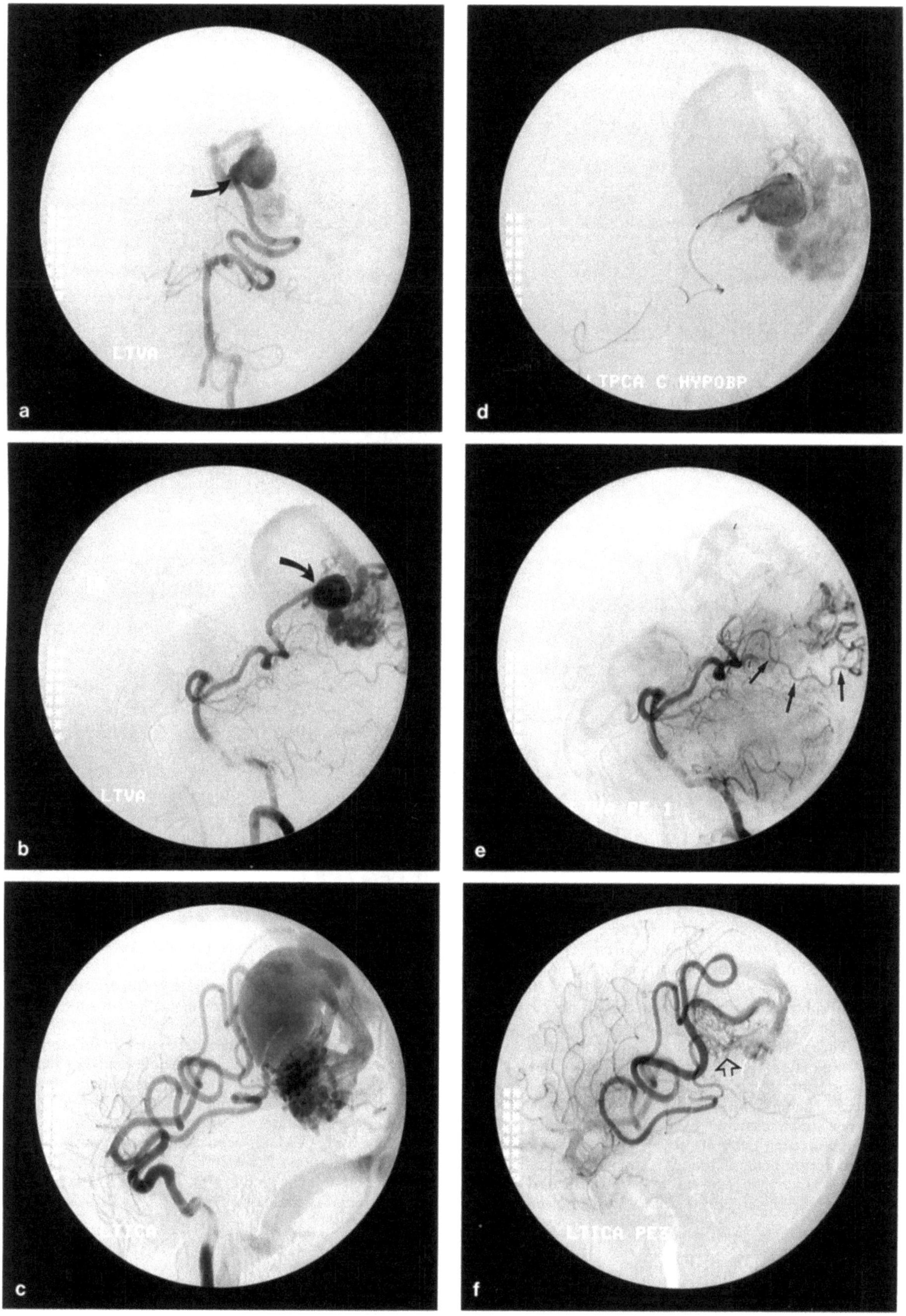
LTVA
a
TPCA C HYPOBP
d
LTVA
b
e
c
LTICA PE3
f

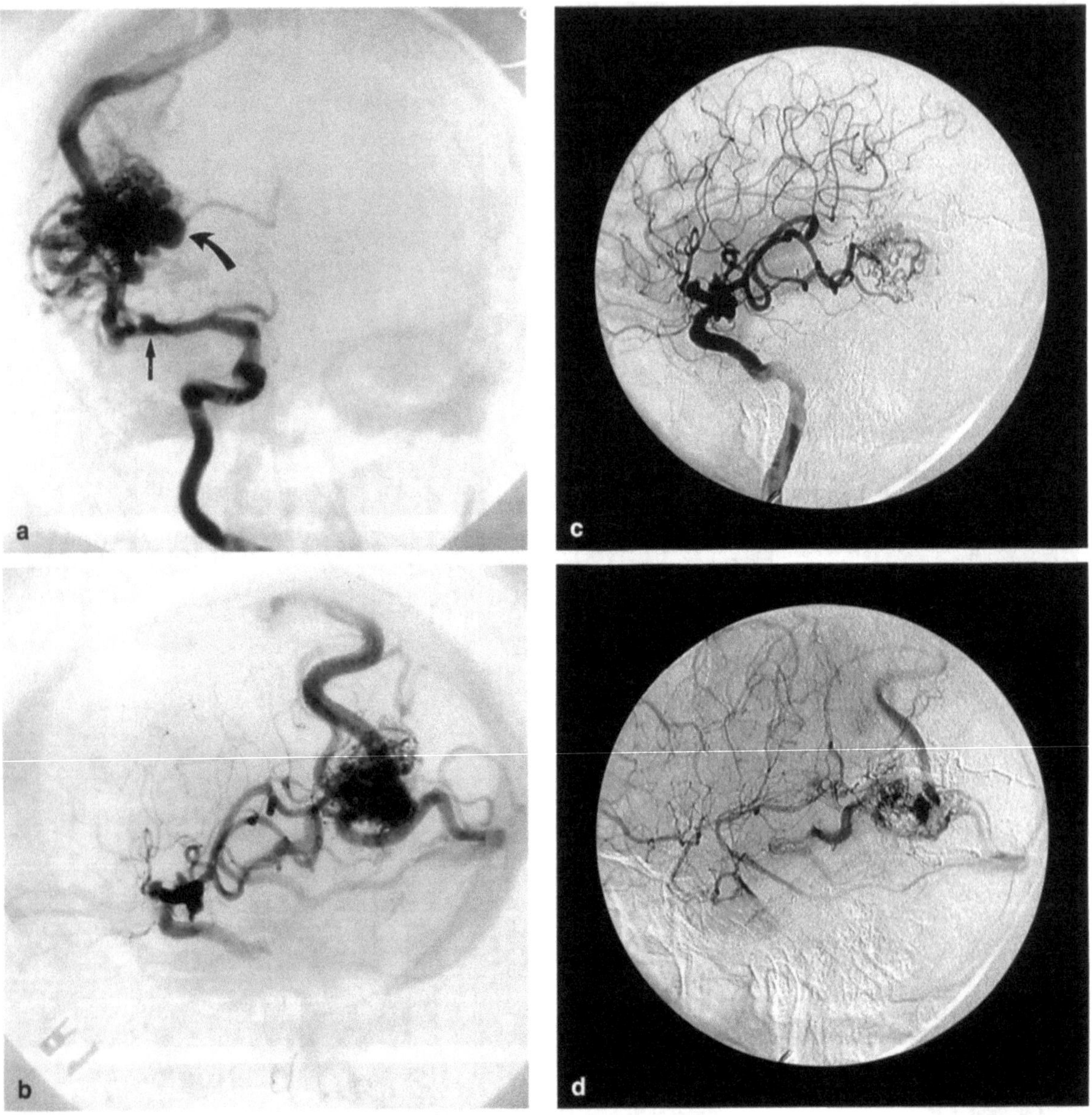

Fig. 6.2a–h. 52-year-old female who presented with two episodes of intracerebral hemorrhage. Preoperative embolization and surgery were planned. **a** Anteroposterior and **b** lateral subtraction angiograms of the left internal carotid artery show an AVM located in the right temporo-occipital area. The posterior temporal and angular branches of the MCA are major feeders. Additional supply is derived from the posterior temporal branch of the PCA. Note, an associated aneurysm (*arrow*) in the MCA and an intranidal aneurysm (*curved arrow*). **c** Arterial and **d** venous phase of postembolization DSA of the left internal carotid artery. One posterior temporal branch is still filling the nidus. This branch was thought to be on the gyral surface, which can be easily seen at surgery; therefore it was not embolized. AV shunting is markedly decreased. **e** Postembolization left vertebral angiogram demonstrates no residual supply from the PCA. **f** CT scan immediately after an ictus. Three days following embolization, while waiting for surgery, the patient suddenly developed severe headache and became comatose with signs of transtentorial brain herniation. CT scan revealed a large intracerebral hematoma. The patient was taken to the operating room immediately and the AVM and hematoma were removed. **g,h** Follow-up angiography of the right internal carotid artery 1 month postoperatively. The AVM has been completely removed. Note persistent dilatation of the feeding artery. The associated aneurysm has not changed in size. Fortunately, the patient recovered almost completely

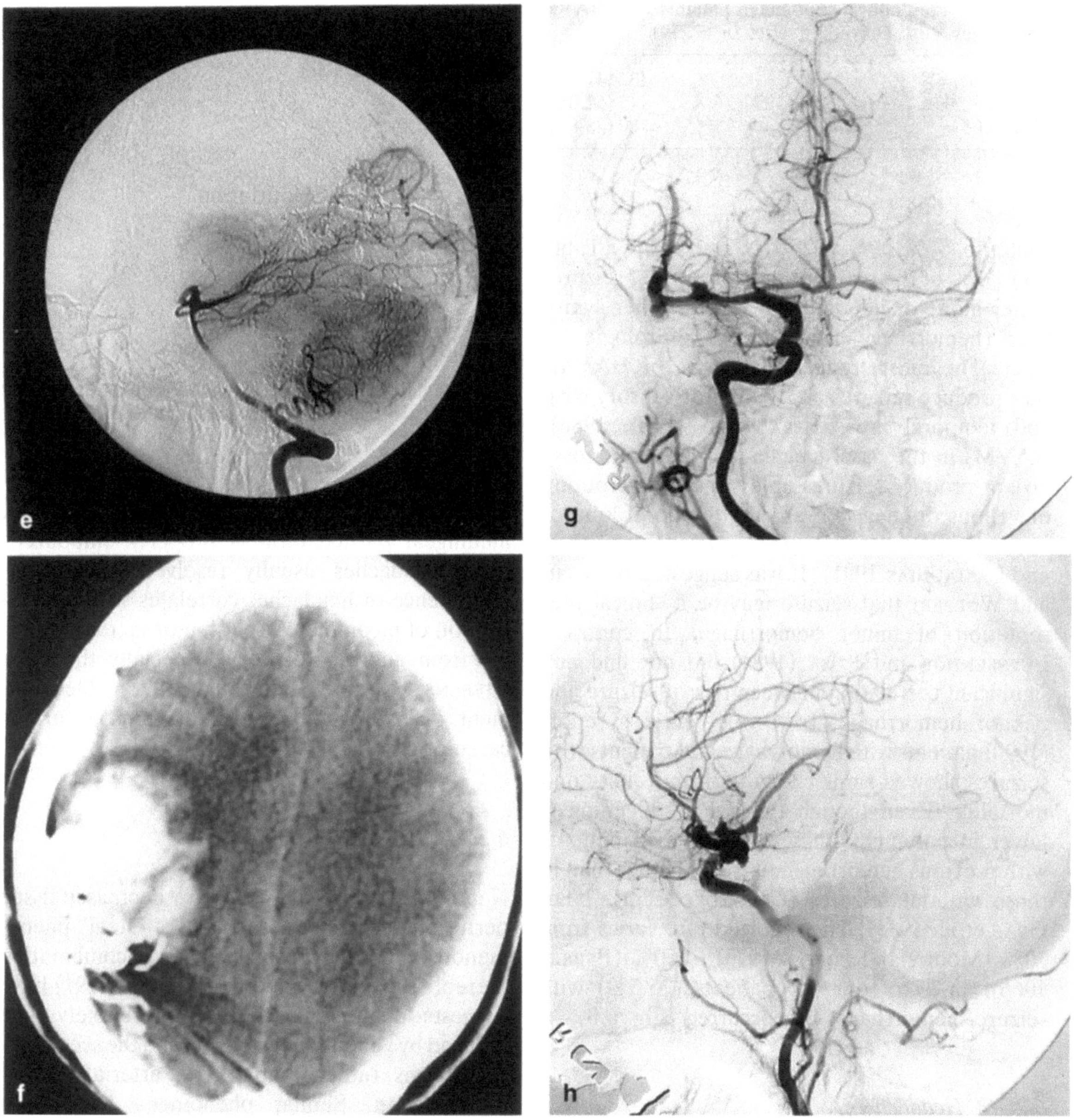

Fig. 6.2 (*continued*). Legend see p. 96

to aneurysm rupture or hypertensive hemorrhage, and may be more closely related to the location of the lesion.

The mortality from the first hemorrhage is approximately 10% and it reaches 20% for subsequent recurrent hemorrhages (WILKINS 1985). ONDRA et al. (1990) reported 1% mortality and 1.7% severe morbidity per year from hemorrhage in the symptomatic population. These rates were constant over the entire course of their study and bore no relation to the original mode of presentation. In total, 85% of those who bled (34% of the entire patient population) suffered major morbidity or died during the 23.7 years of their study.

6.2.1.2 Seizures

Seizure is the second most common presenting symptom in patients with BAVMs, the reported incidence ranging from 28% (PERRET and NISHIOKA

Table 6.1. Presenting symptoms in patients with BAVM in the New York University series (n = 279)

Hemorrhage	132 (47.3%)
Seizure	145 (52.0%)
Headache	100 (38.8%)

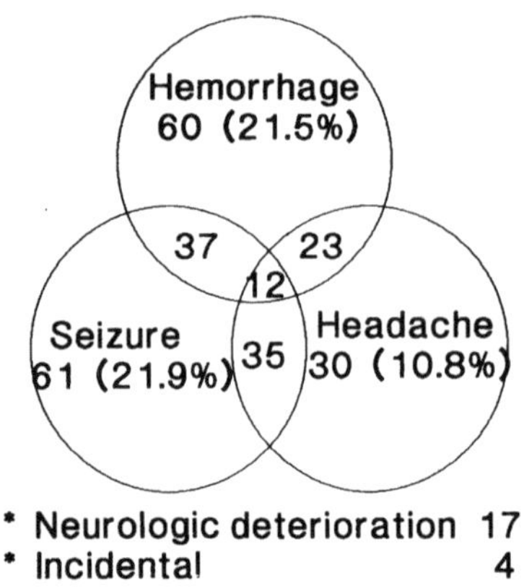

Fig. 6.3. Clinical presentation of BAVM in 279 patients at the New York University Medical Center (1978–1990)

1966) to 67% (PIA 1975). In our series (Table 6.1), 52% of the patients had a history of seizure, either alone or in combination with other symptoms (hemorrhage, headache, or neurologic deficit). The most frequent locations of BAVMs that produce seizures are the motor-sensory strip and temporal areas (CRAWFORD et al. 1986). BAVMs in the basal ganglia and posterior fossa do not produce seizures unless there is rerouting of venous drainage toward the temporal lobe or another supratentorial venous system (BERENSTEIN and LASJAUNIAS 1991). It was suggested by STEIN and WOLPERT that seizure may be a clinical presentation of minor hemorrhage. In contrast, LUESSENHOP and ROSA (1984) did not find any significant correlation between risk of seizure and risk of hemorrhage. In ONDRA et al.'s report (1990) patients with hemorrhage and patients with seizures showed similar long-term morbidity and mortality. Even though the risk of bleeding is lower in patients with seizures than in patients with previous hemorrhage, it is still higher than in those without seizures (CRAWFORD et al. 1986; GRAF et al. 1983). The reported rate varies from 20% (MOODY and POPPEN 1970) to 50% (PERRET 1966). In 37 of our 145 patients (25.5%) with seizure, hemorrhages had occurred (Fig. 6.3).

6.2.1.3 Headache

Headache not associated with hemorrhage (subacute or chronic) can be unilateral or migraine-like and periodic or constant. These headaches may be the result of dilatation of the feeding arteries and possibly of the draining veins near the dura, particularly the tentorium (LUESSENHOP and ROSA 1984). Headache is frequently seen in patients with dural supply, posterior cerebral artery (PCA) supply middle cerebral artery (MCA) supply. Similarly, pulsations of ectatic veins of BAVMs on the dura may produce chronic headache. In our experience, selective injection of hyperosmolar contrast material in the dural arteries can reproduce headaches with the same characteristics as the patients' complaints. When meningeal participation is properly embolized, these headaches usually resolve or diminish. Recurrence of headaches correlates with recanalization of incomplete occlusion or increased supply from another territory, especially the PCA (BERENSTEIN and LASJAUNIAS 1991). Development of hydrocephalus or edema is a further cause of chronic headaches.

6.2.1.4 Neurologic Deficits

Neurologic deficits are caused by decreased tissue perfusion due to arterial stenosis, a "steal" phenomenon, venous hypertension, or a combination thereof. BERENSTEIN and LASJAUNIAS (1991) have suggested that tissue ischemia is more likely to be induced by venous hypertension and the secondary thrombosis rather than by an arterial "steal" phenomenon. Similar phenomena have been observed in cases of dural AVM with cortical venous drainage (LASJAUNIAS et al. 1986). The presence of gliotic areas, of dystrophic calcifications at a distance from BAVMs, and occasionally of neurologic symptoms unrelated to the functional territory of a BAVM supports the thesis of the importance of venous hypertension. We have observed on several occasions that dementia in older patients with BAVMs in the parieto-occipital region without any focal neurologic deficit resolves after partial treatment by embolization if the deep venous system is patent (BERENSTEIN and LASJAUNIAS 1991).

6.3 Indications for Embolization

As discussed in the previous section, not all BAVMs become symptomatic. The incidental discovery of a BAVM does not represent an automatic indication for treatment. Selection of proper treatment (conservative or interventional) is the first step toward accomplishing optimal care for the patient. Various decision analysis schema (FISCHER 1989; STEINMEIER et al. 1989) weighing the risks of treatment have failed to take into consideration the angioarchitecture of the lesion and the value of embolization as part of or as a form of treatment. Complete angiographic investigation, including the supply to the BAVM, the angioarchitecture of the AVM, its venous drainage, associated lesions, the status of the collateral circulation, and the circulation of the remaining brain, plays an important role in establishing the need for treatment and the strategy to be followed. Intranidal aneurysms, venous stenosis, or evidence of venous hypertension indicate potential instability or weakness of a vascular wall which may lead to hemorrhage (WILLINSKY 1988; MARKS et al. 1990; BERENSTEIN and LASJAUNIAS 1991). Based on careful analysis of pancerebral angiography in conjunction with other factors such as age, the location and size of the lesion, and clinical presentation, proper treatment can be recommended.

6.3.1 Age

Arteriovenous malformations of the brain are dynamic, i.e., they undergo continuous anatomic and hemodynamic change. When a BAVM becomes clinically evident, it is believed that the host's capacity to effectively compensate has reached its threshold. Therefore, we can postulate that younger patients with symptoms of BAVMs have a higher chance of future deterioration and eventual hemorrhage. ONDRA et al. (1990) reported the average life expectancy of the BAVM population to be 51 years, compared to 73 years among the general Finnish population. In our opinion, the younger a patient is at the time of initial presentation, the more aggressive the treatment that is warranted.

6.3.2 Sex

In general, sex is not a significant factor in the decision as to the appropriate management, even though many series have indicated a slight male predominance (MOODY and POPPEN 1970; PERRET and NISHIOKA 1966; ONDRA et al. 1990; BERENSTEIN et al. 1990; LASJAUNIAS et al. 1988). There is some controversy as to the increased risk of hemorrhage or other symptoms during pregnancy or labor. In YASARGIL's (1988) analysis of his material, in our study, and in the excellent study by HORTON et al. (1990), pregnancy or labor had no particular effect on the incidence or severity of hemorrhage. The fact that presentation is more common at the child-bearing age may account for the confusion.

6.3.3 Presenting Symptoms

6.3.3.1 Hemorrhage

Hemorrhage is the most serious consequence of BAVMs. It is generally accepted that hemorrhage from an AVM is a strong indication for aggressive treatment. The only sure way of preventing further hemorrhage is the complete and permanent exclusion of the AV shunt from the circulation. As many reports have indicated, the likelihood of severe neurologic deficit and death increases significantly with each recurrence (CRAWFORD et al. 1986; GRAF et al. 1983; BERENSTEIN and LASJAUNIAS 1991). If lesions cannot be cured by any available modality or by combined treatment, partial embolization is indicated; the latter is geared to eliminating the weakness in the angioarchitecture (such as intranidal aneurysms or associated arterial aneurysms) or decreasing hemodynamic stress (closure of AV fistulas). We believe that the likelihood of recurrent hemorrhage can be reduced.

6.3.3.2 Seizures

Improvement in seizure control after embolization has been observed by various authors (LUESSENHOP and PRESPER 1975; WOLPERT et al. 1981). In our opinion, invasive treatment is warranted in patients with difficult or uncontrollable seizures. Treatment is always warranted in young patients with seizures and when cure is possible by means of embolization or a combination of treatments with a low morbidity and mortality.

6.3.3.3 *Headache*

Nonhemorrhagic headaches are subjective symptoms and difficult to quantify. Indications for intervention are therefore individualized. As discussed previously, headaches may correlate with anatomic features, such as participation of the PCA or meningeal arteries in the supply to the AVM. Embolization of this supply can relieve "incapacitating" headaches. In cases where hydrocephalus is a cause of chronic headache, embolization can improve CSF circulation by reducing venous hypertension or correcting mechanical distortion. Therefore, embolization is an important palliative treatment of headache in lesions that otherwise would not be considered for intervention.

6.3.3.4 *Neurologic Deficits*

Neurologic deficits not related to hemorrhage are primarily due to tissue ischemia. Arterial stenosis or occlusion from high flow angiopathy (PILE-SPELLMAN et al. 1989) constitutes an anatomic aspect of decreased tissue perfusion. There are two different explanations for the hemodynamic changes causing ischemia: an arterial "steal" phenomenon and venous hypertension (BERENSTEIN and LASJAUNIAS 1991). Less often, a mass effect from ectatic veins or hydrocephalus may cause neurologic deficits. We have observed that larger, diffuse AVMs present more often with progressive neurologic deficit. When complete eradication is not possible, partial treatment by embolization may stabilize or even improve the neurologic condition.

6.3.4 *Topographic Factors*

The location, size, and deep venous drainage of an AVM are the most important factors in determining the risks of surgical therapy (SPETZLER et al. 1987). When employing an endovascular approach, morbidity is related to our capacity to reach the lesion and to remain strictly within it. It is obvious that a neurologic deficit resulting from inadvertent embolization of normal parenchyma in an "eloquent" area would be a serious eventuality; however, by careful analysis of superselective angiography, meticulous technique, and the sparing of normal, noncontributing arteries, AVMs in "eloquent" areas can be successfully embolized.

6.3.5 *Associated Lesions*

The reported incidence of arterial aneurysms in association with BAVMs varies from 2.7% (PATERSON and MCKISSOCK 1956) to 23% (LASJAUNIAS et al. 1988). There are two types of associated aneurysm: flow-related aneurysms and dysplastic aneurysms. Flow-related aneurysms develop on the pedicle supplying the AVM, more commonly at the proximal segment. Dysplastic aneurysms occur at a location remote from the AVM supply. LASJAUNIAS and co-workers suggested that development of a flow-related aneurysm may be due to a chronically increased diastolic fraction of flow in a feeding pedicle. Reports on the incidence of hemorrhage from associated aneurysms are scanty. DRAKE et al. (1986) found 9 of 12 associated aneurysms (75%) to be the source of hemorrhage among 66 posterior fossa AVMs operated on. BATJER and SAMSON (1986) reported six associated aneurysms (18%) among 23 posterior fossa AVMs, of which two (33%) ruptured. The presence of associated aneurysms does not indicate that these should be treated urgently. Flow-related aneurysms, especially, decrease in size and may even disappear following occlusion of the distal pedicle either by embolization or surgery (TERBRUGGE 1987; YASARGIL 1988). Nevertheless, we give priority to the arterial pedicle with flow-related aneurysms when planning endovascular treatment (Fig. 6.1).

6.3.6 *Lifestyle*

Socioeconomic function and tolerance of symptoms are as important as various other indicators in deciding upon the appropriate treatment. Homonymous hemianopia as a consequence of treatment may not be acceptable to certain professional groups, such as pilots or radiologists. Therefore, each case is assessed bearing such factors in mind, and in consultation with the patient.

6.4 Therapeutic Modality and Objectives

A multidisciplinary approach should be adopted toward therapeutic decision making and sequential planning. Initial assessment, execution of treatment, and evaluation of its results all entail co-operation between various specialists. As single treatment modalities, surgical excision, curative embolization, and radiosurgery (STEINER 1984) have each proved successful in achieving permanent and complete exclusion of some BAVMs. More often, however, combined treatment such as embolization plus surgery or embolization plus radiosurgery can be safer and more effective and provides a better chance of complete cure. Discussion of surgery and radiation is beyond the scope of this chapter. Here we will focus on the objectives of endovascular treatment.

6.4.1 Objectives of Embolization

1. *Preoperative* (Fig. 6.2). Preoperative embolization is used in an attempt to decrease the amount of vascularity in the malformation. Preoperative embolization can stage the hemodynamic changes that will occur in large malformations and will decrease bleeding and operative time. Embolization of large malformations has permitted surgical excision in otherwise difficult, in accessible lesions.

   Preoperative embolization of BAVMs with tantalum-im-pregnated *n*-butyl-cyanoacrylate (NBCA) permits not only the desired preoperative devascularization but will also help in providing landmarks during surgery.
2. *Preradiosurgery* (Fig. 6.4). The combination of embolization and radiosurgery seems to offer a promising new means of completely obliterating otherwise difficult malformations (due to their size and/or location). Embolization can reduce the size of a malformation to convert a lesion that is too large for radiosurgery to one that can be treated by radiosurgery. In

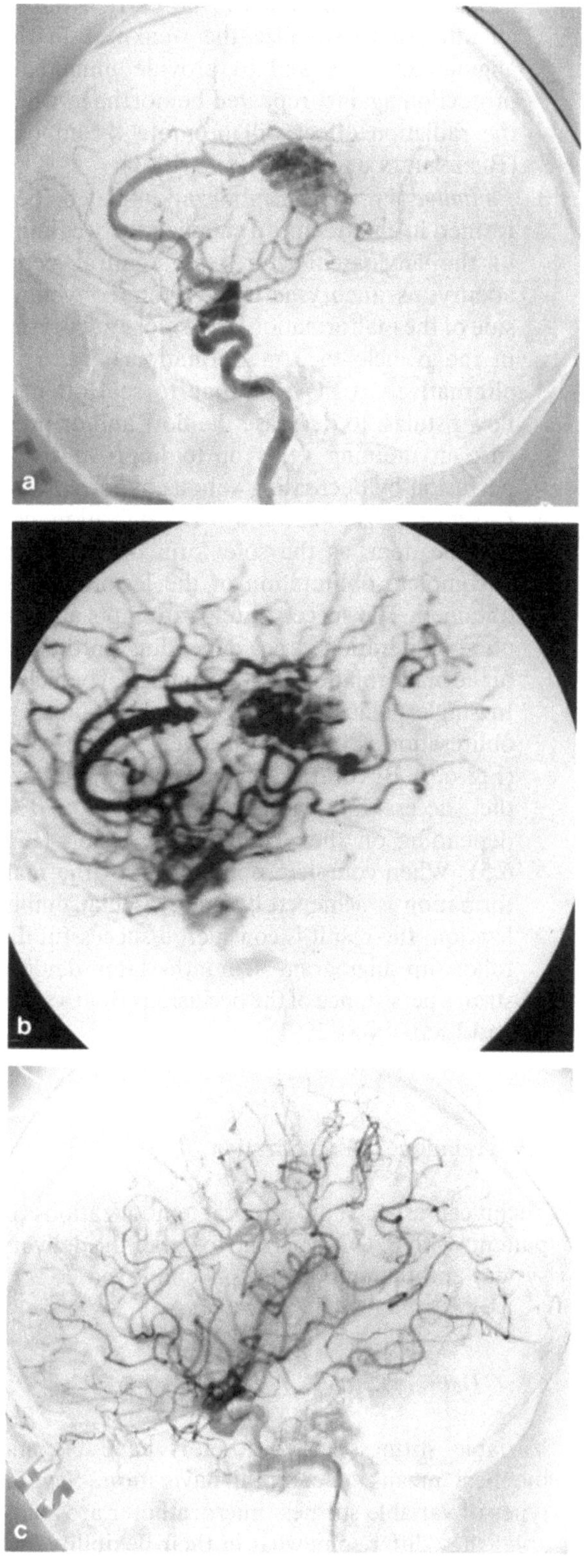

▷

Fig. 6.4a–c. Combined embolization and radiosurgery in a 45-year-old female with hemorrhage. **a** A lateral subtraction angiogram of the left internal carotid artery demonstrated a small AVM in the corpus callosum. **b** Post-embolization DSA (lateral view) of the left internal carotid artery shows a residual nidus. **c** Two-year follow-up angiogram after radiosurgery. The AVM has been completely obliterated and the feeding artery has reduced in size

addition, embolization can be carried out in an attempt to stabilize the weakness in the angioarchitecture and to provide immediate protection against repeated hemorrhage while the radiation effect will promote thrombosis (Berenstein and Lasjaunias 1991).
3. *Palliative* (Fig. 6.1). Embolization may be performed in an attempt to stabilize the weakness in the angioarchitecture (e.g., intralesional aneurysms, aneurysms in the arterial or venous side of the malformation) or to close aneurysms in the pedicle to a malformation (Fig. 6.5); alternatively it may be done to seal off high flow fistulas, to decrease the flow and/or pressure in draining veins or to improve tissue perfusion by decreasing venous hypertension.
4. *Curative* (Figs. 6.5, 6.6). Embolization can also be done as the sole form of treatment if complete obliteration of the lesion can be obtained. The success rate of attempts at complete obliteration varies depending on the size of the malformation and the number of pedicles. In single pedicle AVMs or fistulas, complete obliteration is obtained in over 90% of cases (Fig. 6.6). By contrast, in more extensive lesions the success rate varies from 20% to 20%, depending on the extent of the lesion (Fig. 6.5). When complete obliteration of the malformation is achieved by endovascular embolization, the result is considered successful if a follow-up angiogram 6 months later demonstrates persistence of the occlusion (Berenstein and Lasjaunias 1991).

6.5 Technique of Embolization

Technical aspects of cerebral embolizations in patients with BAVMs pertain to either the delivery system and the embolic agents employed.

6.5.1 Delivery System

Variable stiffness microcatheters have become the best means of cerebral navigation. Several types of variable stiffness microcatheter are available; they differ somewhat in their flexibility and in their suitability for torque catheterization or flow navigation. These microcatheters can be used alone or in combination with calibrated leak microballoon catheters.

6.5.1.1 Flow-Guided Microcatheters

The first catheter for cerebral navigation was designed by Kerber in 1976. This first generation calibrated leak microcatheter was made of silicone tubing with a silicone leak balloon at the tip and required a propelling chamber (Pevsner 1977) or similar device for intracranial navigation (Choi et al. 1988). Subsequent modification of this system (Berenstein 1979; Debrun et al. 1982) improved its reliability. The balloon was changed to a much softer latex balloon. This calibrated leak balloon catheter with the various propelling chambers was used until the new generation of variable stiffness microcatheters were developed in 1986.

6.5.1.2 Variable Stiffness Microcatheters

A major revolution in endovascular treatment occurred with the development of variable stiffness microcatheters. These catheters permit cerebral navigation without the use of cumbersome systems (Kikuchi et al. 1987). When they are used in combination with steerable microwires, distal cerebral arteries can be catheterized by torque control; alternatively, flow-guided catheterization can be achieved by mounting a calibrated leak balloon at the tip of the catheter.

1. *Torque Catheterization* (Fig. 6.7a). Superselective cerebral catheterization using catheter and guidewire technology is best achieved with the variable stiffness microcatheters such as the Tracker catheter (Target Therapeutics, San Jose, CA). These microcatheters can be shaped by steam for cerebral navigation. The use of variable stiffness microguide wires assists in catheter advancement and guiding direction into the desired pedicles.

Fig. 6.5a–f. 24-year-old male who presented with grand male seizure. DSA of the left internal carotid artery (**a** anteroposterior and **b** lateral view) reveals an AVM in the temporal lobe. Two temporal opercular branches supply the AVM. There is no associated aneurysm or venous ectasia. **c,d** Acrylic casts. Each pedicle is selectively embolized with NBCA. The actual cast of NBCA immediately after catheter withdrawal is shown. The radiolucent lines are masks of the catheter after withdrawal. **e,f** Postembolization control angiography (**e** anteroposterior and **f** lateral view). The AVM is completely occluded without any evidence of collaterals ▷

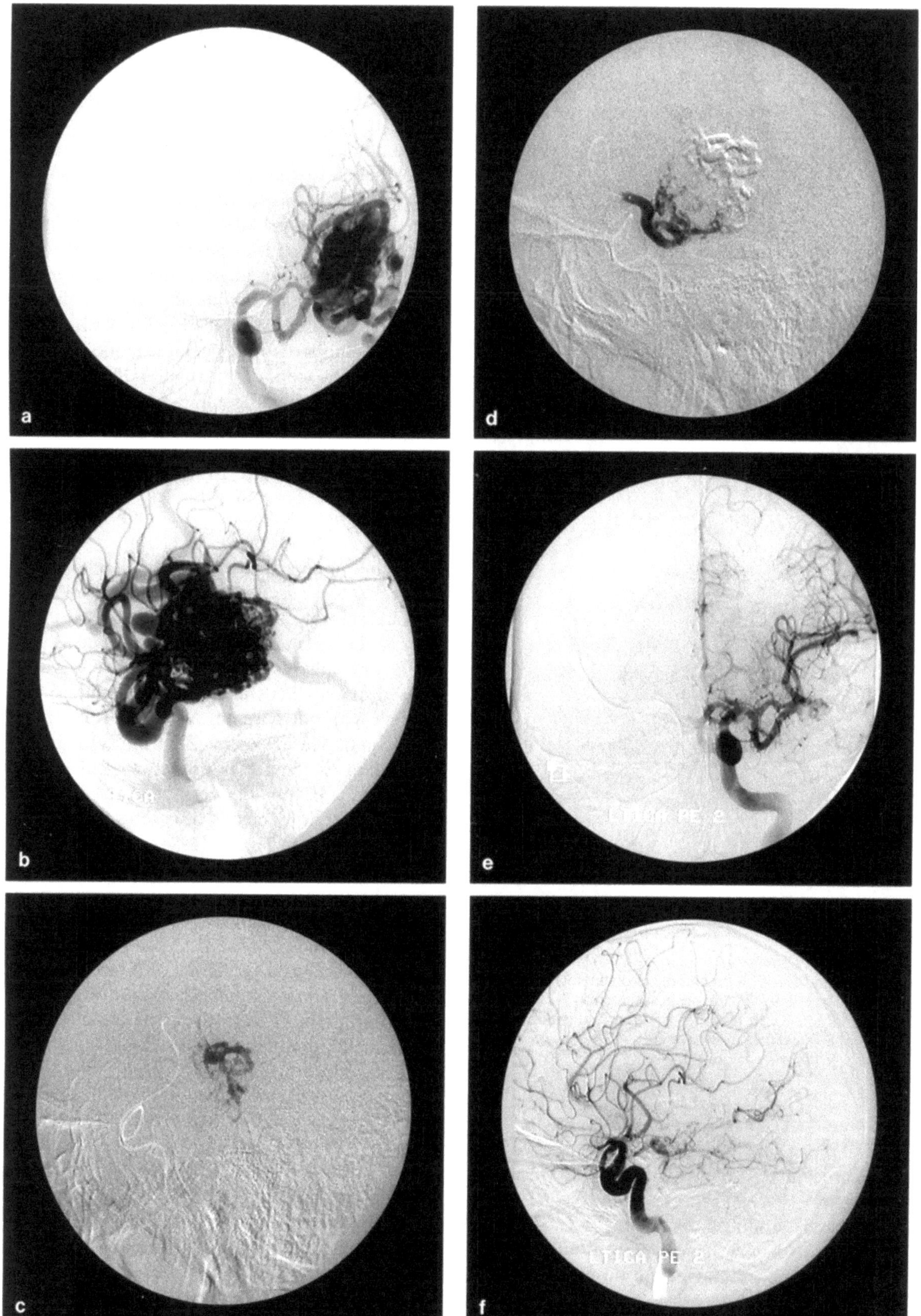
a
d
b
e
c
f

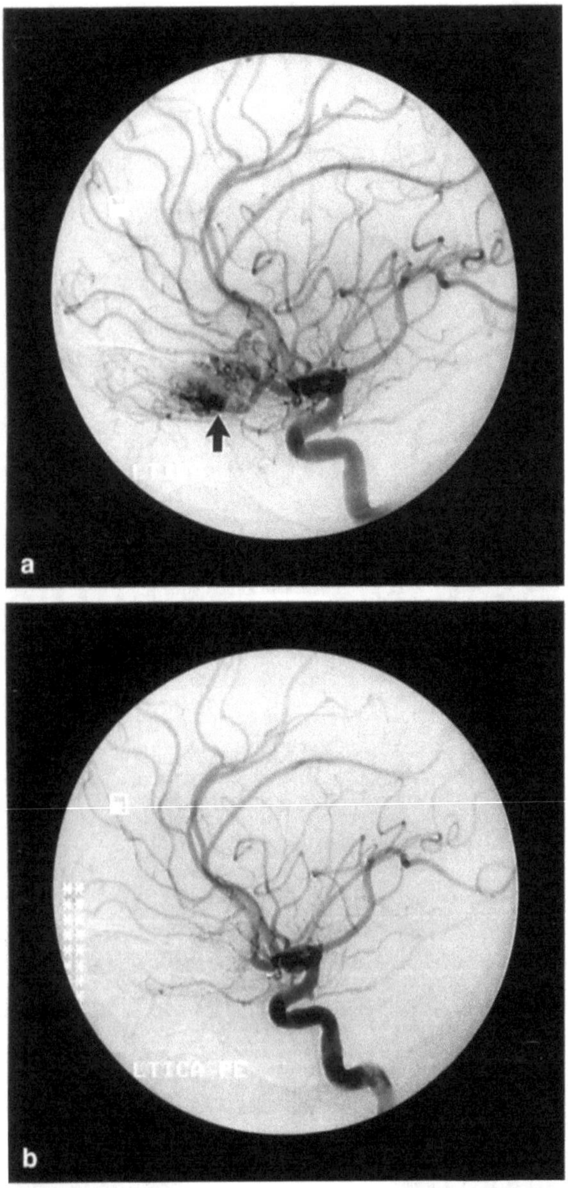

Fig. 6.6 a,b. 41-year-old female with a history of subarachnoid hemorrhage. **a** Preembolization angiogram demonstrates a small AVM in the gyrus rectus. Note a small intranidal aneurysm (*arrow*). **b** Postembolization control angiogram shows no residual nidus

2. *Flow-Guided Catheterization* (Fig. 6.7b,c). There are two other types of variable stiffness microcatheter: the Minitorque produced by Ingenor (Paris, France) and the Magic microcatheter produced by Balt (Paris, France). These catheters have softer distal segments and thus permit navigation through more tortuous vessels (Fig. 6.7b). Their proximal shaft is more rigid than the Tracker catheter. In addition, by shaping the tip of these catheters, pedicles with less flow or with acutely angled origins are readily accessible.

Calibrated leak microballoons can be adapted to any of the variable stiffness microcatheters. By mounting balloons with a small hole at the tip of the catheter, further distal catheterization, flow control, and flow reversal can be obtained (Fig. 6.7c). Soft, thin oval latex balloons which inflate to less than 1–3 mm in diameter are most often used. These balloons adapt to the vessel size and configuration, thus minimizing the likelihood of vessel rupture. A detailed description of the various methods of injecting liquid embolic agents lies beyond the scope of this chapter; the technique requires proper training and experience.

6.5.2 Embolic Agents

6.5.2.1 Particulate Agents

1. *Silicone Sphere*. The particulate materials were the first to be used in the treatment of BAVMs (Luessenhop et al. 1962, 1965, 1967; Kricheff et al. 1972; Hilal 1975; Wolpert et al. 1981). Silicone spheres of various sizes were widely used in the 1960s and 1970s until liquid embolic material became available. Delivery of silicone spheres to the BAVM is solely dependent on the preferential flow. The spheres are injected into the cervical carotid or vertebral artery by means of cutdown or via the femoral route. Hilal (1984) described temporary modification of the hemodynamics of cerebral flow by the occlusion of normal pedicles with nondetachable balloons in order to deliver particles to the BAVM. When silicone spheres are used, preferential flow changes in the later stage of embolization, towards the normal brain; therefore complete obliteration is usually unobtainable. We do not use these agents.
2. *Polyvinyl Alcohol Foam (PVA)*. Since PVA was introduced as an embolic agent by Tadavarthy et al. (1974), it has been the most widely used particulate material in interventional neuroradiology. PVA in pieces or in suspension (Berenstein and Graeb 1982) was delivered in the same way as silicone spheres until variable stiffness catheters were developed. It is now possible to deliver various sizes of PVA particle selectively to the feeding

pedicles of BAVMs (Purdy et al. 1990; Eskridge 1989). PVA is not an absorbable material, but as Quisling et al. (1984) showed, particles produce occlusion by mixing with stagnant blood that coagulates; therefore, recanalization of these vessels occurs more frequently than when liquid embolic agents are used. Embolization with PVA particles is valuable as a preoperative measure (Spetzler et al. 1987). We limit our use of PVA particles to the embolization of head and neck neoplasms or AVMs.

3. *Silk*. Surgical silk was introduced as an embolic agent by Benati et al. (1987). It is biocompatible and thrombogenic and easy to inject through small catheters of various lengths. Silk has been used alone or in combination with other embolic agents for preoperative embolization or to close single hole fistulas (Eskridge 1989). Its long term results and stability require further study.
4. *Coils*. Soft platinum microcoils can be injected through the Tracker catheter to produce thrombosis of BAVM feeders (Hilal 1988). Several different sizes and configurations of microcoil are available. In some of these, Dacron fibers are attached to promote thrombogenicity. In certain high flow arteriovenous fistulas, it is useful to decrease flow by placing coils prior to the injection of liquid material as this reduces the chances of distal migration. Whether preoperative embolization with microcoils is of value in the treatment of BAVMs is doubtful.

6.5.2.2 Liquid Agents

1. *Cyanoacrylate*. Both in our own series and in large series of other authors, cyanoacrylate has been the primary material used in the management of BAVMs. Isobutyl cyanoacrylate (IBCA) and NBCA are the two major types

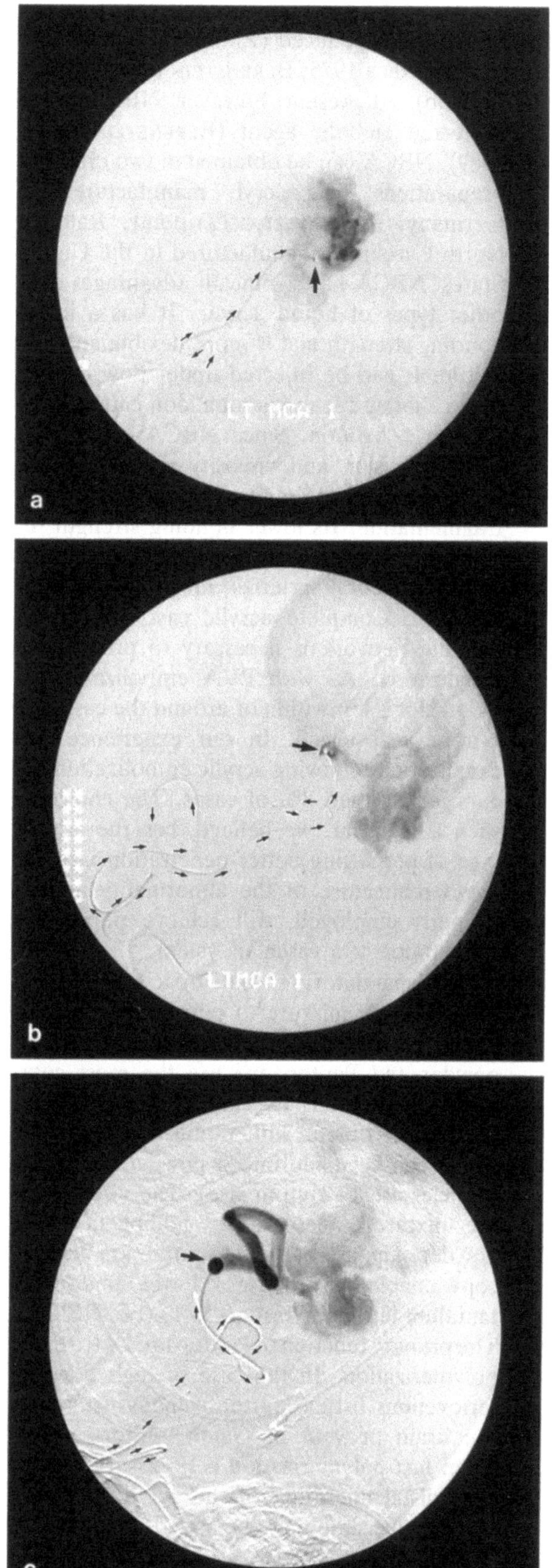

▷

Fig. 6.7. a Use of a Tracker catheter. The Tracker is more useful in catheterization of vessels with relatively smooth curves and a proximal location. Once positioned, it is very stable. **b** Use of a Magic microcatheter. The softer and more flexible distal segment of the Magic microcatheter allows navigation through tortuous and multiple curves. **c** Calibrated leak balloon microcatheter. When a variable stiffness microcatheter is not advancing further or flow arrest is needed at the time of acrylic injection, a small thin latex balloon (*arrow*) is attached employed for embolization. IBCA was the first to be introduced (Zanetti and Sherman 1972; Kerber 1975; Berenstein and Kricheff 1979a,b). At present, however, NBCA is the preferred embolic agent (Berenstein et al. 1989). NBCA can be obtained in two different preparations: Histoacryl, manufactured in Germany, and Avacryl (Tripoint, Raleigh, North Carolina), manufactured in the United States. NBCA has significant advantages over other types of liquid acrylic. It has a lower bonding strength and is more flexible and less brittle. It can be injected under flow control with calibrated leak microballoon catheters or without a balloon. Since NBCA has higher surface tension and viscosity than IBCA, it produces a more uniform column with less fragmentation. Its lower bonding strength reduces the likelihood of gluing the catheter in the cerebral arteries immediately after injection. Complete acrylic cast of a given vascular network is necessary to prevent recanalization. As with PVA embolization, if blood clot is left within or around the cast, this can be reabsorbed. In our experience, recanalization following acrylic embolization occurs in less than 2% of cases. The choice of such a material, we believe, has the advantage of permitting better penetration into the angioarchitecture of the abnormality and, if properly employed, will achieve permanent obliteration of a vascular system.

It is mandatory to add opacifying agents to the acrylic mixture to permit visualization under fluoroscopy (Fig. 6.5c,d). Tantalum powder and Pantopaque are the most commonly used materials. Tantalum is a biocompatible, inert metal with atomic number of 73, which can be made into a powder form (the particles are 1–2 µm in size). The viscosity of the mixture is increased by adding tantalum powder. The use of digital subtraction fluoroscopy enabled us to use a lower amount of tantalum in the mixture (0.5–1 g/1 cc NBCA). The primary function of Pantopaque is to retard polymerization. In the case of high flow arteriovenous fistulas (arteriovenous fistulas of the brain or vein of Galen mulformation), when fast polymerization is necessary to prevent distal migration of the acrylic mixture, Pantopaque should not be added. The amount of Pantopaque added is varied depending upon the flow pattern and the operator's experience and judgment. We customarily add 50%–60% of Pantopaque to the mixture.

2. *Avatine–PVA–Ethanol Combination*. Various combinations of avatine, PVA, and ethanol have recently been introduced for the embolization of BAVMs (Fox et al. 1988; Hehta 1989). We have limited experience of this "cocktail," having employed it only in external carotid artery embolization. We have observed significant inflammatory reactions and a higher incidence of recanalization. Like PVA particles, it may represent an alternative material for preoperative embolization of BAVMs.

6.6 Perioperative Measures

Although the specifics may vary, the basic principles of catheterization, embolization, and patient care are the same among different teams. In general, we perform all procedures via the transfemoral route under neuroleptic analgesia. Systemic blood pressure is monitored throughout the procedure by an arterial line. All coaxial catheter systems are continuously flushed with heparinized saline solution. In embolization of BAVMs in the motor or sensory cortex, the brain stem, or the thalamus, somatosensory evoked potential monitoring is employed. Two measures, the Sodium Amytal test and systemic hypotension, are worth discussion in this section.

6.6.1 Sodium Amytal Test

Sodium Amytal is a short-acting barbiturate widely used to determine the dominance of a hemisphere prior to a surgical intervention (Wada and Rasmussen 1960). Between 100 and 150 mg Sodium Amytal is injected into each internal carotid artery to produce immediate and complete anesthesia of the corresponding hemisphere. Its effect lasts for approximately 10–15 min. This measure is applied to provoke any neurologic deficit which might result from embolization of a specific artery (Fig. 6.8). When the pedicle to be embolized is in an "eloquent" area or the pedicle is suspected of supplying normal territory, 50–70 mg Sodium Amytal is injected in the same manner as the embolic material; neurologic function is then monitored in accordance with its location (Berenstein et al. 1984; Horton et al. 1988). If an important neurologic deficit develops,

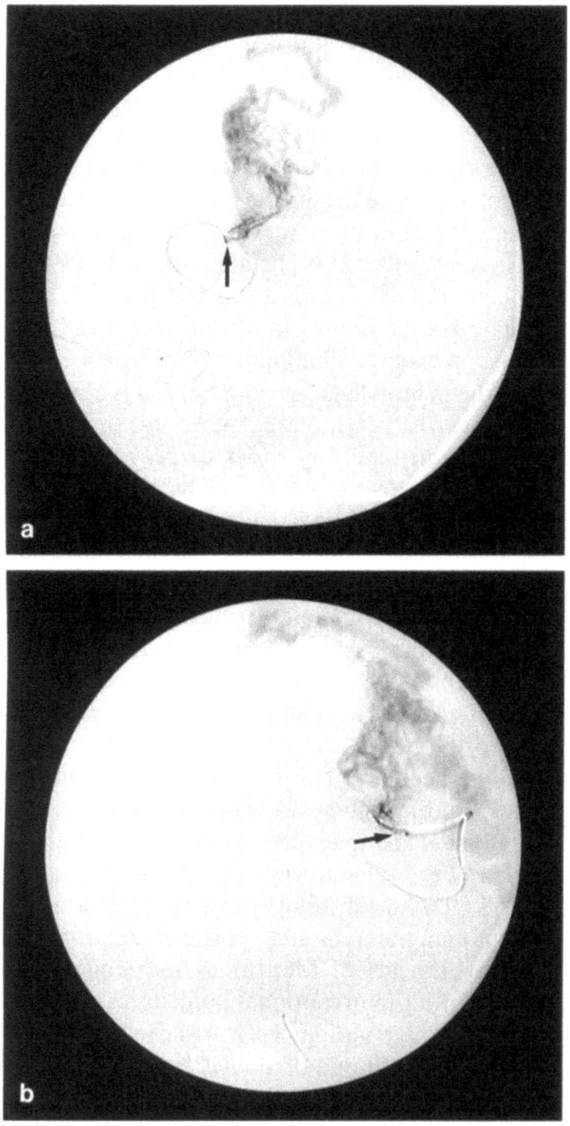

Fig. 6.8 a,b. Superselective DSA of the posterior frontal branch of the MCA (**a** anteroposterior and **b** lateral view). The patient developed central facial palsy and paresis of the right hand after injection of 50 mg Sodium Amytal. The catheter was advanced further and this pedicle was embolized with NBCA following negative repeated Sodium Amytal test

it is advisable to catheterize more distally beyond normal branches or to find an alternative route. However, false negative studies are occasionally observed. The high flow shunting in an AVM produces an uneven infusion of Sodium Amytal, and an inadequate amount in the normal parenchyma will fail to provoke any neurologic deficit. We consequently rely more on the anatomic analysis of the superselective angiography.

6.6.2 Systemic Hypotension

Since flow in the AVM depends solely on the systemic blood pressure, by lowering systemic blood pressure the flow can be slowed and the nidus better filled. Thus, one can achieve better control of the injection of embolic material in high flow lesions, and better penetration into the nidus. It is important that the catheter should be closer to the malformation when hypotension is used, because normal arteries undergo vasodilatation with the result that emboli can easily penetrate into them. The reduction in blood pressure is maintained for 10–20 min after occlusion of a large fistula, to permit gradual adaptation to the new hemodynamic situation.

6.7 Results and Complications

6.7.1 Results

As our knowledge of BAVMs and the technique, the catheter systems, and the embolic materials employed in their treatment have evolved over the last 15 years, so the results and complication rate have improved. In the age of free-flow embolizations with particulate materials, complete cure by embolization alone was unthinkable. Since the introduction of liquid embolic agents (IBCA, and recently NBCA), complete exclusion of the AVM has become feasible. In addition, the recent development of variable stiffness microcatheters has revolutionized our ability to reach closer to the nidus with simpler techniques and less risk.

The goal of treatment is complete exclusion of AVMs. As a result of a multidisciplinary approach involving surgery, endovascular treatment, and radiosurgery, more patients with BAVMs are benefitting from complete cure. Of our 279 patients, 45 were treated by embolization and surgery (Fig. 6.2), 45 by embolization and radiosurgery (Fig. 6.4), and 189 by embolization alone. Most of the patients treated by embolization alone had large AVMs or AVMs in inaccessible areas or were nonsurgical candidates for various other reasons. When an AVM is extensive with multiple feeding pedicles and involvement of several territories, complete occlusion is not possible. For these lesions, the strategy is palliative treatment to exclude the weak angioarchitecture so that recurrence of hemorrhage or deterioration of the neurologic deficit can be prevented (Fig. 6.1). It is currently too early to assess the long-term effect of palliative treatment.

For small AVMs with one or several feeding pedicles, by contrast, there is a higher chance of achieving total obliteration (Figs. 6.6, 6.7). We have achieved complete occlusion in 11% of 189 patients with AVMs of various sizes and at various locations by means of embolization alone.

In our series hemorrhage occurred in 27 patients (9.6%); 19 had rehemorrhage and eight a first hemorrhage unrelated to the embolization. Of the 27 patients, 22 had silicone sphere embolization or proximal occlusion, and only five had an apparently good embolization (BERENSTEIN and LASJAUNIAS 1991). We have observed a much lower rate of rehemorrhage in patients treated with IBCA or NBCA.

Among patients with seizure disorder, 68% were seizure free following embolization. New seizures developed in 3% of all patients. Embolization is not the only factor responsible for better seizure control. Proper seizure medication, maintenance of optimal level, and awareness of AVM in the family are also contributory factors. Headaches have diminished or disappeared in a large number of patients. Recurrence of headaches has correlated with dural or PCA repermeation.

6.7.2 Complications (Table 6.2)

The most serious complications related to embolization of BAVMs are hemorrhage and cerebral ischemia. Hemorrhage can occur during the procedure or in the postembolization period (up to 72 h) (Table 6.2). Overdistention of an artery by a calibrated leak balloon is the most common cause of intraprocedural hemorrhage. Rupture of an associated aneurysm, of an intranidal aneurysm, or of an AVM is another cause. We experienced 17 hemorrhages in the last 13 years. Only one patient has suffered a serious intracerebral hemorrhage since 1987; during this period all catheterizations have been performed with variable stiffness microcatheters, which gives better torque control and more flexibility. Puncture of an artery by a guidewire or microcatheter has been reported by HALBACH et al. (1991) and PURDY et al. (1990). We have not experienced this complication. Immediate recognition of the hemorrhage and proper management will minimize the consequences. Once the hemorrhage is recognized, it is advisable to occlude the rupture area using coils or cyanoacrylate immediately in order to prevent further hemorrhage.

Hemorrhage during the postembolization period is difficult to explain. We postulate that there are two mechanisms which can induce delayed hemorrhage, incomplete occlusion of the feeding arteries or occlusion of venous outflow. Of our 279 patients, five suffered delayed hemorrhage.

Of the other serious complications, probably the most common are cerebral ischemia and infarction. Technical failure such as dissection of a major cerebral artery, injection of blood clots or air bubbles, and inadvertent embolization of normal vessels are major causes of these complications. Technical failures can be prevented by careful manipulation and constant attention during catheterization. Meticulous technique is essential for all interventional procedures.

Even though various measures can be taken to reduce the likelihood of inadvertent embolization of normal territory, in some instances it may be unavoidable. In spite of superselective angiography, provocative tests with Sodium Amytal, and functional monitoring with EEG or somatosensory evoked potentials, small functional territories may not be detected. In addition, injection

Table 6.2. Complications of embolization in 279 adults treated at New York University. (BERENSTEIN and LASJAUNIAS 1991)

	1977–1982	1983–1985	1985–1990	Total
No. of patients	44	47	188	279 (100%)
Death	6[a] (13.6%)	1 (2.1%)	1 (0.5%)	8 (2.8%)
Severe deficit	2 (4.5%)	2 (4.2%)	3 (1.5%)	7 (2.5%)
Mild deficit[b]	6 (13.6%)	6 (12.7%)	17 (9.0%)	29 (10.3%)
Transient deficit	11 (25%)	7 (14.8%)	20 (10.6%)	38 (13.6%)

[a] One intraoperative embolization.
[b] By "mild deficit" we mean a mild aggravation of a previous deficit that does not affect the patient's lifestyle, or an expected deficit in the visual field.

of embolic agent cannot be compared with that of contrast medium since their viscosity, rate of flow, polymerization, and degree of reflux are different. Embolic material may penetrate normal arteries noticeably or unnoticeably. Once neurologic symptoms are detected, every effort should be made to minimize the consequences of ischemic brain damage (BERENSTEIN 1991). Volume expansion or vasopressors can improve the capillary circulation of the ischemic area but they may increase the risk of hemorrhage. We believe that decreasing the viscosity of whole blood (isovolemic hemodilution) offers the best chance of improving capillary circulation (STRAND 1984; BERENSTEIN and LASJAUNIAS 1991). At present our overall mortality and severe morbidity rates are 0.5% and 1.5% respectively – figures similar to the annual mortality and major morbidity reported by ONDRA et al. (1990) in respect of unoperated symptomatic AVMs. Proper training, accumulation of experience, better understanding of BAVMs, and improvement of technology will help us to obtain better results and to reduce complications.

References

Batjer H, Samson D (1986) Arteriovenous malformations of the posterior fossa. J Neurosurg 64:849–856

Benati A, Beltramello A, Maschio A, Perini S, Rosta L, Piovan E (1987) Combined embolization of intracranial AVMs with multi-purpose mobile-wing microcatheter system; indications and results in 71 cases. AJNR 8:938

Berenstein A (1981) Technique for catheterization and embolization of the lenticulostriate arteries. J Neurosurg 54:783–789

Berenstein A, Graeb D (1982) Convenient preparation of ready-to-use particles in polyvinyl alcohol foam suspension for embolization. Radiology 145:846

Berenstein A, Kricheff II (1979a) Catheter and material selection for transarterial embolization: technical considerations. I. Catheters. Radiology 132:619–630

Berenstein A, Kricheff II (1979b) Catheter and material selection for transarterial embolization: technical considerations. II. Materials. Radiology 132:631–639

Berenstein A, Lasjaunias P (1991) Surgical neuroangiography, vol 4. Springer, Berlin Heidelberg New York (in press)

Berenstein AB, Krall R, Choi IS (1989) Embolization with *n*-butyl-cyanoacrylate in management of CNS lesions (abstr). AJNR 10:883

Berenstein A, Young W, Ransohoff J, Benjamin V, Merkin H (1984) Somatosensory evoked potentials during spinal angiography and therapeutic transvascular embolization. J Neurosurg 60:777–785

Berenstein A, Choi IS, Neophitydes A, Benjamin V (1990) Endovascular treatment of spinal cord arteriovenous malformations (SCAVMs) (abstr). AJNR 10:898

Choi IS, Berenstein A, Flamm E (1988) Superselective catheterization and embolization of cerebral AVMs. In: Pluching F, Broggi G (eds) Advanced technology in neurosurgery. Springer, New York Berlin Heidelberg, pp 183–192

Crawford PM, West CR, Chadwick DW, Shaw MDM (1986) Arteriovenous malformations of the brain: natural history in unoperated patients. J Neurol Neurosurg Psychiatry 49:1–10

Debrun GM, Vinuela FV, Fox AJ, Kan S (1982) Two different calibrated leak balloons: experimental work and application in humans. AJNR 3:407

Drake CG, Friedman A, Peerless S (1986) Posterior fossa arteriovenous malformations. J Neurosurg 64:1–10

Eskridge JM (1989) Interventional neuroradiology. Neuroradiology state of the art. Radiology 172:991–1006

Fischer WS (1989) Decision analysis: a tool of the future: an application to unruptured arteriovenous malformations. Neurosurgery 24:129–136

Forster DMC, Steiner L, Hakanson S (1972) Arteriovenous malformations of the brain. A long-term clinical study. J Neurosurg 37:562–570

Fox AJ, Lee DH, Pelz DM, Brothers MF, Deveikis JP (1988) Thrombotic mixture as a polymerizing agent (abstr). AJNR 9:1029

Graf CJ, Perret GE, Torner JC (1983) Bleeding from cerebral arteriovenous malformations as part of their natural history. J Neurosurg 58:331–337

Halbach V, Higashida R, Dowd C et al. (1991) Management of Vascular performations that occur during neurointerventional procedures. AJNR 12:319–327

Hilal SK, Michelsen JW (1975) Therapeutic percutaneous embolization for extraaxial vascular lesions of head, neck and spine. J Neurosurg 43:275–287

Hilal SK (1984) Endovascular treatment of AVMs of CNS. In: Wilson CB, Stein BN (eds) Intracranial arteriovenous malformations. Williams and Wilkins, Baltimore, London, pp 259–273

Hilal SK, Khandji AG, Chi TL, Stein BM, Bello JA, Silver AJ (1988) Synthetic fiber-coated platinum coils successfully used for endovascular treatment of arteriovenous malformations and direct arteriofistulas of CNS (abstr). AJNR 9:1030

Horton JA, Dawson RC (1988) Retinal Wada test. AJNR 9:1167

Horton JC, Chambers WA, Lyons S, Adams RD, Kjellberg RN (1990) Pregnancy and risk of hemorrhage from AVM. Neurosurgery 27:867–872

Kerber C (1975) Intracranial cyanoacrylate: a new catheter therapy for arteriovenous malformation. Invest Radiol 10:536–538

Kerber C (1976) Balloon catheter with a calibrated leak. A new system for superselective angiography and occlusive catheter therapy. Radiology 120:547–550

Kikuchi T, Strother CM, Boyar M (1987) New catheter for endovascular interventional procedures. Radiology 165:870–871

Kricheff II, Madayag M, Braunstein P (1972) Transfemoral catheter embolization of cerebral and posterior fossa arteriovenous malformations. Radiology 103:107–111

Lasjaunias P, Chiu M, Terbrugge K (1986) Neurological manifestations of intracranial dural arteriovenous malformations. J Neurosurg 64:724–730

Lasjaunias P, Piske R, Terbrugge K, Willinsky R (1988) Cerebral arteriovenous malformations and associated arterial aneurysms. Acta Neurochir (Wien) 91:29–36

Lasjaunias P, Garcia-Monaco R, Rodesch G (1991) Vein of Galen malformation. Endovascular management of 43 cases. Childs Nerv Syst (in press)

Luessenhop AJ, Presper JH (1975) Surgical embolization of cerebral arteriovenous malformations through internal carotid and vertebral arteries. Long-term results. J Neurosurg 42:443–451

Luessenhop AJ, Rosa L (1984) Cerebral arteriovenous malformations. Indications for and results of surgery, and the role of intravascular techniques. J Neurosurg 60:14–22

Luessenhop AJ, Gibbs M, Velasquez AC (1962) Cerebrovascular response to embolic. Observations in patients with arteriovenous malformations. Arch Neurol 7:264–274

Luessenhop AJ, Kachmann R, Shevlin W et al. (1965) Clinical evaluation of artificial embolization in the management of large cerebral arteriovenous malformations. J Neurosurg 23:400–417

Marks MP, Lane B, Steinberg G, Chay P (1990) Hemorrhage in intracerbral AVMs: angiographic determinants. Radiology 176:807–813

McKenzie I (1953) The clinical presentation of the cerebral angioma. A review of 50 cases. Brain 76:184–214

Mehta BA, Sanders WP, Malik G, Burke TH, Spickler EM, Patel SC (1989) Detroit cocktail, new embolic agent for preoperative embolization of cerebral AVM (abstr). AJNR 10:902

Michelsen WJ (1979) Natural history and pathophysiology of arteriovenous malformations. Clin Neurosurg 26: 307–313

Moody RA, Poppen JL (1970) Arteriovenous malformations. J Neurosurg 23:503–511

Ondra SL, Troupp H, George ED, Schwab K (1990) The natural history of symptomatic arteriovenous malformations of the brain: a 24 year follow up assessment. J Neurosurg 73:387–391

Paterson JH, McKissock W (1956) A clinical survey of intracranial angiomas with special reference to their mode of progression and surgical treatment: a report of 110 cases. Brain 79:233–266

Perret G, Nishioka H (1966) Report on the cooperative study of intracranial aneurysms and subarachnoid hemorrhage. Section VI. Arteriovenous malformations. An analysis of 545 cases of cranio-cerebral arteriovenous malformations and fistulae reported to the cooperative study. J Neurosurg 25:467–490

Pevsner PH (1977) Microballoon catheter for superselective angiography and therapeutic occlusion. AJR 128:225–230

Pia HW (1975) The acute treatment of cerebral arteriovenous malformations associated with hematomas. In: Pia HW, Gleaveg JRW, Grote E, Zierski J (eds) Cerebral angiomas: advances in diagnosis and therapy. Springer, New York Berlin Heidelberg, p 155

Pile-Spellman JMD, Baker KF, Lisczak TM et al. (1989) High-flow angiopathy: cerebral blood vessel changes in experimental chronic arteriovenous fistula. AJNR 7:811

Purdy PD, Samson D, Batjer HH et al. (1990) Preoperative embolization of cerebral arteriovenous malformations with polyvinyl alcohol particles: experience in 51 adults. AJNR 11:501–510

Quisling RG, Mickle JP, Ballinger WB, Carver CC, Kaplan B (1984) Histopathologic effects of intraarterial polyvinyl alcohol microemboli in rat cerebral cortex. AJNR 5:101

Spetzler RF, Martin RNA, Carter LP et al. (1987) Surgical management of large AVMs by staged embolization and operative excision. J Neurosurg 67:17–28

Stein BM, Wolpert SM (1977) Surgical and embolic treatment of cerebral arteriovenous malformations. Surg Neurol 7:359–369

Stein BM, Wolpert SM (1980) Arteriovenous malformations of the brain II: current concepts and treatment. Arch Neurol 37:69–75

Steiner L (1984) Treatment of arteriovenous malformations by radiosurgery. In: Wilson CB, Stein BM (eds) Intracranial arteriovenous malformations. Williams and Wilkins, Baltimore, pp 295–314

Steinmeier R, Schramm J, Muller HG, Fahlbusch R (1989) Evaluation of prognostic factors in cerebral arteriovenous malformations. Neurosurgery 24:193–200

Strand T, Splund K, Eriksson S et al. (1984) A randomized controlled trial of hemodilution therapy in acute ischemic stroke. Stroke 15:980–989

Svien HJ, McRae JA (1965) Arteriovenous anomalies of the brain. Fate of patients not having definitive surgery. J Neurosurg 23:23–28

Tadavarthy SM, Knight L, Ovitt TW, Snyder C, Amplatz K (1974) Transcatheter arterial embolization. Radiology 112:13–16

TerBrugge KG, Lasjaunias P, Chiu P (1987) Surgical neuroangiography of intracranial vascular malformations. Can J Neurol Sci 14:70–74

Troupp H, Marttila L, Halonen V (1970) Arteriovenous malformations of the brain. Acta Neurochir (Wien) 22:125–128

Wada JT, Rasmussen T (1960) Intracarotid injection of sodium amytal for the lateralization of cerebral speech dominance. J Neurosurg 17:266–282

Waltimo O (1973a) The relationship of size, density and localization of intracranial arteriovenous malformations to the type of initial symptom. J Neurol Sci 19:13–19

Waltimo O (1973b) The change in size of intracranial arteriovenous malformations. J Neurol Sci 19:21–27

Wilkins RH (1985) Natural history of intracranial vascular malformations. A review. Neurosurgery 16:421–430

Willinsky R, Lasjaunias P, TerBrugge K et al. (1988) Brain arteriovenous malformations. Analysis of the angio-architecture in relationship to hemorrhage. J Neuroradiol 15:225–237

Willinsky R, Lasjaunias P, Terbrugge KN, Hurth M (1990) Angiography in the investigation of spinal dural arteriovenous fistula. A protocol with application of the venous phase. Neuroradiology 32:114–116

Wolpert SM, Barnett FJ, Prager RJ (1981) Benefits of embolization without surgery for cerebral arteriovenous malformation. AJNR 2:535

Yamada S (1982) Arteriovenous malformations in the functional area: surgical treatment and regional cerebral blood flow. Neurol Res 4:283–322

Yasargil MG (1988) AVM of the brain in microsurgery, vol IIIb. Thieme, Stuttgart New York

Zanetti P, Sherman F (1972) Experimental evaluation of a tissue adhesive as an agent for the treatment of aneurysms and arteriovenous anomalies. J Neurosurg 36:72–79

7 Endovascular Treatment of Intracranial Aneurysms with Detachable Coils and Electrothrombosis

GUIDO GUGLIELMI

CONTENTS

The technique of intra-aneurysmal electrothrombosis via an endovascular approach was conceived about a decade ago (GUGLIELMI et al. 1983), integrating the observations of SAWYER (SAWYER and PATE 1953a,b; SAWYER et al. 1953), MULLAN (MULLAN 1974; MULLAN et al. 1964, 1965, 1969), and PITON (PITON et al. 1978). Not until recently, however, has the technology become available to produce microcatheters and microguidewires soft enough to navigate atraumatically into cerebral aneurysms. A novel device, consisting of a soft detachable platinum coil soldered to a stainless steel delivery wire, was developed and tested during animal experimental research performed at U.C.L.A. in 1989 (GUGLIELMI et al. 1991a). The goal was to find an endovascular occlusive agent that would adopt the shape of intracranial aneurysms without distorting their fragile walls.

GUIDO GUGLIELMI, M.D., Department of Radiological Sciences, Service of Endovascular Therapy, UCLA Medical Center, 10833 Le Conte Avenue, Los Angeles, CA 90024-1721, USA and Department of Neurological Sciences, Service of Therapeutic Neuroangiography, University of Rome Medical School, Viale Dell'Universita'30/A, 00185 Roma, Italy

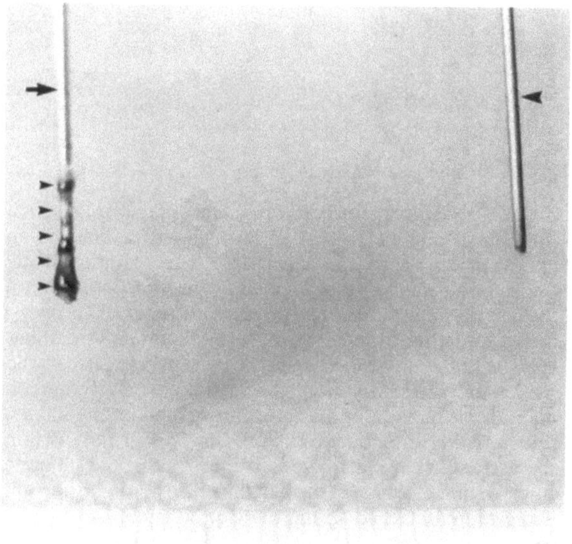

Fig. 7.1. In vitro experiment performed to test electrothrombosis. Two stainless steel 0.038-in. guidewires (*arrow* and *arrowhead*) were simultaneously immersed in a metallic cup containing heparinized blood. A 0.5 mA positive direct electric current was passed through the guidewire on the left (*arrow*) for 10 min, while no current was passed through the other guidewire. At the end of the experiment a thrombus (*arrowheads*) was seen covering the guidewire through which the current had been passed while none was seen around the other guidewire

Due to the encouraging results of the research, this technique has been applied in selected clinical cases (GUGLIELMI et al. 1991b).

The technique of aneurysm occlusion with detachable coils is based upon two electrochemical principles: electrothrombosis and electrolysis. Electrothrombosis occurs because white blood cells, red blood cells, platelets, and fibrinogen are negatively charged. If a positively charged electrode is positioned in blood, it will attract these negatively charged blood components, thus promoting clot formation (SAWYER and PATE 1953a) (Fig. 7.1). Electrolysis occurs when two iron electrodes connected to a source of direct electric current are dipped into a solution. Under these

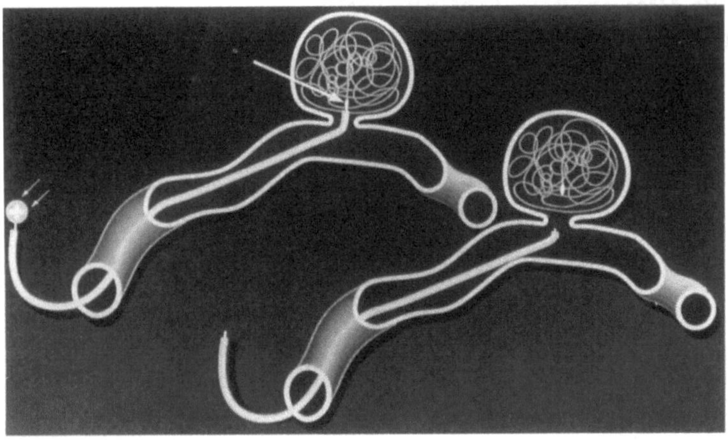

Fig. 7.2. Diagrams representing the steps in electrothrombosis and electrolysis of saccular aneurysms via an endovascular approach. *Upper left*: The platinum distal portion of a stainless steel delivery wire is introduced into the aneurysmal sac through a microcatheter. The *arrow* points to the junction between the platinum and the stainless steel. A positive direct electric current is applied to the guidewire (*double arrows*) so that the positively charged platinum attracts the negatively charged blood components, thus initiating thrombus formation. *Lower right*: In 4–12 min the current has also dissolved, by electrolysis, the stainless steel portion proximal to the junction. The platinum portion is therefore detached within the clotted aneurysm

conditions, the immersed end of the positive wire dissolves, and the other wire recruits the migrating ferrous ions from the anode to the cathode. Noble metals, such as platinum, are not affected by this phenomenon (Potter 1956). Electrolysis is the process that detaches the platinum coil from the stainless steel delivery wire within an aneurysm (Fig. 7.2).

7.1 History of Electrothrombosis

Electrothrombosis consists in the production of an endovascular thrombus by a positively charged endovascular metallic electrode. Velpeau in 1831 and Phillips in 1832 were the first to introduce needles into the lumen of vessel, producing an intraluminal clot and withdrawing the needle after the thrombus had formed. The same authors suggested that the introduction of metals with a high dissociation constant of positively charged ions (Fe^{2+}, Cu^{2+}, and Be^{2+}) might be useful in the treatment of aneurysms. Moore and Murchison in 1864 were the first to introduce a permanent wire into the sac of an aortic aneurysm in order to produce an intra-aneurysmal thrombus. In 1847 Ciniselli had been the first to apply a positive electric current, passing it through needles temporarily positioned into the sac of an aneurysm.

In 1952, Bigelow and De Foyes demonstrated that washed platelets migrated to the positive pole of an electrophoretic cell. Abramson (1924) had demonstrated earlier that a similar phenomenon occurred with white blood cells. In 1953 Sawyer and Pate showed that the use of direct electric current through citrated or heparinized blood led to precipitation of blood elements around the positively charged electrode (anode) (Sawyer and Pate 1953a). These elements were red blood cells, white blood cells, platelets, and fibrinogen. They used 0.2–10 mA for approximately 30 min.

7.2 Electrolysis

Miller et al. (1978) utilized 5–10 mA direct electric current to produce a thrombus in the citrated blood of dogs; stainless steel or platinum electrodes were employed. They proved that platinum is three to four times more thrombogenic than stainless steel, that stainless steel dissolves during the passage of current by electrolysis, and that there is no difference in the size of the clot if the diameter of the platinum electrode is changed from 0.25 to 0.9 mm. They also observed that the size of the clot is directly proportional to the time of the application of the current. Piton et al. (1978) tested various metals in saline. They applied 10 mA direct electric current to silver, copper, platinum, and stainless steel electrodes, all 0.6 mm in diameter, and showed that the silver electrode underwent electrolysis in 22 min and the stainless steel electrode in 12 min; the copper electrode was rapidly affected by oxidation and the platinum was not electrolyzed.

7.3 Endothelial Current

In 1953 SAWYER and PATE performed a series of experiments in dogs and showed that the intima of vessels has a constant negative charge (between −3 and −15 mV) when compared to the adventitia (SAWYER and PATE 1953b). Due to this negative charge the negatively charged blood elements are normally repelled from the intima, decreasing the possibility of organization of an intravascular thrombus. If the intima is injured, immediate reversal of the electrical polarity takes place so that it becomes positively charged, attracting the negatively charged blood elements. This phenomenon may play an important role in posttraumatic vascular clotting.

7.4 Electrothrombosis

In 1961, SALAZAR produced complete thrombosis of the coronary arteries in dogs by applying a very small intravascular positive electric current (0.5 mA, 3 V) for 2 h. ARAKI et al. (1965) studied electrical thrombosis applying 3 mA positive direct electric current for 1 h. They showed that, using this technique, a thrombus could be formed in the carotid artery of dogs in 90% of cases. Thrombus formation was reduced if the artery was infused with heparin. Subsequently, PITON et al. (1978) elicited electrothrombosis of the aorta, femoral artery, and common carotid artery in rabbits by applying electric current (10 mA, 9 V) to a platinum or stainless steel endovascular electrode (anode). GUGLIELMI et al. (1983) reported intra-aneurysmal thrombus formation in saccular aneurysms created ont he common carotid artery of ten rabbits. Using an endovascular approach, they introduced a stainless steel electrode through a transfemoral microcatheter into the aneurysms and applied 10 mA positive direct electric current to initiate intra-aneurysmal thrombosis.

Based upon the in vitro and in vivo experiments described above, it is possible to say that: (a) if a positive direct electric current is used within a vessel, a thrombus will precipitate on the positive electrode (anode); (b) the size and weight of a thrombus are directly proportional to the coulombs (mA × min) of electricity delivered; (c) platinum appears to produce the largest clots and is not affected by electrolysis; and (d) stainless steel electrodes are electrolyzed within a few minutes.

7.5 Clinical Application of Electrothrombosis: Extravascular Approach

MULLAN was the first to use electrothrombosis to occlude saccular intracranial aneurysms in a large number of patients. His technique consisted of stereotactic insertion through a burr hole of fine copper-plated steel needles, 0.2 mm in diameter, across the neck of the aneurysm at 1.0-mm intervals. Thrombosis was initiated by passing a positive direct electric current through each needle for 5 min. Postembolization angiograms were obtained every 30 min until satisfactory thrombosis was achieved. With this technique, satisfactory occlusion of the aneurysm was achieved in 49 patients; incomplete occlusion resulted in eight patients, all of whom died 1–66 days postembolization due to recurrent intracranial hemorrhage. MULLAN concluded that stereotactic copper electrothrombosis offered a risk comparable to that associated with conservative management followed by surgical clipping. This technique has not become very popular because the aneurysm has to be punctured, extensive equipment is required, it is necessary to penetrate cerebral tissue in order to reach the aneurysm with the probe, and it is unsuitable for a wide spectrum of aneurysms.

7.6 Clinical Application of Electrothrombosis: Endovascular Approach

Between March 1990 and July 1991 surgically difficult intracranial saccular aneurysms in 33 patients were treated by electrothrombosis via an endovascular approach. Twenty-one patients were women and 12 were men. The patients ranged in age from 21 to 73 years (mean 49 years). Eighteen patients presented with subarachnoid hemorrhage (SAH), 11 with a mass effect, and two with other symptoms. In the remaining two patients the aneurysm was discovered incidentally. All patients presenting with SAH were in grades I–II except for three who were in grade V (HUNT and HESS 1968). Eleven aneurysms involved the basilar bifurcation, four the intracavernous carotid, and three the vertebrobasilar junction. The

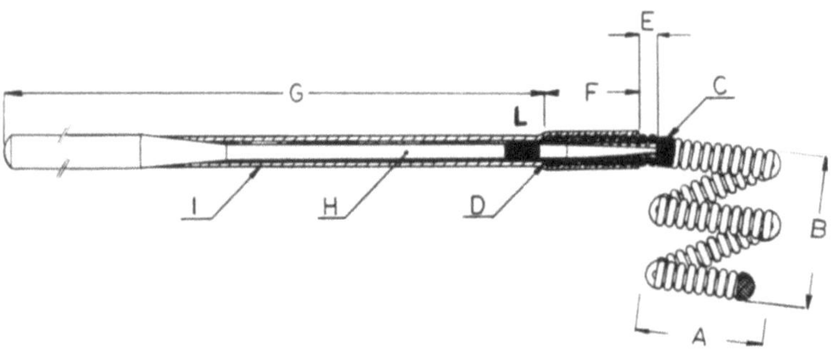

Fig. 7.3. Diagram of the detachable platinum coil. *A*, diameter of the circular memory; *B*, the distal portion (10–40 cm in length) made of coiled platinum wire; *C*, microsolder connecting the distal portion to the intermediate stainless steel portion; *D*, microsolder connecting the intermediate stainless steel portion to the intermediate platinum portion; *E* and *F*, the intermediate stainless steel portion (3 cm in length) made of coiled stainless steel wire (*E*, the uninsulated part of the intermediate stainless steel portion); *G*, the proximal stainless steel portion (175 cm in length); *H*, the tapering stainless steel core wire; *I*, Teflon lamination; *L*, the intermediate platinum portion (0.5 cm in length) made of coiled platinum wire, which serves as a marker

remaining 13 aneurysms involved: the posterior inferior cerebellar artery, the internal carotid artery bifurcation, the anterior communicating artery, and the trigeminal, carotid (at the origin of the ophthalmic artery), middle cerebral, superior cerebellar, and posterior communicating arteries. Sixteen aneurysms were small (<12 mm), seven were large (12–25 mm), and ten were giant (>25 mm).

7.6.1 Occlusion Technique

All procedures are performed with the patient awake and under systemic heparinization (3000 units at the beginning and subsequently 1000 units per hour). The transfemoral approach and digital subtraction angiography with "road-mapping" capability are always used. The proximal parent artery is catheterized with a No. 6 French non-tapered polyethylene guiding catheter. A Tracker-GDC microcatheter is then advanced coaxially into the aneurysm sac with the aid of a micro-guidewire (Tracker 10 GDC, Tracker 18 GDC, Seeker 10 Lite, Seeker 14; Target Therapeutics, San Jose, CA, USA). In the case of lateral aneurysms (i.e., aneurysms arising at a 90° angle to the parent vessel) it is necessary to curve the tip of the microcatheter with steam. The Tracker GDC microcatheters have two radiopaque markers: one is at the distal end and the other is 3 cm proximal to the first one. The guidewire is removed once the microcatheter tip is inside the aneurysm sac in order to avoid aneurysm perforation. Continuous pressurized flushing with heparinized saline of both coaxial systems is utilized during the whole procedure to decrease friction, to eliminate the possibility of clot formation, and to avoid electric current dispersion. An intra-aneurysmal angiogram may be performed to make sure of proper microcatheter positioning. The detachable coil (GDC, Target Therapeutics, San Jose, CA, USA) is then introduced into the microcatheter with the aid of a special introducer.

7.6.2 Detachable Coils

The "detachable coils" can be 0.010 in. or 0.015 in. in diameter (this 50% increment in diameter leads to a 100% increment in volume). The former size is used for small aneurysms and is compatible with the Tracker 10 GDC microcatheter; the latter size is utilized for giant aneurysms and is compatible with the Tracker 18 GDC microcatheter. The detachable coil has four components (Fig. 7.3): the proximal part (175 cm in length) is made of stainless steel core wire; the intermediate platinum portion is a 5 mm long platinum marker; the intermediate stainless steel portion (3 cm in length) is made of a very soft stainless steel coil; the distal component varies from 4 to 40 cm and is a coil made of platinum. It has a circular memory that allows its deposit in the dome of aneurysms without traumatizing their fragile walls.

The distal 30 cm of the proximal portion, the platinum marker, and most of the intermediate part of the stainless steel delivery system are laminated with Teflon to achieve electrical insulation. The distal 2 mm of the stainless steel coiled portion is uninsulated to allow electrolytic detachment (Fig. 7.4).

Currently, eight types of coil are available and are selected depending upon the aneurysm sac and neck size. They are:

1. A helix, 8 cm long with a 2-mm circular memory
2. A coil 10 cm long with a 4-mm circular memory
3. A coil, 15 cm long with a 5-mm circular memory
4. A coil, 15 cm long with a 6-mm circular memory
5. A coil, 20 cm long with an 8-mm circular memory
6. A coil, 40 cm long with an 8-mm circular memory
7. A coil (0.015 in. in diameter), 20 cm long with an 8-mm circular memory
8. A coil (0.015 in. in diameter), 40 cm long with an 8-mm circular memory (Fig. 7.5)

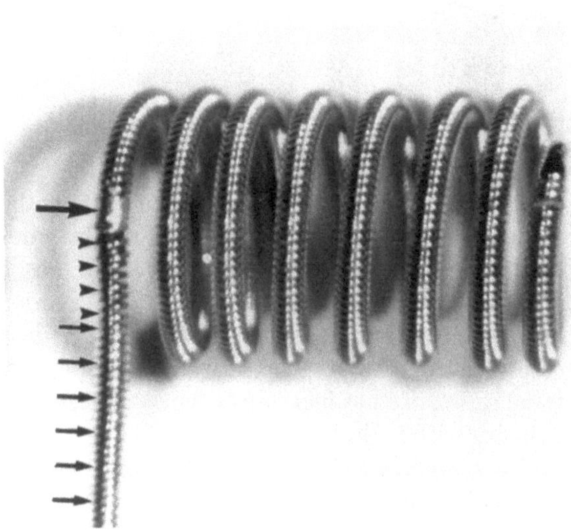

Fig. 7.4. A platinum spiral with circular memory. The microsolder that connects the connects the platinum to the stainless steel is visible (*large arrow*). The uninsulated stainless steel coil (2 mm in length) is seen (*arrowheads*): this is the part that is dissolved by electrolysis. The opalescent Teflon lamination is also visible (*arrows*)

7.6.3 Delivery of the Detachable Coils

When the platinum coil is positioned in the microcatheter, it adopts a straight shape that allows it to be advanced toward the aneurysm without significant friction. As soon as the platinum coil emerges from the microcatheter it adopts a circular formation and folds upon itself, decreasing the possibility of migration outside the aneurysmal neck and adapting to the aneurysmal lumen without causing aneurysmal wall distortion.

Platinum is more radiopaque than stainless steel, so that the platinum distal component is easy to see under fluoroscopy. This property allows

Fig. 7.5. Photograph of detachable platinum coils for aneurysm occlusion: a platinum coil, 40 cm long with an 8-mm circular memory (*double arrows*); a platinum coil, 15 cm long with a 5-mm circular memory (*arrow*). The solder between the platinum and the stainless steel components of the detachable coil is indicated (*long arrow*). The platinum marker, 0.5 cm in length, is also visible (*arrowheads*)
▽

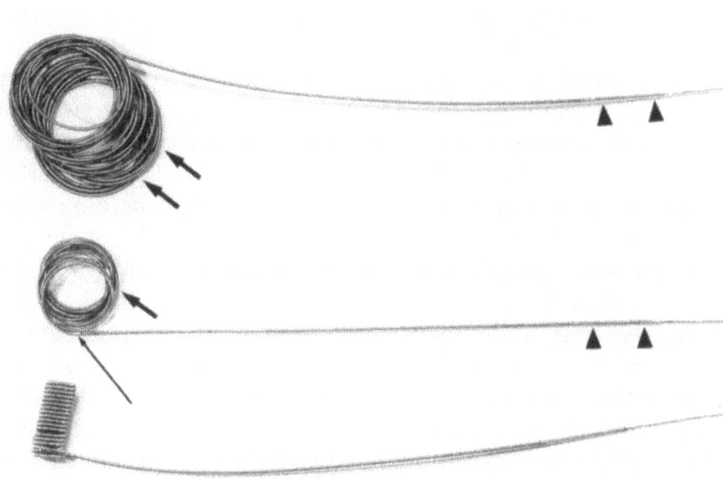

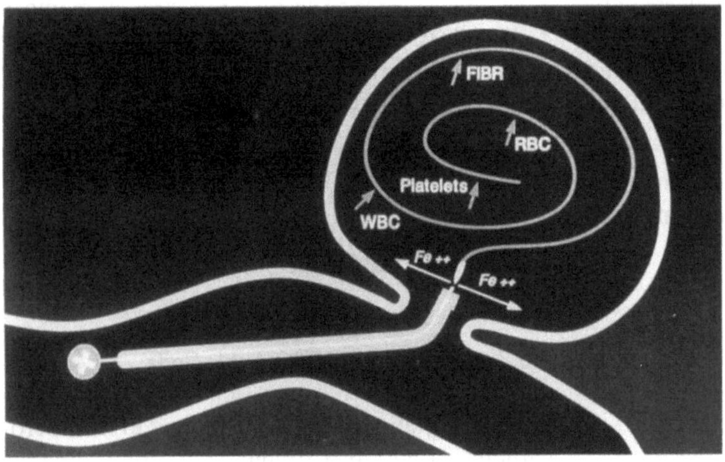

Fig. 7.6. Diagram representing the effects of electric current in an aneurysm. The positively charged intra-aneurysmal platinum attracts the negatively charged red blood cells (*RBC*), white blood cells (*WBC*), platelets, and fibrinogen (*FIBR*), thus initiating thrombus formation. At the same time the electric current induces migration of ferrous ions from the stainless steel, thus dissolving it and detaching the platinum component within the aneurysm

control of the coil deposited in the aneurysm and ensures that none is placed in the parent vessel. When such a migration was observed, the coil was withdrawn and repositioned inside the aneurysm or exchanged with a different sized one. This maneuver is performed by pulling back the delivery guidewire and advancing it again through the microcatheter.

When the detachable platinum coil is seen to be in a suitable position inside the aneurysm and with the platinum–stainless steel junction zone 3 mm beyond the tip of the microcatheter, intra-aneurysmal electrothrombosis and electrolysis are generated by applying a 0.5/0.7-mA, 2.2/2.9-V positive direct electric current to the proximal end of the stainless steel guidewire using a battery-operated current generator. The negative ground pole is connected to a surface or needle electrode at the groin. In this way the intra-aneurysmal platinum becomes positively charged and attracts the negatively charged white blood cells, red blood cells, platelets, and fibrinogen, thus electrically inducing thrombus formation (Fig. 7.6).

By the time a thrombus forms around the platinum coil, the current has also dissolved the uninsulated intra-aneurysmal stainless steel coil closest to platinum coil by electrolysis (Fig. 7.6). The detachment of the coil occurs within 4–12 min. By taking advantage of this phenomenon, it is possible to detach the platinum coil within the aneurysm without any need for pulling. In order to detect the detachment, the generator has a milliampere meter and a voltmeter. A sudden drop in current or a sudden rise in voltage indicates that detachment has occurred (i.e., the electrical resistance has increased). The stainless steel delivery wire is then withdrawn.

The platinum coils represent a packing material that holds the intra-aneurysmal thrombus and prevents both its displacement into the parent artery and its fragmentation. It is possible to introduce, deliver, and detach more than one coil in the aneurysm, depending on the size of the lesion. In 16 small aneurysms (<12 mm) an average of 59 cm of platinum coils was detached. This length increased for larger aneurysms.

After detachment of the first coil it is no longer possible to see under fluoroscopy the distal intra-aneurysmal marker of the microcatheter and the platinum–stainless steel junction of the subsequent coil(s) emerging from the microcatheter. This is because the radiopaque intra-aneurysmal platinum covers the microcatheter tip, preventing the correct visualization of the platinum–stainless steel junction. The visualization of the proximal radiopaque markers located on the microcatheter (3 cm before its tip) and on the detachable coils (2.8 cm before the junction) allows safe delivery of the coils subsequent to the first one: when the two markers (inside the parent artery and 3 cm proximal to the aneurysm) match, it means that the platinum–stainless steel junction is 2–3 mm beyond the microcatheter tip, i.e., in the correct position to be detached. It is imperative that the platinum–stainless steel junction emerges from the microcatheter for no more than 2–3 mm. In fact, the

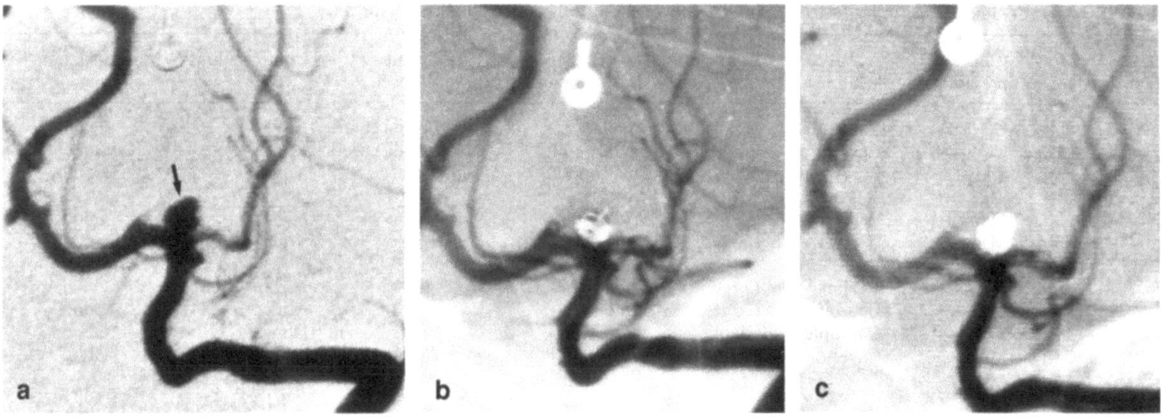

Fig. 7.7a–c. Case 22. **a** Vertebral angiogram, anteroposterior view, demonstrating a small basilar bifurcation aneurysm (*arrow*). **b** Vertebral angiogram obtained during the procedure, showing partial occlusion of the aneurysm with one 15 cm long coil. Another coil, 8 cm in length, was then detached to achieve complete aneurysm occlusion (not shown). **c** Vertebral angiogram obtained 6 days postembolization showing complete aneurysm obliteration. Note that the coils assume the original shape and size of the aneurysm without deforming it. A follow-up angiogram 4 months after the procedure demonstrated complete occlusion of the aneurysm

stainless steel coil proximal to the platinum portion is relatively stiff and might perforate the aneurysm if pushed against its wall.

After the detachment of each coil an angiogram is performed in order to assess the amount of occlusion achieved and to decide whether to use more coils or not. At the end of the embolization procedure, the microcatheter is slowly removed from the aneurysm. A postembolization angiogram is obtained to assess the final result, the proper placement of the detached coil(s), and the patency of the parent artery and adjacent vessels. The heparinization is reversed by protamine sulfate. The patients are hospitalized for 3 days. Follow-up angiography is performed at 1 week, 3 months, and 12 months.

7.6.4 Results

Table 7.1 (see p. 118) summarizes the treatment, complications, results, and outcome in this series of 33 patients. It was possible to enter all aneurysms with a microcatheter–guidewire combination. It was always possible to retrieve the coil(s) from the aneurysm if inappropriate in size or position. Failure of electrolytic detachment never occurred. Intra-aneurysmal thrombosis ranging from 70% to 100% was achieved in all cases. Incomplete aneurysm occlusion resulted from partial coil filling of the aneurysm. The portions of the aneurysm filled with coils underwent thrombosis in 100% of cases. The immediate postthrombosis angiogram demonstrated partial thrombosis and occlusion of aneurysms insufficiently packed with coils. Nevertheless, even with such insufficient packing, progressive thrombosis took place, within the mesh of coils, in the hours that followed the procedure.

A complete aneurysm occlusion can be achieved in small neck aneurysms (Figs. 7.7, 7.8). Such results are more difficult to achieve in wide neck aneurysms because of the danger of parent vessel occlusion or coil migration.

In this series there was one transient neurologic deficit (aphasia in case 5, with complete regression within 2 days) and one permanent neurologic deficit (hemianopia in case 21). The three patients who were originally in grade V (cases 19, 23, and 29) died.

7.7 Critical Evaluation and Conclusions

Two percent of the population of North America will have an intracranial aneurysm; such an intracranial aneurysm will rupture in less than 1% of the population and will be the cause of death in 0.5%. In North America, 25000 intracranial aneurysms rupture every year followed by bleeding into the subarachnoid space or cerebral tissue (Weir 1985). The primary purpose of treatment for ruptured intracranial aneurysms is to prevent rebleeding, which in most cases would be catastrophic.

Table 7.1. Profile of 33 patients treated with the GDC aneurysm occlusion system[a]

Case no.	Age, sex	Clinical presentation	Aneurysm location	Aneurysm size[a]	Neck size[b]	Coil Length (cm)	Result (% occl.)	Complications	Outcome
1	28F	CC fist.	Cavernous	Small	Small	35	Fistula cured	None	Good
2	21M	CC fist.	Cavernous	Large	Small	20	Fistula cured	None	Good
3	33F	SAH	PICA	Small	Small	16	80%	None	Good (surgery)
4	60F	Mass	Bas. bif.	Giant	Wide	265	80%	None	Good
5	45M	Mass	ICA bif.	Large	Wide	80	70%	Transient aphasia, resolved in 2 days	Good
6	58M	SAH	VB junct.	Large	Wide	140	95%	None	Good
7	46M	SAH	Bas. bif.	Large	Wide	120	80%	None	Good
8	47F	SAH	Car. ophth.	Giant	Wide	55	70%	None	Good
9	58F	Mass	Cavernous	Giant	Wide	120	Cured	Incomplete coil delivery. Balloon ICA occlusion	Good
10	56F	SAH	Bas. bif.	Small	Wide	168	95% (3 embos)	None	Good
11	50M	SAH	ACoA	Small	Wide	38	90%	None	Good
12	43F	Mass	Trig. art.	Giant	Wide	220	70%	None	Good
13	69F	SAH	Bas. bif.	Small	Wide	15	95%	None	Good
14	67F	Mass	MCA	Giant	Wide	384	98% (3 embos)	None	Good
15	57F	SAH	Bas. bif.	Small	Small	55	100%	None	Good
16	32M	SAH	PCom	Large	Wide	360	80%	None	Good (surgery)
17	45F	Mass	Bas. bif.	Giant	Wide	155 (0.015 in.)	90%	None	Good
18	51F	Incidental finding	Paraophth.	Small	Wide	15	Cured	Incomplete coil delivery. Balloon ICA occlusion	Good
19	48F	SAH (grade V)	ICA bif.	Small	Small	95	100%	None	Dead (grade V)
20	70F	SAH	SCA	Small	Wide	115	90%	None	Good
21	56M	SAH	Bas. bif.	Small	Wide	120	100%	Thrombus progression resulting in PCA occlusion	Hemianopia
22	29F	Incidental finding	Bas. bif.	Small	Small	23	100%	None	Good
23	67F	SAH (grade V)	PICA	Small	Small	8	N/A	Aneurysm rupture with microcatheter after 1st coil delivery	Dead (grade V)
24	32F	SAH	Car. ophth.	Small	Small	125	100%	None	Good
25	34M	Mass	Bas. bif.	Giant	Wide	200 (0.015 in.)	90%	None	Good
26	42F	SAH	VB junct.	Small	Wide	14	95%	None	Good
27	70M	Mass	Bas. bif.	Giant	Wide	53	95%	None	Good
28	56F	Mass	Bas. bif.	Large	Wide	255	98%	None	Good
29	44M	SAH (grade V)	MCA	Small	Small	70	100%	None	Dead (grade V)
30	38M	Mass	VB junct.	Giant	Wide	400 (0.015 in.)	85%	None	Good
31	73F	Mass	Cavernous	Giant	Wide	200 (0.015 in.)	90%	None	Good
32	61M	SAH	ICA bif.	Large	Wide	260 (0.015 in.)	95%	None	Good
33	30F	SAH	Car. ophth.	Small	Small	68	100%	None	Good

CC fist., carotid–cavernous fistula; SAH, subarachnoid hemorrhage; Mass, mass effect; PICA, posterior inferior cerebellar artery; Bas. bif., basilar bifurcation; ICA, internal carotid artery; VB junct., vertebrobasilar junction; ACoA, anterior communicating artery; MCA, middle cerebral artery; PCom, posterior communicating artery; SCA, superior cerebellar artery; embos, embolizations; PCA, posterior cerebral artery; N/A, not applicable.

[a] Small: <12 mm; large: 12–25 mm; giant: >25 mm.

[b] Small: <3 mm; wide: >3 mm.

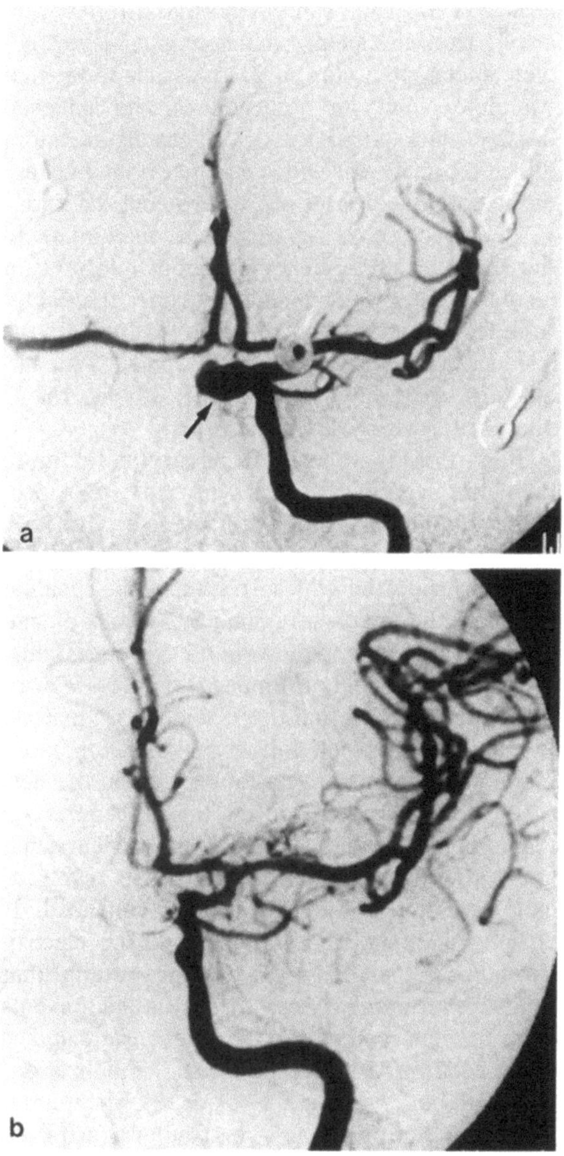

Fig. 7.8 a,b. Case 24. **a** Left internal carotid angiogram, anteroposterior view, demonstrating a paraophthalmic aneurysm (*arrow*). **b** Left internal carotid angiogram obtained 4 days postembolization showing aneurysm obliteration with one 40 cm long coil, two 20 cm long coils, and three 15 cm long coils

7.7.1 Surgery

Microsurgical treatment of aneurysms, preserving the parent artery, is currently the treatment of choice for most intracranial saccular aneurysms. The methods of surgical treatment include: a metallic surgical clip placed across the aneurysmal neck, a suture ligation of the neck, or aneurysm wrapping. All these procedures are performed without entering the interior of the aneurysm (extravascular treatment). In order to reach the aneurysm, general anesthesia, craniotomy, brain retraction and manipulation, and arachnoid dissection are required. For surgically difficult aneurysms, other methods of treatment have been proposed.

7.7.2 Extra-endovascular Approach

The aneurysm is surgically exposed or stereotactically reached with a probe. Its wall is then perforated and various techniques are used to occlude it. The techniques proposed are: electrical thrombosis, isobutyl-cyanoacrylate (IBCA) embolization, and ferromagnetic thrombosis.

Mullan's (1974) experience with electrically induced thrombosis has already been described.

Isobutyl-cyanoacrylate is a liquid adhesive which rapidly on contact with blood to form a firm mass. Zanetti and Sherman (1972) and Debrun et al. (1984) performed experimental studies on IBCA embolization of surgically created aneurysms in dogs. Both groups of authors injected IBCA in the aneurysm by puncturing its sac with a small needle. To avoid the spillage of IBCA into the parent artery during IBCA injection, Zanetti and Sherman momentarily reduced or interrupted the blood flow, while Debrun inflated a balloon into the parent artery, blocking the neck of the aneurysm before injecting IBCA into it. In spite of this, injection of IBCA into saccular aneurysms has not become a clinical method of treatment owing to the risk of spillage into the parent artery.

In the past some authors tried to treat intracranial aneurysms by stereotactic placement of a magnetic probe against the sac of the aneurysm followed by the injection of iron microspheres into the aneurysm by puncturing its wall with a small needle. The aim was to create an intraaneurysmal thrombus by the attraction of iron microspheres to the extravascular magnet. However, the fragmentation of the metallic thrombus, after removal of the probe, was a significant problem. In 1980 Alksne and Smith reported their experience with 22 consecutive cases of anterior communicating artery aneurysms treated by stereotactic iron-acrylic occlusion; they suspended the iron powder in methyl-methacrylate to prevent fragmentation. This technique has not become very popular.

7.7.3 Endovascular Approach

The desire to avoid craniotomy and to take advantage of the fact that arteries are natural channels through which aneurysms can be reached led some researchers to seek a way of treating cerebral aneurysms via an endovascular approach. The endovascular approach to aneurysm occlusion has in the past been limited to balloon embolization (HIESHIMA et al. 1986; ROMODANOV and SHCHEGLOV 1982; SERBINENKO 1974). Balloon embolization has the advantages of avoiding general anesthesia, craniotomy, and brain manipulation. However, it has an important disadvantage in that the fragile wall of the aneurysm undergoes stress while adapting to the shape of the balloon, thus carrying the risk of aneurysm rupture. This risk may be higher in the acute posthemorrhagic phase. HIGASHIDA et al. (1990), in a series of 84 inoperable patients treated by balloon embolization with preservation of the parent artery, reported 17.9% mortality and 10.7% morbidity directly related to the embolization procedure.

A less traumatic approach which consists in using a very soft detachable platinum coil soldered to a stainless steel delivery wire has been developed. It has the advantages of the endovascular approach and it is also usable in the acute posthemorrhagic phase.

In this series of 33 patients treated with endovascular electrothrombosis by means of detachable coils, all aneurysms were considered to be difficult and to carry a high surgical risk. Balloon embolization was not used because it is believed that detachable coils are less traumatic than balloons and that endovascular electrothrombosis consequently entails less risk of rupturing an aneurysm, especially in the acute phase after SAH. Furthermore in four instances (cases 4, 5, 13, and 25) balloon embolization would have led to occlusion of normal vessels arising from the aneurysmal base.

In this preliminary clinical experience one transient (case 5) and one permanent (case 21: hemianopia) neurologic deficit have been observed after embolization. Three patients (cases 19, 23, and 29) who were devastated by the original bleeding eventually died.

It has been possible to achieve complete aneurysm occlusion in seven cases (15, 19, 21, 22, 24, 29, and 33) and satisfactory aneurysm occlusion in nine more cases (6, 11, 14, 17, 26, 27, 28, 31, and 32). In the remaining cases the aneurysmal neck was too wide (and/or normal arteries were arising from the aneurysmal sac) to achieve complete aneurysm occlusion. It is possible to say that complete aneurysm occlusion can be achieved in small neck aneurysms. Such results are more difficult to achieve in wide neck aneurysms because of the potential danger of parent vessel occlusion.

Detachable coils are very soft; they adapt to the shape of the aneurysm without a significant increase in intra-aneurysmal pressure; the risk of rupturing an aneurysm seems to be low. In six instances (cases 3, 16, 19, 23, 29, and 33) the aneurysms were treated in the acute posthemorrhagic phase, i.e., within 48 h after SAH.

It is possible to occlude aneurysms in more than one session (cases 10 and 14), thus progressively embolizing the aneurysmal sac. In mostly thrombosed aneurysms, coils do not seem to migrate inside the clot surrounding the residual lumen of the aneurysm (cases 8, 14, and 27 had repeated angiograms showing no coil migration).

Intra-aneurysmal thrombosis progresses with time. It is believed that this is due to two factors: (a) in the hours that follow embolization more blood components are entrapped within the network of coils, and (b) during the procedure systemic heparinization impedes intra-aneurysmal clot formation – as soon as heparin is reversed, clot formation within the coils is enhanced. It is believed that, aside from producing electrothrombosis, the coils are a packing material that holds the intra-aneurysmal thrombus and prevents both its displacement into the parent artery and its fragmentation. This prevents distal embolization.

In all but two cases (9 and 18), the parent vessel has been preserved. This result was achieved mainly because it is possible to retrieve the coil into the microcatheter if a satisfactory position in the aneurysm has not been reached. It is then possible to try to achieve a better intra-aneurysmal coil position using the same coil or a different sized one.

In two cases (3 and 16) the aneurysms were surgically clipped 3 months after occlusion of the dome and most of the sac of the aneurysms with detachable coils.

A major goal in the management of ruptured intracranial aneurysms is to treat the patient as soon as possible after his admission to the hospital, preferably within 2 days after SAH. The recently published results of the International Cooperative Study on the Timing of Aneurysm Surgery (KASSELL et al. 1990a,b) confirm that early surgery

(1–3 days post-SAH) carries more operative risk than a delayed intervention. A delayed intervention carries lower morbidity and mortality. On the other hand, many patients die while waiting for the best surgical timing (subsequent to day 10 post-SAH) because of rebleeding. With the described device, implantable at the time of the diagnostic angiogram, it may be possible to avoid early rebleeding.

In this preliminary experience with 33 patients, the follow-up period is short. This is due to the fact that the technique has been applied only recently in the clinical setting (as of 6 March 1990). Long-term angiographic and clinical follow-up is necessary to achieve an accurate idea of the advantages and limitations of this newly developed aneurysm occlusion device.

References

Abramson HA (1924) A possible relationship between the current of injury and the white-blood cell in inflammation. Am J Med Sci 167:702–710

Alksne JF, Smith RW (1980) Stereotaxic occlusion of 22 consecutive anterior communicating artery aneurysms. J Neurosurg 52:760–763

Araki C, Handa H, Yoshida K et al. (1966) Electrically induced thrombosis for the treatment of intracranial aneurysms and angiomas. In: deVet AC (ed) Proceedings of the Third International Congress of Neurological Surgery, Copenhagen, 1965. Excerpta Medica, Amsterdam, vol 110, pp 651–654

Bigelow FS, De Foyes JF (1952) Cited by in reference Sawyer and Pate 1953a

Ciniselli L (1847) Sulla elettropuntura nella cura degli aneurismi. Gazz Med Ital Lomb Milano 6:9–14

Debrun GM, Varsos V, Liszczak TM et al. (1984) Obliteration of experimental aneurysms in dogs with isobutyl-cyanoacrylate. J Neurosurg 61:37–43

Guglielmi G, Guerrisi R, Guidetti B et al. (1983) L'elettrotrombosi intravasale nelle malformazioni vascolari sperimentalmente provocate. In: Carella A (ed) Proceedings of IIIrd Congress of the Italian Society of Neuroradiology. Associazione Italiana di Neuroradiologia, Bari, pp 139–146

Guglielmi G, Viñuela F, Sepetka I et al. (1991a) Electrothrombosis of saccular aneurysms via endovascular approach. Part 1: Electrochemical basis, technique, and experimental results. J Neurosurg 75:1–7

Guglielmi G, Viñuela F, Dion J, Duckwiler G (1991b) Electrothrombosis of saccular aneurysms via endovascular approach. Part 2: Preliminary clinical experience. J Neurosurg 75:8–14

Hieshima GB, Higashida RT, Wapenski J et al. (1986) Balloon embolization of a large distal basilar artery aneurysm. Case report. J Neurosurg 65:413–416

Higashida RT, Halbach VV, Barnwell SL et al. (1990) Treatment of intracranial aneurysms with preservation of the parent vessel: results of percutaneous balloon embolization in 84 patients. AJNR 11:633–640

Hunt WE, Hess RM (1968) Surgical risk as related to time of intervention in the repair of intracranial aneurysms. J Neurosurg 28:14–20

Kassell NF, Torner JC, Haley EC Jr et al. (1990a) The International Cooperative Study on the Timing of Aneurysm Surgery. Part 1: Overall management results. J Neurosurg 73:18–36

Kassell NF, Torner JC, Jane JA et al. (1990b) The International Cooperative Study on the Timing of Aneurysm Surgery. Part 2: Surgical results. J Neurosurg 73:37–47

Miller MD, Johnsrude IS, Limberakis AJ et al. (1978) Clinical use of transcatheter electrocoagulation. Radiology 129:211–214

Moore CH, Murchison C (1864) On a new method of procuring the consolidation of fibrin in certain incurable aneurisms: with the report of a case in which an aneurism of the ascending aorta was treated by the insertion of wire. Proc R Med Chir Soc Lond 4:327–335

Mullan S (1974) Experiences with surgical thrombosis of intracranial berry aneurysms and carotid cavernous fistulas. J Neurosurg 41:657–670

Mullan S, Beckman F, Vailati G et al. (1964) An experimental approach to the problem of cerebral aneurysms. J Neurosurg 21:838–845

Mullan S, Raimondi AJ, Dobben G et al. (1965) Electrically induced thrombosis in intracranial aneurysms. J Neurosurg 22:539–547

Mullan S, Reyes C, Dawley J et al. (1969) Stereotactic copper electric thrombosis of intracranial aneurysms. Prog Neurol Surg 3:193–211

Phillips B (1832) A series of experiments performed for the purpose of showing that arteries may be obliterated without ligature, compression or the knife. Longman, London, p 66 (pamphlet)

Piton J, Billerey J, Constant P et al. (1978) Selective vascular thrombosis induced by a direct electrical current: animal experiments. J Neuroradiol 5:139–152

Potter EC (1956) Electrochemistry, principles and applications. Cleaver-Hume, London, pp 1–19, 124–165

Romodanov AP, Shcheglov VI (1982) Intravascular occlusion of saccular aneurysms of the cerebral arteries by means of a detachable balloon catheter. Adv Tech Stand Neurosurg 9:25–48

Salazar AE (1961) Experimental myocardial infarction. Induction of coronary thrombosis in the intact closed chest dog. Circ Res 9:1351–1356

Sawyer PN, Pate JW (1953a) Bio-electric phenomena as an etiologic factor in intravascular thrombosis. Am J Physiol 175:103–107

Sawyer PN, Pate JW (1953b) Electric potential differences across the normal aorta and aortic grafts of dogs. Am J Physiol 175:113–117

Sawyer PN, Pate JW, Weldon CS (1953) Relations of abnormal and injury electric potential differences to intravascular thrombosis. Am J Physiol 175:108–112

Serbinenko FA (1974) Balloon catheterization and occlusion of major cerebral vessels. J Neurosurg 41:125–145

Velpeau A (1831) Mémoire sur la piqûre ou l'acupunture des artères dans le traitement des anévrismes. Gaz Med Paris 2:1–4

Weir B (1985) Intracranial aneurysms and subarachnoid hemorrhage: an overview. In: Wilkins RH, Rengachary SS (eds) Neurosurgery, vol 2. McGraw-Hill, New York, pp 1308–1329

Zanetti PH, Sherman FE (1972) Experimental evaluation of a tissue adhesive as an agent for the treatment of aneurysms and arteriovenous anomalies. J Neurosurg 36:72–79

8 Angioplasty of Vasospasm

JOSEPH M. ESKRIDGE

CONTENTS

8.1 Introduction

The morbidity and mortality from subarachnoid hemorrhage are extraordinarily high. In the first 3 months following a hemorrhage the mortality exceeds 50% (ALLCOCK and DRAKE 1965; GRAF and NIBBELINK 1974). Among those who survive, fully two-thirds never regain the quality of life that they had prior to the hemorrhage (MULLAN 1975; ROPPER and ZERVAS 1984; SAH et al. 1969). Symptomatic vasospasm occurs in one-third of those who survive the initial hemorrhage (ALLCOCK and DRAKE 1965; MULLAN 1975). In 1984, ZUBKOV et al. first reported the successful treatment of vasospasm by transluminal angioplasty. Additional reports subsequently confirmed these initial encouraging results (ESKRIDGE 1989; NEWELL et al. 1989; HIGASHIDA et al. 1989).

Angioplasty represents a significant breakthrough in the treatment of vasospasm. Before the advent of angioplasty, a great variety of pharmacologic agents and techniques to minimize spasm had been tried. A number of these had been shown to reduce the incidence of symptoms from vasospasm, but once neurologic deficit occurred, no treatment was entirely effective (HUNT and HESS 1968; MIZUKAMI et al. 1982; OWADA et al. 1977, 1979; SUNDT 1975; WILKINS 1979). Angioplasty represents a technique to actually reverse a neurologic deficit after it has occurred secondary to vasospasm.

8.2 History

Almost 150 years ago the English physician GULL described the death of a young woman due to an intracranial catastrophe. Four days following the onset of her illness, she was able to utter a few words. The next day, however, she deteriorated and died. At autopsy GULL found a ruptured middle cerebral aneurysm imbedded in a large clot and the adjacent hemisphere showed massive softening. His description is consistent with a cerebral infarct caused by the vasospasm (GULL 1859). During this early period the infarction that resulted from vasospasm was often referred to as the second stroke (ECHLIN 1965).

ZUCKER in 1944 described smooth muscle contraction secondary to substances in blood serum and also observed the vasoconstrictive activity of lysed red blood cells. He suggested that the infarction was due to temporary spasm of the blood vessels rather than compression of the arteries by the aneurysm.

In 1951 ECKER and RIEMENSCHNEIDER provided the first description of angiographic spasm of the intracranial vessels and established the relationship to ruptured intracranial aneurysms. They noted that the spasm was greatest near the ruptured aneurysm and was most marked in the intracranial portion of the artery. They reasoned that the vasospasm could become excessive and produce infarction secondary to lowering of the blood flow to the area of brain supplied by the affected artery. They suggested that vasospasm probably plays an important role following the spontaneous rupture of saccular aneurysms arising from the

JOSEPH M. ESKRIDGE, M.D., Associate Professor of Radiology, Department of Neurological Surgery RI-20, University of Washington Medical Center, 1959 NE Pacific Street, Seattle, WA 98195, USA circle of Wills. It would be another 10 years before the widespread skepticism regarding ECKER and RIEMENSCHNEIDER's work would dissipate. By the mid-1960s papers were starting to suggest that vasospasm was the crucial determinate of the outcome in patients with aneurysm and subarachnoid hemorrhage (STORNELLI and FRENCH 1964). The 1965 study by ALLCOCK and DRAKE impressed upon the medical establishment that vasospasm was the primary cause of postoperative morbidity and mortality following the rupture of intracranial aneurysms.

8.3 Pathology of Vasospasm

Despite over 40 years of extensive clinical and experimental investigation, controversy over the basic pathophysiology of cerebral vasospasm following subarachnoid hemorrhage persists. The primary controversy centers around whether there is spasm per se of the vessel or whether there is thickening of the intima and media that results in the vasoconstriction (FOLKOW 1982; ZERVAS et al. 1982). Changes noted in the arterial morphology associated with vasospasm include thickening and edema of the intima and media, necrosis and proliferation of the media, and inflammation in the adventitia (TANABE et al. 1978; TANISHIMA 1980; ALKSNE and GREENHOOT 1974; MAYBERG et al. 1978; ECHLIN 1971). In the later stages of vasospasm, the media demonstrates fibrosis (ALKSNE 1974; FEIN et al. 1974).

There is considerable indirect evidence indicating that the agent responsible for inducing vasospasm is contained in the erythrocyte component of whole blood and is most likely hemoglobin (LISZCZAK et al. 1983; DUFF et al. 1987). There are also clinical and experimental data suggesting that the degree of vasospasm is related to the amount of blood that the vessel adventitia is exposed to as well as the duration of this exposure (LISZCZAK et al. 1983; VARSOS et al. 1983; FISHER et al. 1980; HUGHES and SCHIANCHI 1978). Unfortunately, to date there has not been a good histopathologic study of the effects of angioplasty on vasospasm, the reason being that there is not a good animal model in which the same balloon system and inflation pressures as are used in humans can be studied.

8.4 Clinical Features

Vasospasm typically develops from the 4th through roughly the 8th day following subarachnoid hemorrhage (HEROS et al. 1983; KWAK et al. 1979; SAITO and SANO 1980). It is unusual for patients to become symptomatic from vasospasm before day 4. It is also unusual for patients to manifest symptoms after day 12.

Usually the first symptom of vasospasm is an altered sensorium (FISHER 1975; HEROS et al. 1983). The patient becomes drowsy and confused. Hemiparesis and aphasia can result if the dominant middle cerebral artery is primarily involved. Coma can result if there is spasm of the distal basilar and proximal posterior cerebral arteries (PLUM and POSNER 1980). Bicerebral coma can result as well from involvement of both middle cerebral arteries. Vasospasm involving the proximal basilar artery can result in respiratory arrest and death.

8.5 Diagnosis and Management

Computed tomography (CT) has proved to be the most reliable technique for predicting vasospasm. Using a method originally described by FISHER et al. (1980) and later confirmed by a prospective study from KISTLER et al. (1983), patients can be divided into four groups with predictable outcomes:

- Group I: no blood visible on CT; no severe spasm predicted
- Group II: diffuse blood, not dense enough to represent thick clot; no severe spasm predicted
- Group III: dense accumulation of blood with clot thicker than 1–3 mm in the interhemispheric fissure, insular cisterns, or basilar cisterns; severe spasm predicted
- Group IV: intracerebral or intraventricular clot with or without diffuse blood but no clot in the basilar cisterns; no severe spasm predicted

The International Cooperative Study on Timing of Aneursym Surgery on almost 1000 patients found the initial CT appearance to be the single best prognostic indicator of delayed ischemia (ADAMS et al. 1987). A normal CT scan obtained within 5 days of subarachnoid hemorrhage was associated with a low risk of ischemic deficit from vasospasm. Focal or thick collections of clot in the basilar cisterns indicated a high risk of developing ischemia. The CT findings of intraventricular hemorrhage, intracerebral hemorrhage, and hydrocephalus were not valuable predictors of the later development of ischemia secondary to vasospasm. Again, a well-defined clot within the subarachnoid cisterns is the single best predictor that symptomatic vasospasm will develop.

The recent development of transcranial Doppler ultrasonography (TCD) has made it possible to noninvasively access the degree of vasospasm and to follow its development and resolution over time (AASLID et al. 1982, 1984). TCD provides the earliest clue that vasospasm is developing. Once this is known, medical therapy can be instituted. If the patient becomes symptomatic from vasospasm despite maximal medical therapy, there is no excuse for postponing angioplasty. The sooner one attempts to reverse a neurologic deficit, the more likely one is to be successful. If TCD monitoring is not available, there is often a tendency to start medical therapy after the patient becomes symptomatic. There then is a tendency to wait and see whether this will be effective, before attempting angioplasty. This delay only serves to reduce the effectiveness of angioplasty.

Transcranial Doppler ultrasonography utilizes pulsed Doppler transmissions which allow recording of velocity signals at preselected depths. This is essential for transcranial use because it permits differentiation of the arteries at the base of the brain. Another unique feature of TCD is the use of a 2-MHz ultrasonic frequency which allows the ultrasound to penetrate the thin portions of the temporal bone to access the intracranial arteries. With TCD the systolic, diastolic, and average mean velocities can be recorded. Stenosis caused by vasospasm, atherosclerosis, or other lesions will increase the blood flow velocity through the stenosis in proportion to the reduction in the cross-sectional area of the artery.

The range of normal blood flow velocity in the middle cerebral artery is between 30 and 80 cm/s with an average of 62 cm/s (AASLID et al. 1982). Middle cerebral arteries with a velocity of 120 cm/s or more are in spasm. Mean velocities greater than 200 cm/s correspond to severe angiographic spasm with greater than 50% narrowing of the involved vessel.

The definitive method to diagnose vasospasm is cerebral angiography. Vasospasm typically involves the supraclinoid carotid, proximal anterior cerebral, proximal middle cerebral, distal vertebral, basilar, and proximal posterior cerebral arteries. The cisterns around these vessels accumulate the largest quantities of blood.

The degree of spasm is obviously important as an indicator of whether or not the patient will become symptomatic. With luminal diameter narrowing of at least 50%, there is significant reduction in cerebral blood flow (SIMEONE and TREPPER 1972). Also the longer the segment of narrowing, the more severe the reduction in flow. This is particularly important in vasospasm since frequently the narrowing occurs over a long segment.

Once the presence of vasospasm has been confirmed, medical therapy is instituted. This consists of hypertensive and hypervolemic therapy to increase the cerebral blood flow through the narrowed intracranial vessels. Calcium channel blockers are also utilized. The primary beneficial effect of hypertensive and hypervolemic therapy, as well as calcium channel blockers, is to reduce the number of patients who become symptomatic from vasospasm (ALLEN et al. 1983; PHILIPPON et al. 1986; MORAWETZ et al. 1979). They are not able to consistently reverse the symptoms of vasospasm once they occur (HUNT and HESS 1968; MIZUKAMI et al. 1982; OWADA et al. 1977, 1979; SUNDT 1975; WILKINS 1979; ALLEN et al. 1983).

8.6 Patient Selection

Certain guidelines are useful when determining which patients with symptomatic vasospasm are candidates for angioplasty. These criteria include: (a) recent onset of a neurologic deficit following subarachnoid hemorrhage that cannot be attributed to other causes such as hydrocephalus or mass effect; (b) a neurologic deficit that does not reverse with hypertensive and hypervolemic therapy; (c) no infarction on a recent CT scan; and (d) angiographically apparent vasospasm in a location that would explain the deficit.

Angioplasty should be performed as soon as possible after the onset of symptoms (ESKRIDGE et al. 1990). The most dramatic neurologic improvements occur when the procedure is performed within 6–12 h of symptom onset (NEWELL et al. 1989). However, complete recoveries have occurred when as long as 48 h has elapsed between neurologic deterioration and angioplasty

(Eskridge et al. 1990). The obvious reason for early intervention is to reverse the ischemia before infarction occurs. The longer the delay, the greater the risk that infarction will develop. It is also vitally important to obtain a CT scan prior to performing angioplasty to rule out infarction. If angioplasty is performed in the presence of an infarction, a bland infarct may be turned into a hemorrhagic infarct following the reestablishment of normal cerebral perfusion.

A problem arises when one waits to see whether the neurologic deficit will reverse with hypertensive and hypervolemic therapy. At our institution the use of TCD alerts us to the onset of vasospasm at an early stage and hypertensive and hypervolemic therapy is instituted. If the patient then develops a deficit with hypertensive and hypervolemic therapy, it is considered a failure and we proceed immediately with angioplasty. As already pointed out, if TCD is not available, there is often a tendency to start hypertensive and hypervolemic therapy after the patient becomes symptomatic and then to wait 12–24 h to see whether this therapy is effective. Unfortunately, this delay often increases the risk that the patient will develop an infarction which precludes angioplasty.

The aneurysm that caused the original subarachnoid hemorrhage should probably be obliterated prior to performing angioplasty (Newell et al. 1989). In our series of 30 patients, only two patients underwent angioplasty when the aneurysm had not been treated. Both of these patients rebled and died while awaiting surgery or balloon embolization. There is a marked increase in cerebral perfusion following angioplasty and this serves to increase the risk of rehemorrhage from an unprotected aneurysm.

Overall the most important criteria for the success of angioplasty is early treatment. Angioplasty should be instituted as soon as possible after the onset of symptoms.

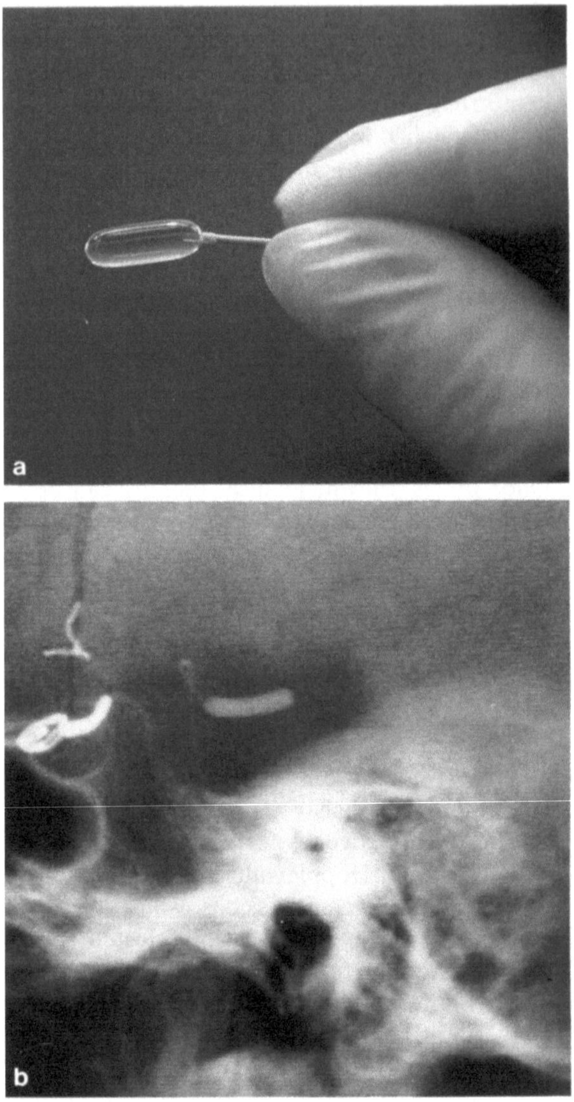

Fig. 8.1. a Silicone angioplasty balloon fully inflated (courtesy of Interventional Therapeutics Corporation, South San Francisco, CA). **b** Lateral view of the skull shows the balloon inflated in the proximal posterior cerebral artery. The catheter is in the basilar artery

8.7 Technique

There are a number of microballoons available for performing vasospasm angioplasty. A latex balloon was originally described for this purpose by Zubkov et al. (1984). More recently a silicone balloon (Interventional Therapeutics Corporation, South San Francisco, California) has been developed which measures 3 mm in diameter and 12 mm in length when fully inflated (Fig. 8.1). The advantage of this microballoon is that it requires a low inflation pressure (0.5 atm) and readily conforms to the shape of the vessel lumen. With overinflation, the balloon elongates and does not increase in diameter. This low inflation pressure and the tendency to elongate rather than overdilate reduce the risk of vessel rupture. The low inflation pressure is particularly valuable because with lower inflation pressure there is less risk of damage to the vessel. Also the balloon can be navigated through the intracranial circulation

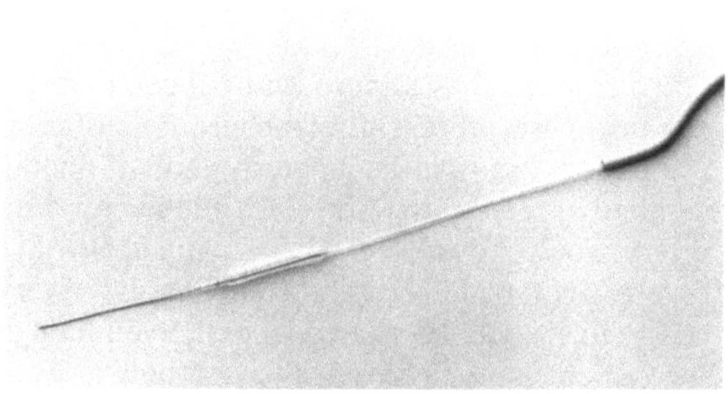

Fig. 8.2. Steerable polyethylene microballoon. The steerable microguidewire passes through the center of the balloon. (Courtesy of Target Therapeutics Corporation, San Jose, CA)

without the need of a guidewire. This further reduces the risk of endothelial damage.

A polyethylene microballoon (Target Therapeutics Corporation, San Jose, California) has recently been developed. The inflated diameter of this balloon is 2.5 mm with a length of 15 mm (Fig. 8.2). This balloon utilizes a higher inflation pressure (up to 5 atm), which is sometimes necessary in chronic vasospasm when there is more fibrosis within the vessel wall. These more fibrotic vessels sometimes do not respond to the lower pressure silicone balloon. The polyethylene balloon also uses a steerable microguidewire for navigation and this can be quite useful when trying to enter vessels arising at right angles from the parent artery. This system has been particularly valuable for entering branches such as the A-1 segment of the anterior cerebral artery (Fig. 8.3).

Both balloons are attached to a 150 cm variable stiffness microcatheter which allows for transfemoral catheterization. Larger balloons (> than 3 mm in diameter) are available, but these larger diameters are not necessary for intracranial vessels and are much more hazardous because of the increased risk of overdistention and vessel rupture.

As mentioned earlier, latex balloons also work for vasospasm angioplasty. Latex balloons typically have higher inflation pressures than silicone balloons. To counteract this, some work has been done with calibrated leak latex balloons. The calibrated leak allows for lower pressure inflation. Latex balloons have a tendency to increase in diameter, rather than elongate, with overinflation, and care must be taken not to rupture the vessel.

The basic transfemoral technique consists in a large introducer catheter being placed in the

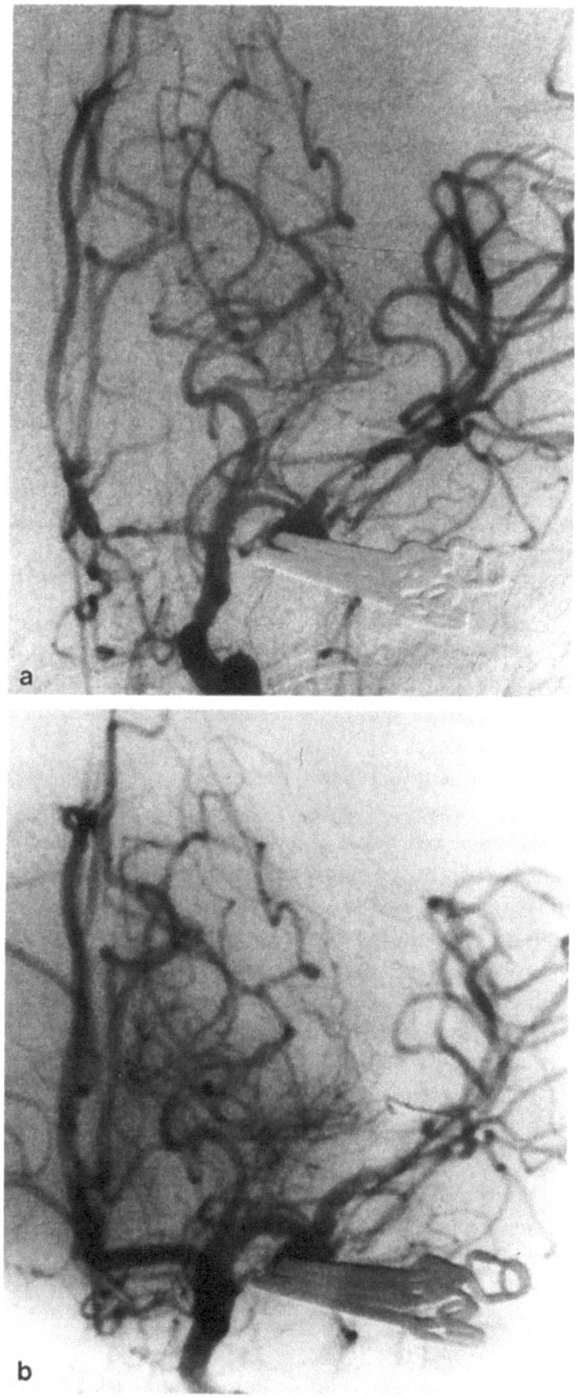

Fig. 8.3. **a** Angiography shows severe spasm of the proximal anterior and middle cerebral arteries. Clips are present on the middle cerebral artery aneurysm. The steerable balloon was needed to enter the anterior cerebral artery and the middle cerebral artery distal to the aneurysm. **b** Following angioplasty, there is marked improvement in the caliber of the anterior and middle cerebral arteries

internal carotid or vertebral artery. Through this introducer catheter, the microballoon can be passed. High resolution digital fluoroscopic equipment with digital road-mapping capabilities is essential for the safe performance of the procedure. Through the large introducer catheter repeated road-maps can be obtained during the course of angioplasty. Utilizing the road-mapping technique, a balloon can be kept out of small side branches that would rupture with balloon inflation. The technique consists in multiple rapid (less than 5 s) inflations and deflations along the course of the vessel in spasm, usually beginning in the most proximal segment and extending distally. Heparinization is used if the aneurysm has been clipped. Immediately after the procedure, the heparin is reversed by protamine sulfate. If the patient is able to remain stationary, the procedure can be done under neuroleptic analgesia. But if there is motion, general anesthesia should be used. Any patient motion reduces the effectiveness of road-mapping techniques and increases the danger of small vessel rupture. Vessel rupture in these cases is almost always fatal.

The question often arises about how far distally in the vessel should angioplasty be performed. Basically with present balloon technology, angioplasty cannot be safely performed beyond the M-2 segment of the middle cerebral artery or the P-1 segment of the posterior cerebral artery; anterior cerebral artery catheterization should not extend much beyond the A-1 segment. Once the microballoon passes these points, the balloon becomes much larger than the vessel and obviously if inflation is performed with a balloon diameter that exceeds the vessel diameter, there is a very high risk of vessel rupture. Until smaller balloons are developed, catheterization and angioplasty beyond these points will not be safe.

8.8 Approach to the Patient

Following a subarachnoid hemorrhage, the offending aneurysm is usually treated. TCD is then used to monitor for the earliest signs of vasospasm. Once the velocities start to increase, medical therapy, including hypertensive and hypervolemic therapy as well as calcium channel blockers, is started. If the patient becomes symptomatic a head CT scan is immediately performed. If there is no explanation on the CT scan for the new deficit, it is assumed that vasospasm is the etiology. The patient then undergoes angiography to evaluate the total extent of vasospasm.

To date, the basic approach has been to dilate any vasospasm present intracranially. For instance, if a patient has right hemiparesis and left middle cerebral artery spasm, the left middle cerebral artery would be dilated. If the patient also has severe right middle cerebral and basilar artery spasm this would be dilated as well, even though the patient is not necessarily symptomatic from these arteries. There have been two cases in our experience where we did not do this and we had to repeat the angioplasty on the asymptomatic vessels 2 days later when the patient became symptomatic. Also the degree of spasm in the asymptomatic vessels would be a factor. If the spasm is mild, the vessels would not be dilated. If the spasm is severe, even though the patient is asymptomatic at that time, angioplasty would be performed.

In the patient with an isolated hemiparesis and aphasia, the spasm is usually located in the supraclinoid carotid and middle and anterior cerebral arteries. Typically in these cases, it is sufficient to dilate the supraclinoid and middle cerebral arteries (Fig. 8.4). If possible, it is good to dilate the proximal anterior cerebral artery as well, but this is often difficult to do. Many times dilatation of the supraclinoid carotid and middle cerebral arteries alone will dramatically increase the flow in the anterior cerebral artery despite not dilating the proximal anterior cerebral artery (Fig. 8.5).

The approach to the comatose patient is slightly more complicated. The coma center of the brain is in the ascending reticular activating system which extends from the medial midbrain up through the dorsal thalamus (Plum and Posner 1980). This critical area is supplied by the thalamoperforating arteries arising from the P-1 segments of the posterior cerebral arteries. In over 85% of people, the thalamoperforators arising from each proximal posterior cerebral artery anastomose in the midline. Because of this anastomosis it usually requires occlusion of both posterior cerebrals to induce coma. Therefore when treating the comatose patient, one should dilate the vertebrobasilar system and at least one proximal posterior cerebral artery. It would be best to dilate both posterior cerebral arteries, but this is often not possible or safe. Based on anatomic studies, dilatation of one posterior cerebral artery will be sufficient in the majority of patients.

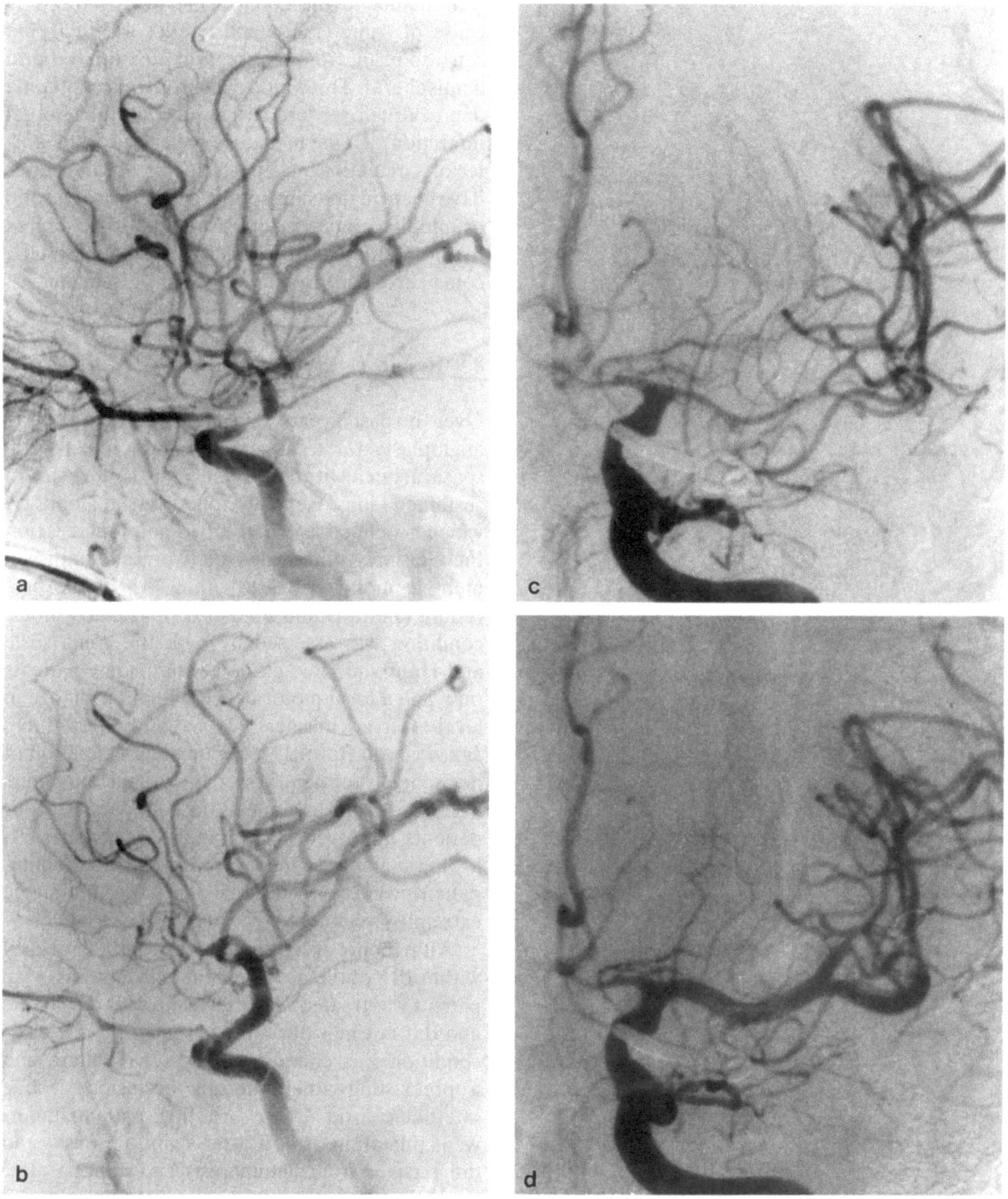

Fig. 8.4. a Lateral angiogram shows severe spasm of the supraclinoid carotid. The patient was hemiparetic and aphasic. **b** Following angioplasty, the supraclinoid carotid and proximal middle cerebral arteries are widely patent. Over the next 2 days the patient completely recovered from hemiparesis and aphasia. There is subtraction artifact from the sella turcica superimposed over the cavernous carotid artery. **c** Angiography shows severe middle cerebral artery spasm. The patient was hemiparetic. **d** Following angioplasty the middle cerebral artery is widely patent. The hemiparesis had completely resolved by the next morning

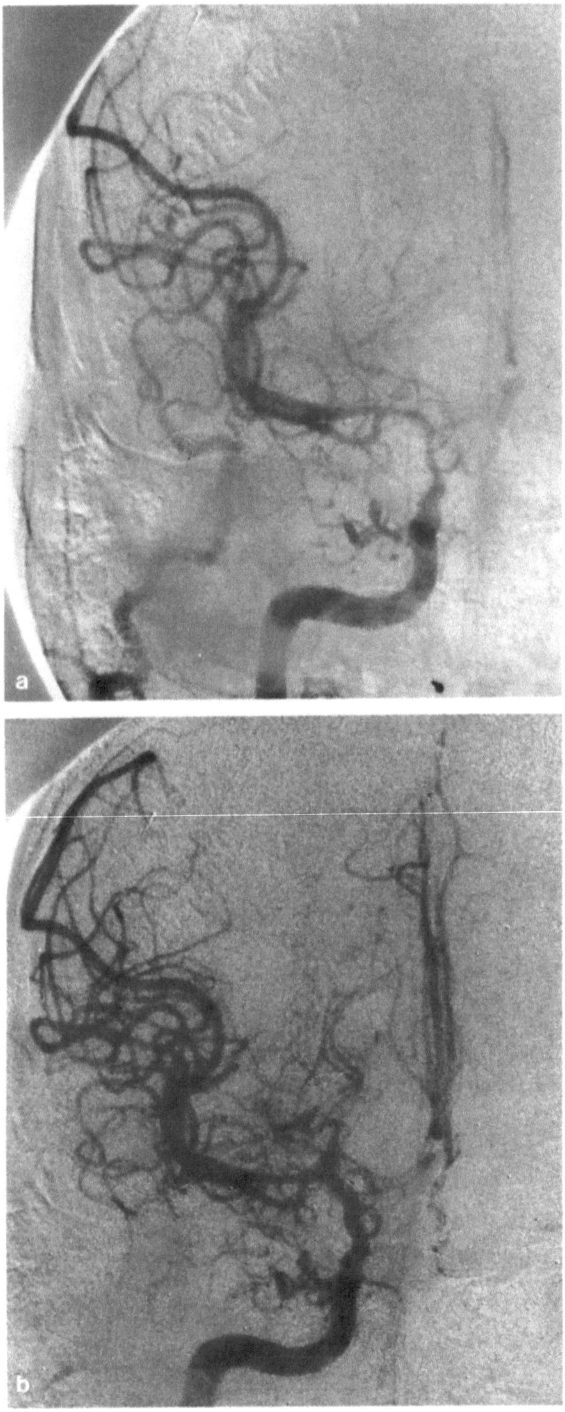

Fig. 8.5. a Angiography reveals spasm of the supraclinoid carotid and proximal anterior and middle cerebral arteries. The patient had 0/5 strength on the left. b Angioplasty was performed on the supraclinoid carotid and proximal middle cerebral arteries. The anterior cerebral artery could not be entered, but there is marked improvement of flow in the anterior cerebral artery distribution. During groin compression following the procedure, the patient was able to move his left foot. The following morning the patient was normal neurologically

Ischemia to the coma center is not the only cause of coma (Plum and Posner 1980). Coma can also result from diffuse injury to both cerebral hemispheres. This would explain instances of coma due to drug overdose and large bilateral cerebral infarctions. In the comatose patient after the posterior circulation and posterior cerebral arteries have been dilated, any spasm in the internal carotid or middle cerebral arteries should also be dilated to make sure that the coma is not a bihemispheric coma secondary to bilateral cortical ischemia.

8.9 Results

Over the past 3 years, 30 patients have undergone angioplasty for treatment of symptomatic vasospasm at our institution. Twenty (66%) have shown sustained improvement following angioplasty, which is defined as either a two-point increase on the Glasgow coma scale or a two-grade improvement in motor strength within 48 h of the procedure (Jennett and Bond 1975). The neurologic condition was assessed by both the coma scale and Hunt and Hess grade because some patients only had a focal motor deficit without a change in level of consciousness (Hunt and Hess 1968; Jennett and Bond 1975). Complete resolution of hemiparesis occurred in six patients and four others improved from hemiplegia to hemiparesis. Four patients improved from grade IV to normal following angioplasty and there were two other similar patients whose only residual deficit was mild single extremity weakness.

All patients except two underwent angioplasty within 18 h of the development of symptoms. One patient was treated 72 h after symptoms developed and did not improve and subsequently died. His condition was complicated by renal failure and a preexisting atherosclerotic occlusion of one internal carotid artery. Another patient underwent dilatation at 48 h after symptom onset and did recover from hemiparesis and aphasia after angioplasty of the left supraclinoid carotid and middle cerebral arteries (Fig. 8.4). Again, our most and dramatic improvements occurred when angioplasty was performed within 12 h of development of symptoms. It is unlikely that patients will have significant improvement when symptoms have been present for longer than 48 h.

Six patients died in our series. Two died from rehemorrhage from unprotected aneurysms. One patient had had a prior unsuccessful attempt at

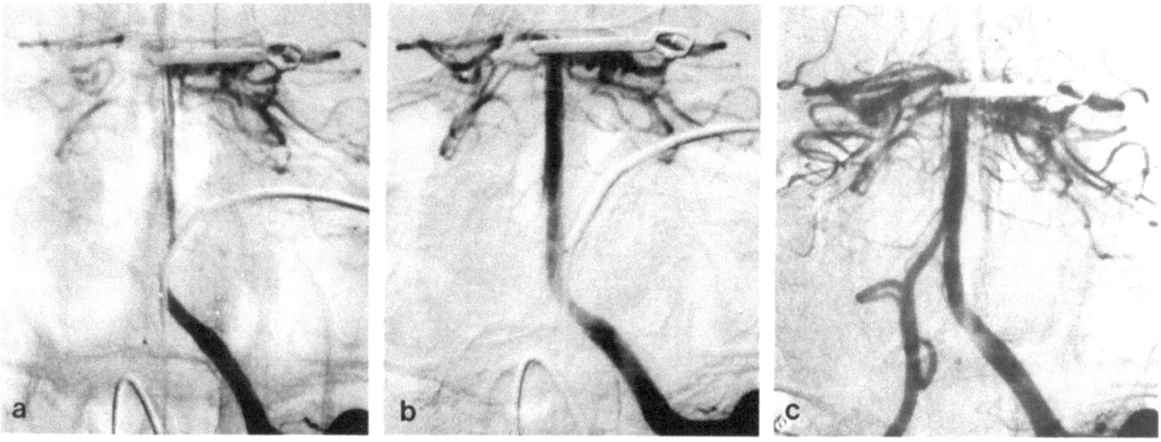

Fig. 8.6. a Angiography following clipping of a basilar tip aneurysm shows severe spasm of the basilar artery. The patient was comatose. b Angiogram immediately after angioplasty of the basilar and left posterior cerebral arteries. The patient made a full recovery over the next 72 h. c Angiography 18 months after angioplasty demonstrates a normal vertebral basilar system. The patient remains normal neurologically

clipping of an aneurysm and was awaiting balloon embolization. While recovering from a second hemorrhage, the patient rebled a third time and died before balloon embolization could be performed. Another patient died from hemorrhage of a mycotic aneurysm arising from the distal posterior cerebral artery. In this patient, angioplasty had been performed on the carotid arteries, but not on the posterior circulation. One patient died during the procedure from a massive hemorrhage. The patient's aneurysm had been only partially clipped. It is not certain whether the patient died from rehemorrhage from the aneurysm or from rupture of the internal carotid artery during balloon dilatation. Three other patients were decerebrate before angioplasty and never recovered and eventually died.

There was one delayed complication. Six weeks following angioplasty, this patient returned with a small middle cerebral infarct and repeat angiography revealed that a middle cerebral branch that had been dilated had occluded. The occluded branch had been dilated with a rigid high pressure balloon that actually ruptured in the vessel. This rigid balloon is no longer used for vasospasm angioplasty. The patient presented with mild hemiparesis from this small branch occlusion, but the hemiparesis completely resolved in 1 week.

Long-term follow-up has been performed for up to 3 years in these patients and all are stable and doing well without any delayed adverse effects. Two patients have undergone repeat angiography 18 months following angioplasty and the vessels are normal without evidence of long-term damage (Figs. 8.6, 8.7). Long-term follow-up with TCD has been done in eight patients and the velocities are normal without evidence of restenosis or vessel damage.

8.10 Complications

Vessel rupture is the most serious complication and this occurs when the balloon is larger in diameter than the vessel. This can occur when the vessel is overdistended with the balloon or when the balloon is placed too distal in the vessel. As mentioned earlier, there is rarely any need to use a balloon larger than 3 mm in diameter. Also going beyond the proximal segments of the anterior, middle, and posterior cerebral arteries is too dangerous with present balloon technology. Again, vessel rupture during angioplasty is usually fatal.

Another complication to be avoided is balloon rupture. As mentioned earlier, there was a delayed branch occlusion 6 weeks after the procedure. The damage that occurs to a vessel during balloon rupture can cause long-term adverse effects. This can usually be avoided when balloon inflation is monitored carefully.

8.11 Conclusion

The pathogenesis of vasospasm following subarachnoid hemorrhage remains poorly understood. Some combination of increased muscular tone, edema, and fibrosis within the vessel wall

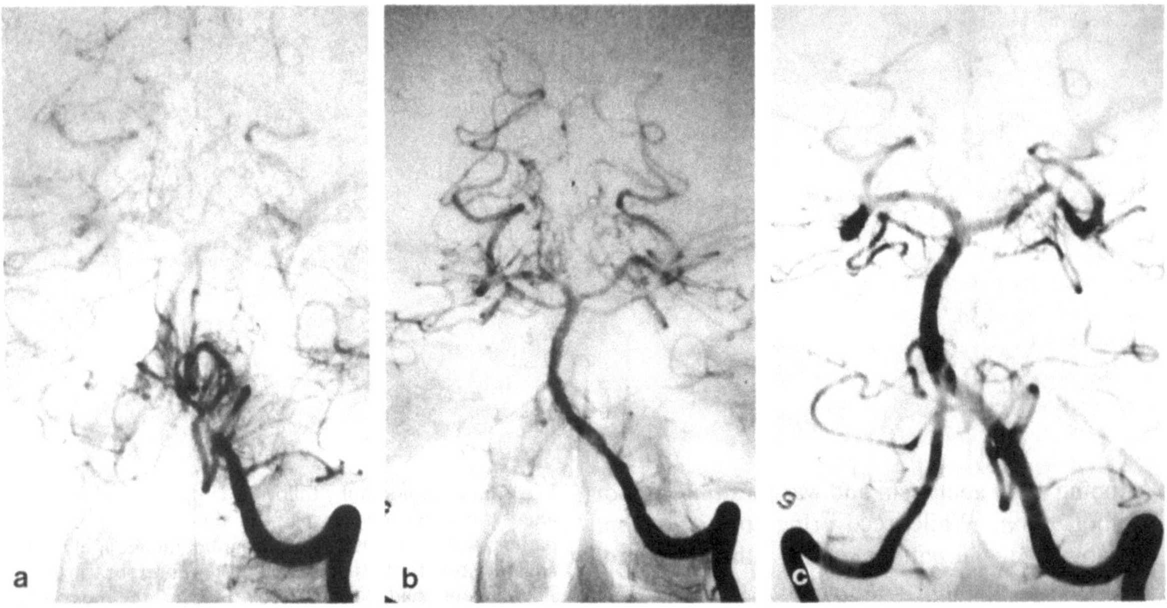

Fig. 8.7. **a** Angiography shows severe spasm of the distal vertebral and proximal basilar arteries. The patient was comatose. **b** Immediately following the angioplasty, the vessel is normal in caliber. Eight hours later the patient had made a full recovery and was normal. **c** Angiography 18 months after angioplasty shows the vertebral basilar system to be normal. The patient remains normal neurologically

must play a role (ECHLIN 1971; ESKRIDGE et al. 1990). Mere mechanical stretching of the vessel would overcome any of these factors. The balloon could easily overcome adhesions from fibrosis within the vessel wall. Also stretching the vessel would counteract the effects of muscular contraction, as well as edema. The effect of angioplasty is persistent, because vasospasm has not been known to recur after angioplasty unless there is another hemorrhage. Also the effect that angioplasty has on the vessel seems to be atraumatic because with up to 3 years' follow-up there has been no evidence of long-term damage to the vessel from this procedure.

The most important factor in the effectiveness of angioplasty is early intervention. The chances of reversing a deficit are obviously greater with early intervention.

There is little doubt, based on the clinical response, angiographic data, and TCD results that angioplasty of vasospasm can markedly improve cerebral perfusion. This restoration of normal perfusion can rapidly reverse neurologic deficits. The preliminary results of angioplasty for symptomatic vasospasm are encouraging. When proper technique is utilized, the technique is effective and has a low complication rate. All major intracranial vessels are amenable to this technique. Angioplasty should prove to be a major advance in the management of subarachnoid hemorrhage.

References

Aaslid R et al. (1982) Noninvasive transcranial Doppler ultrasound recording of flow velocity in basal cerebral arteries. J Neurosurg 57:769–774

Aaslid R et al. (1984) Evaluation of cerebrovascular spasm with transcranial Doppler ultrasound. J Neurosurg 60:37–41

Adams HP et al. (1987) Predicting cerebral ischemia after aneurysmal subarachnoid hemorrhage: influences of clinical condition, CT results, and antifibrinolytic therapy. A report of the cooperative aneurysm study. Neurology 37:1586–1591

Alksne JF (1974) Myonecrosis in chronic experimental vasospasm. Surgery 76:1–7

Alksne F, Greenhoot M (1974) Experimental catecholamine-induced chronic cerebral vasospasm: myonecrosis in vessel wall. J Neurosurg 41:440–445

Allcock JM, Drake CG (1965) Ruptured intracranial aneurysms – the role of arterial spasm. J Neurosurg 22:21–29

Allen GS et al. (1983) Cerebral arterial spasm – a controlled trial of nimodipine in patients with subarachnoid hemorrhage. N Engl J Med 308:619–624

Barker FG, Heros RC (1990) Clinical aspects of vasospasm. Neurosurg Clin North Am 1:277–288

Duff TA et al. (1988) Erythrocytes are essential for development of cerebral vasculopathy resulting from

subarachnoid hemorrhage in cats. Stroke 1:68–72
Echlin FA (1965) Spasm of basilar and vertebral arteries caused by experimental subarachnoid hemorrhage. J Neurosurg 23:1–11
Echlin FA (1971) Experimental vasospasm, acute and chronic, due to blood in the subarachnoid space. J Neurosurg 35:646–656
Ecker A, Riemenschneider PA (1951) Arteriographic demonstration of spasm of the intercranial arteries with special reference to saccular arterial aneurysms. J Neurosurg 8:660–667
Eskridge JM (1989) Interventional neuroradiology. Radiology 172:991–1006
Eskridge JM et al. (1990) Transluminal angioplasty for treatment of vasospasm. Neurosurg Clin North Am 1:387–400
Fein JM et al. (1974) Sequential changes of vascular ultrastructure in experimental cerebral vasospasm. J Neurosurg 41:49–58
Fisher CM (1975) Clinical syndromes in cerebral thrombosis, hypertensive hemorrhage, and ruptured saccular aneurysm. Clin Neurosurg 22:117–147
Fisher CM et al. (1980) Relation of cerebral vasospasm to subarachnoid hemorrhage visualized by computerized tomographic scanning. Neurosurgery 6:1–9
Folkow B (1982) Physiologic aspects of primary hypertension. Physiol Rev 62:347–503
Graf CJ, Nibbelink DW (1974) Cooperative study of intracranial aneurysms and subarachnoid hemorrhage: report on a randomized treatment study. Stroke 5: 559–601
Gull W (1859) Cases of aneurism of the cerebral vessels. Guy's Hosp Rep 5:281–304
Harders AG, Gilsbach JM (1987) Time course of blood velocity changes related to vasospasm in the circle of Willis measured by transcranial Doppler ultrasound. J Neurosurg 66:718–728
Heros RC et al. (1983) Cerebral vasospasm after subarachnoid hemorrhage: an update. Ann Neurol 14:599–608
Higashida RT et al. (1989) Transluminal angioplasty for treatment of intracranial arterial vasospasm. J Neurosurg 71:648–653
Hughes JT, Schianchi PM (1978) Cerebral artery spasm: a histological study at necropsy of the blood vessels in cases of subarachnoid hemorrhage. J Neurosurg 48: 515–525
Hunt WE, Hess RM (1968) Surgical risk as related to time of intervention in the repair of intracranial aneurysms. J Neurosurg 28:14–20
Jennett B, Bond M (1975) Assessment of outcome after severe brain damage. Lancet I:480–484
Kistler JP et al. (1983) The relation of cerebral vasospasm to the extent and location of subarachnoid blood visualized by CT scan: a prospective study. Neurology 33:424–436
Kwak R et al. (1979) Angiographic study of cerebral vasospasm following rupture of intracranial aneurysms: part I. Time of the appearance. Surg Neurol 11:257–262
Liszczak TM et al. (1983) Cerebral arterial constriction after experimental subarachnoid hemorrhage is associated with blood components within the arterial wall. J Neurosurg 58:18–26
Mayberg MR et al. (1978) Ultrastructural changes in feline arterial endothelium following subarachnoid hemorrhage. J Neurosurg 48:49–57
Mizukami M et al. (1982) Prevention of vasospasm by early operation with removal of subarachnoid blood. Neurosurgery 10:301–307
Morawetz RB et al. (1979) Regional cerebral blood flow thresholds during cerebral ischemia. Fed Proc 38: 2493–2494
Mullan S (1975) Conservative management of the recently ruptured aneurysm. Surg Neurol 3:27–32
Newell DW et al. (1989) Angioplasty for the treatment of symptomatic vasospasm following subarachnoid hemorrhage. J Neurosurg 71:654–660
Owada K et al. (1977) Cervical sympathectomy for cerebral ischemic lesions; a follow-up study. Tohoku Med J (Sendai) 90:183
Owada K, Hori S, Suzuki J (1979) Results of cervical sympathectomy for cerebral vasospasm following aneurysmal rupture. In: Suzuki J (ed) Cerebral aneurysms. Neuron, Sendai, p 435
Philippon J et al. (1986) Prevention of vasospasm in subarachnoid haemorrhage. A controlled study with nimodipine. Acta Neurochir (Wien) 82:110–114
Plum F, Posner J (1980) Diagnosis of stupor and coma 3rd edn. FA Davis, Philadelphia
Robertson E (1949) Cerebral lesions due to intracranial aneurysms. Brain 72:150–185
Ropper AH, Zervas NT (1984) Outcome 1 year after SAH from cerebral aneurysm. J Neurosurg 60:909–915
Sah A et al. (1969) Intracranial aneurysms and subarachnoid hemorrhage. Philadelphia, JB Lippincott
Saito I, Sano K (1980) Vasospasm after aneurysm rupture: incidence, onset, and course. In: Wilkins RH (ed) Cerebral arterial spasm: proceedings of the Second International Workshop, Amsterdam, the Netherlands 1979. Williams & Wilkins 1980, pp 294–301
Simeone FA, Trepper P (1972) Cerebral vasospasm with infarction. Stroke 3:449–455
Stornelli SA, French JD (1964) Subarachnoid hemorrhage – factors in prognosis and management. J Neurosurg 21:769–780
Sundt TM Jr (1975) Chemical management of cerebral vasospasm. In: Whisnant JP, Sandoc BA (eds) Cerebral vascular disease, proceedings of the 9th Princeton Conference, 1974. Grune & Stratton, New York, p 77
Tanabe Y et al. (1978) Cerebral vasospasm and ultrastructural changes in cerebral arterial wall. J Neurosurg 49:229–238
Tanishima T (1980) Cerebral vasospasm: contractile activity of hemoglobin in isolated canine basilar arteries. J Neurosurg 53:787–793
Varsos VG et al. (1983) Delayed cerebral vasospasm is not reversible by aminophylline, nifedipine or papavarine in a "two-hemorrhage" canine model. J Neurosurg 58:11–17
Wilkins RH (1979) Attempted prevention or treatment of intracranial arterial spasm: a survey. In: Wilkins RH (ed) Cerebral arterial spasm. Williams and Wilkins, Baltimore, p 542
Zervas NT et al. (1982) Cerebrospinal fluid may nourish cerebral vessels through pathways in the adventitia that may be analogous to systemic vasa vasorum. J Neurosurg 56:475–481
Zubkov YN et al. (1984) Balloon catheter technique for dilatation of constricted cerebral arteries after aneurysmal SAH. Acta Neurochir (Wien) 70:65–79
Zucker MB (1944) A study of the substances in blood serum and platelets which stimulate smooth muscle. Am J Physiol 142:12–26

9 Embolization of Arteriovenous Malformations of the Spinal Cord

GEORGES RODESCH, PIERRE LASJAUNIAS, and ALEX BERENSTEIN

CONTENTS

9.1 Introduction

Arteriovenous malformations of the spinal cord (SCAVMs) are rare lesions of congenital origin (HURTH et al. 1978) that represent only about one-tenth of cerebral AVMs (COGEN and STEIN 1983). Their natural history (AMINOFF and LOGUE 1974a,b; BAILEY and SPERL 1969; HURTH et al. 1978; TOBIN 1976) and their physiopathology (AMINOFF et al. 1974; ARSENI and SAMITCA 1959; GROSS and RALSTON 1959; HURTH et al. 1978; SPETZLER et al. 1989; WYBURN MASON 1943) are still poorly understood, and the treatment required is often difficult, controversial, and challenging (AUSMAN et al. 1977; COGEN and STEIN 1983; DJINDJIAN 1975, 1976; DJINDJIAN and MERLAND 1978; DOPPMAN et al. 1971; HORTON et al. 1986; HOUDART et al. 1974; KITO et al. 1983; KRAYENBUHL et al. 1969; LATCHAW and GOLD 1979; MALIS 1979; MARGOLIS and BIRCHFIELD 1974; MARGOLIS et al. 1979; MORGAN et al. 1986; NEWTON and ADAMS 1968; OMMAYA et al. 1969; PATTERSON and VOORHIES 1978; RICHE et al. 1983; STEIN 1979; THERON et al. 1986; YASARGIL et al. 1975). This lack of knowledge stems from the small size of the published series and the different classifications used by different authors, based on surgical (ROSENBLUM et al. 1987; SPETZLER et al. 1989) or angiographic (RICHE et al. 1983a,b, 1985) considerations. We believe that the distinction between intra- and extramedullary location, widely used in the literature and regarded as a determinant of further treatment, is anatomically inappropriate since all the lesions are subpial, as is also the case with their cerebral homologues (HASSLER et al. 1989; MAILLOT 1991; NICHOLAS and WELLER 1988). This distinction is relevant in respect of surgical data and concerns, but it cannot be applied to endovascular approaches. For example, SCAVMs fed by the anterior spinal axis and previously described as intramedullary may in fact be purely extramedullary, embedded in the anterior spinal sulcus without involvement of the spinal cord itself, like sulcal AVMs of the brain. We shall therefore concentrate our analysis primarily on the anatomic (GARCIA-MONACO and LASJAUNIAS 1990; LASJAUNIAS and BERENSTEIN 1990) and angioarchitectural aspects of SCAVMs (BERENSTEIN and LASJAUNIAS 1992; LASJAUNIAS and BERENSTEIN 1990; RODESCH et al. 1991). Spinal cord angiography at present remains the gold standard for evaluation of these lesions; MRI, although providing diagnostic indications in respect of SCAVMs and excellent information on the spinal cord itself, is unable to reveal the exact location and type of AV shunt involved (DI CHIRO et al. 1985; DOPPMAN et al. 1987; MASARYK et al. 1987; MODIK et al. 1989; RODESCH et al. 1991). Currently MRI and MR angiographic study are unable to provide any of the answers required in order to reach decisions on therapy and technique.

GEORGES RODESCH, M.D.; PIERRE LASJAUNIAS, M.D., Ph.D., Professor of Radiology and Neurosurgery; Unité de Neuroradiologie Vasculaire Diagnostique et Thérapeutique, Hôpital Bicêtre, Université Paris Sud, 78, Rue du Général Leclerc, 94275 Kremlin-Bicêtre, France

ALEX BERENSTEIN, M.D., Professor of Radiology and Neurosurgery, Department of Radiology, New York University Medical Center, 560 First Avenue, New York, NY 10016, USA

9.2 Spinal Cord Angiography – Technique

About 200 spinal vascular examinations have been performed in our department in the last 15 years. The youngest patient in whom we performed spinal cord angiography was 6 months old and the oldest was 82 years old. We believe that there is a priori no contraindication to spinal angiography if one attentively follows specific technical rules and angiographic protocols (BERENSTEIN and LASJAUNIAS 1992; GARCIA-MONACO and LASJAUNIAS 1990; LASJAUNIAS and BERENSTEIN 1990; WILLINSKY et al. 1990).

Diagnostic angiograms and, by extension, embolization procedures, are performed under general anesthesia without the use (even for endovascular occlusion) of peroperative functional testing [evoked potentials (BERENSTEIN et al. 1984) or other tests]; a femoral sheath with straight saline coaxial flushing is always placed first.

Exploration of the cervical spinal cord is done with a 4F catheter (Nycomed Ingenor) that allows superselective catheterization of both the vertebral and the ascending and deep cervical arteries. Low osmolar contrast material is routinely used (Hexabrix 320, Laboratoires Guerbet) and contrast injection rates in adults are 4 cc/s over 3 s (total 12 cc) for vertebral arteries and 1 cc/s over 4 s for each cervical artery (total 4 cc). These amounts can be significantly reduced in the pediatric population, where a total dose of 4–6 cc/kg body weight is generally accepted. In our opinion conventional angiograms still provide the best detail when dealing with this pathology. In general, only anteroposterior (AP) views are used, although lateral projections are employed exceptionally.

Exploration of the thoracolumbar spinal cord is performed with a spinal cord catheter (5F-4F, Nycomed Ingenor). Each intercostal and iliolumbar artery is catheterized selectively and explored using fluoroscopy. When on visualizes a radiculomedullary artery (or a radiculopial artery), a series of films is taken with injection of 9 cc contrast at a rate of 1 cc/s. Thirteen conventional films are taken, paying special attention to the venous phase of the series (17th, 20th, and 22nd seconds). In all the cases in which this protocol was used, we obtained good visualization of all the arteries and veins of the spinal cord. Failure to visualize a normal venous phase despite a correct protocol (selective injection, venous opacification proving that the catheter is not wedged) is the best indication of venous congestion. Visualization of the veins on the last three films of the run confirms the absence of a venous constraint (GARCIA-MONACO and LASJAUNIAS 1990; WILLINSKY et al. 1990). The main view used in this exploration is again the AP projection. We consider that global injection (aortography) as a primary modality of exploration is inappropriate. We only perform it when selective study has proved not to be feasible (3% of our cases).

Exploration of the sacral region is performed with a 4F catheter (Nycomed Ingenor) and selective catheterization of the median and lateral sacral arteries is performed. About 6 cc of contrast is injected at a rate of 3 cc/s. These vessels are generally explored when there is suspicion of a dural fistula: one should begin with the analysis of these pedicles in order to avoid filling of the bladder with contrast, which could mask the region of interest. In most cases, proper injection of the median sacral artery opacifies the lateral sacral artery systems bilaterally.

Morbidity due to diagnostic angiography is less than 0.5% (no morbidity in our series). Choice of contrast material is important since a 2% neurologic complication rate has been observed in a similar number of patients at the Mayo Clinic. Non-ionic contrast material has not been shown to provide any specific advantage.

9.3 Classification and Angioarchitecture of Arteriovenous Malformations of the Spinal Cord (SCAVMs)

The concept of angioarchitecture has been discussed previously in the study of the relationship between brain AVMs and hemorrhage (LASJAUNIAS et al. 1986; WILLINSKY et al. 1988). Our analysis of SCAVMs is based on the same ideas and data. As assessed by HURTH et al. (1978), SCAVMs have a congenital origin but several acquired phenomena alter the aspect of this primary defect. They constitute the response of the vascular system to the chronicity of the AV shunt. We believe that most of these features are time related, despite the personal susceptibility of individuals. This combined (inborn and acquired) angioarchitecture of the SCAVM expresses the equilibrium established between the lesion and the remaining normal vasculature, and therefore the surrounding parenchyma. This establishes the role of the "host": The traditional statistical reviews and concepts of aggressiveness of lesions postulate that every vasculature responds in the same way, and ignore the fact that patients' biology varies. Based on retrospective information, obtained by analysis of the angioarchitecture, an analysis of projected risks will determine whether the patient is at risk and whether treatment should be proposed. Currently we consider the endovascular approach to be the primary treatment modality, this being guided by the angioarchitectural information and the functional status of the tissue (information provided by angiography and MRI). Therefore the distinction between an intra- and an extramedullary location of the lesion is not of primary importance for the treatment and will only be discussed if surgery is chosen (which chiefly occurs when the endovascular approach has failed or is thought not to be feasible).

9.3.1 Types of SCAVMs

Over the last 10 years we have treated 59 patients with SCAVMs. On the basis of the anatomic specimens and angiographic studies, several types of SCAVM can be described:

1. *Arteriovenous fistulas* (AVFs) (Fig. 9.1) (12 cases = 20%). In these cases a direct communication exists between a spinal cord artery and a spinal cord vein, without interposition of any vașcular network (AMINOFF et al. 1988; BERENSTEIN and LASJAUNIAS 1992). These lesions are always superficial to the cord. They are frequently encountered in children and Rendu-Osler-Weber disease.
2. *Arteriovenous malformations* (AVMs) (45 cases = 76%). In this type a network of pathologic vessels is interposed between the arterial feeders and the venous drainage. A true nidus with direct or indirect supply can then be identified, as in brain AVMs. In two of our cases direct fistulas also existed in the depth of the nidus itself. Anatomically this type of SCAVM can be superficial or buried in the cord.
3. *Micro arteriovenous malformations* (mAVMs). These lesions consist of a small nidus or fistulous point fed by a "normal sized" artery and draining into a "normal sized" vein. In fact the draining vein of the mAVM is enlarged and corresponds to a small pial vein usually not seen at angiography. These lesions are not visualized by MRI: they can only be detected by angiography and their only mode of presentation is hemorrhage.
4. *Multiple AVMs* (7 cases = 12%). SCAVMs may be associated with cerebral AVMs (one case), with vascular phakomatoses (EHLERS-DANLOS, VON HIPPEL-LINDAU, and KLIPPEL-TRENAUNAY syndromes) (BENHAIEM-SIGAUX et al. 1985), or with osseous localizations of AVMs. The involvement of skin, vertebra, and spinal cord by vascular malformations at the same metameric level constitutes the Cobb syndrome (metameric angiomatosis). One should remember that the dura is never involved in this syndrome. We have never encountered multiple AVMs purely involving the spinal cord at several segments, even in Rendu-Osler-Weber disease.

9.3.2 Angioarchitectural Analysis and Related Symptomatology

Symptoms can be related to arterial steal and/or venous congestion. Our knowledge in respect of dural arteriovenous shunts (KENDALL and LOGUE 1977; LASJAUNIAS et al. 1986; MERLAND et al. 1980) (see below) and brain AVMs indicates that the venous drainage and its consequences for the spinal cord parenchyma are most likely responsible for the subacute and chronic symptomatology.

Spontaneously progressive changes resulting from the chronicity of the arteriovenous shunt (high flow angiopathy) will be detected. Hemorrhagic complications will also create additional features to look for. Traumatic, iatrogenic, or other changes will finally have to be recognized. Therefore the image of the lesion itself will be distinct from the images of events that have occurred.

One can distinguish:

1. *Arterial stenoses*. Arterial stenoses are located on the feeding vessel of the malformation, but may be detected remote from it. They represent a manifestation of the high flow angiopathy and have to be distinguished from the normal transdural stenosis of the spinal arteries (Fig. 10.1k). These flow-related changes are most often seen at the cervical level, while dysplastic (fusiform) changes are more likely to be noted at the thoracolumbar level.
2. *Arterial aneurysms* (AAs) (Figs. 9.2, 9.3). Arterial aneurysms are to be considered differently according to their localization (Table 9.1). Cervical AAs are also part of the high flow angiopathy (like intracranial flow-related

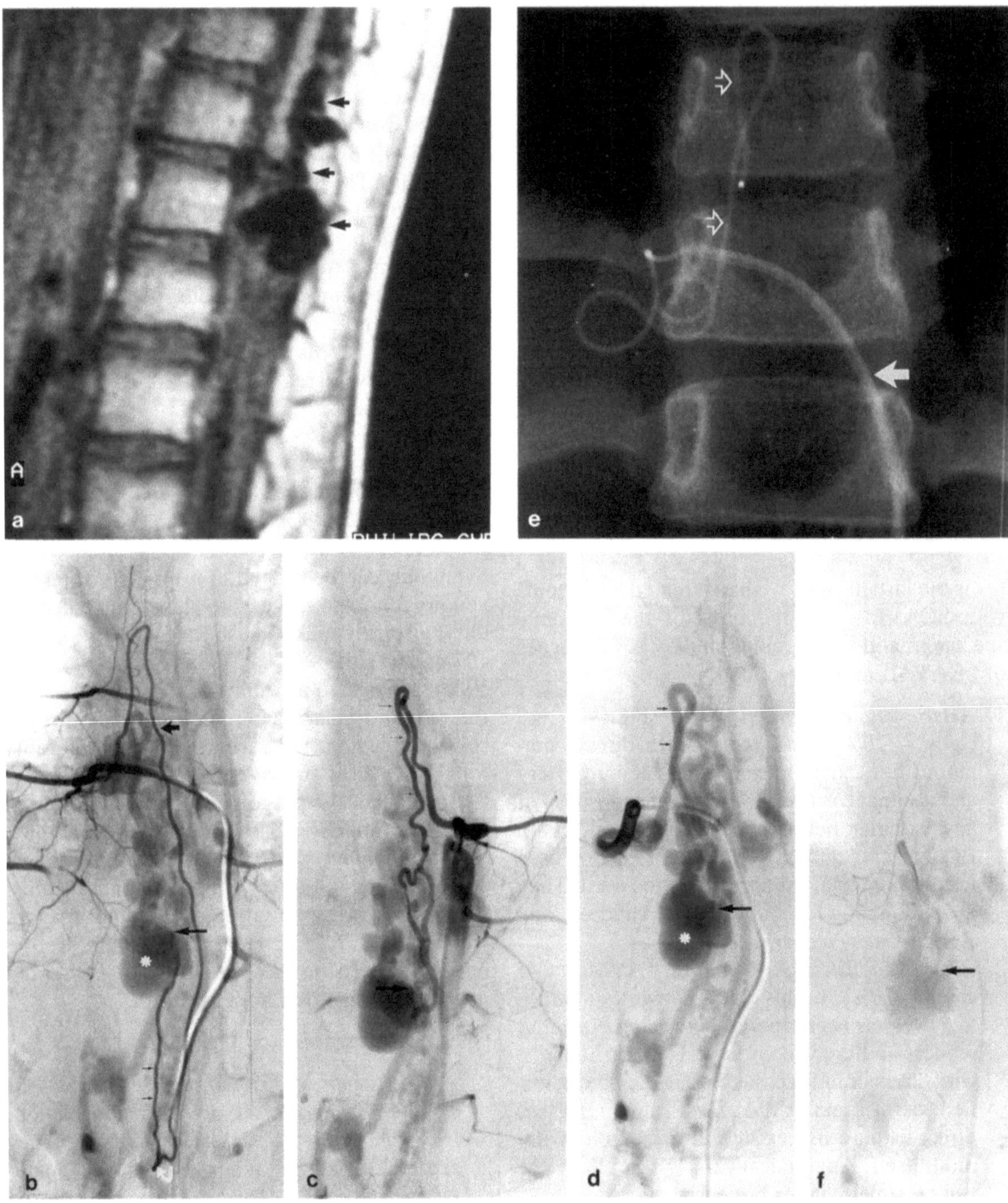

Fig. 9.1a–n. 9½-year-old boy presenting with acute abdominal and dorsal pain associated with neck stiffness. A lumbar puncture was performed and showed hemorrhagic CSF. Neurologic examination was normal except for spasticity of both lower limbs of long duration. **a** MRI of the thoracolumbar junction. Sagittal view, T1-weighted image. Structures of low signal intensity (*arrows*) are detected at the posterior surface of the dorsal spinal cord, suggesting large vascular channels. The precise localization and exact nature of this vascular lesion could not be assessed and angiography was performed. **b** Selective injection of the right T9 intercostal artery shows the anterior spinal axis. Its descending branch (*large arrow*) reaches the basket (*curved arrow*) and opacifies a radiculopial artery (*small arrows*) that terminates in a large venous ectasia (*asterisk*) through a fistulous point (*long arrow*). From this pouch, ascending and descending venous drainage can be assessed. **c** Selective injection of the left T9 intercostal artery shows a radiculopial artery (*small arrows*), reaching the SCAVM through the same fistulous point (*long arrow*). **d** Selective injection of the right T10 intercostal artery opacifies a large radiculopial artery (*small arrows*) opening into the venous ectasia previously described (*asterisk*) through the same fistulous point (*long arrow*).

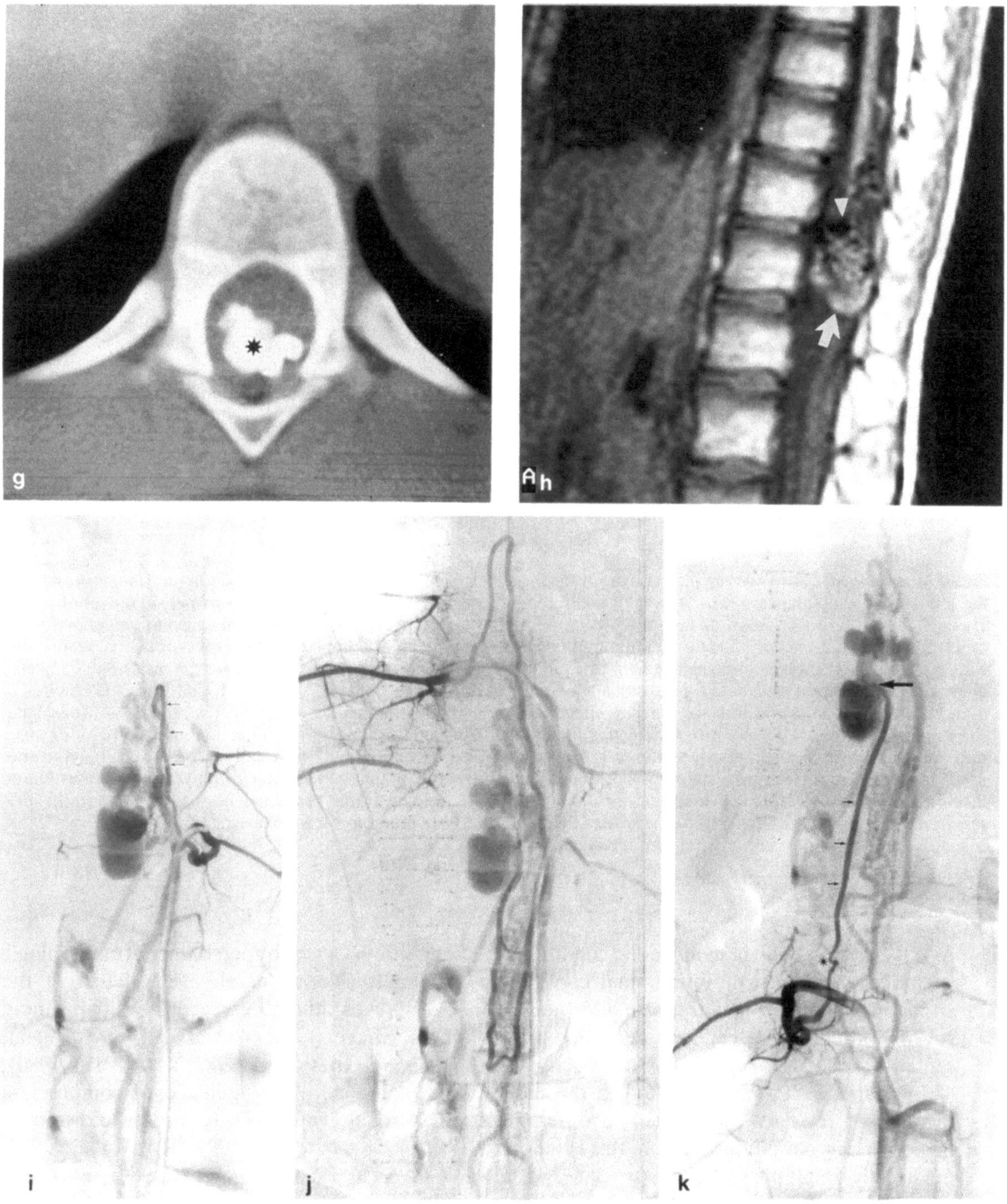

◁ **Fig. 9.1** (*continued*). The SCAVM is a single hole direct fistula AVF located at the posterior surface of the dorsal spinal cord at the T11 level. The venous pouch is responsible for a mass effect that displaces the spinal cord laterally (see **b**). **e** Endovascular treatment of the AVF was decided upon; through a 5F thin-walled catheter (*arrow*) a Mini-torquer (Nycomed Ingenor) (*open arrows*) was introduced into the right T10 radiculopial artery. **f** Pre-embolization injection of contrast (Hexabrix 320, Laboratoire Guerbet) opacifies clearly the arteriovenous shunt (*arrow*) and the venous ectasia. In this position 0.4 ml of a 20% mixture of NBCA and Lipiodol, added to tantalum powder, was injected. Partial occlusion of the pouch was obtained. The child remained neurologically unchanged. **g** Nonenhanced CT scan at the T11 level shows the cast of glue in the venous pouch (*asterisk*). **h** MRI of the thoracolumbar region. Sagittal view. T1-weighted image. The pathologic vascular channels now show a mottled aspect with signals of low intensity (rapid flow; *arrowhead*) and high intensity (slow flow and/or thrombosis; *arrow*). **i** Repeat angiography 2 months later. A moderate reduction in the size of the venous ectasia is noted; the AVF is still open.

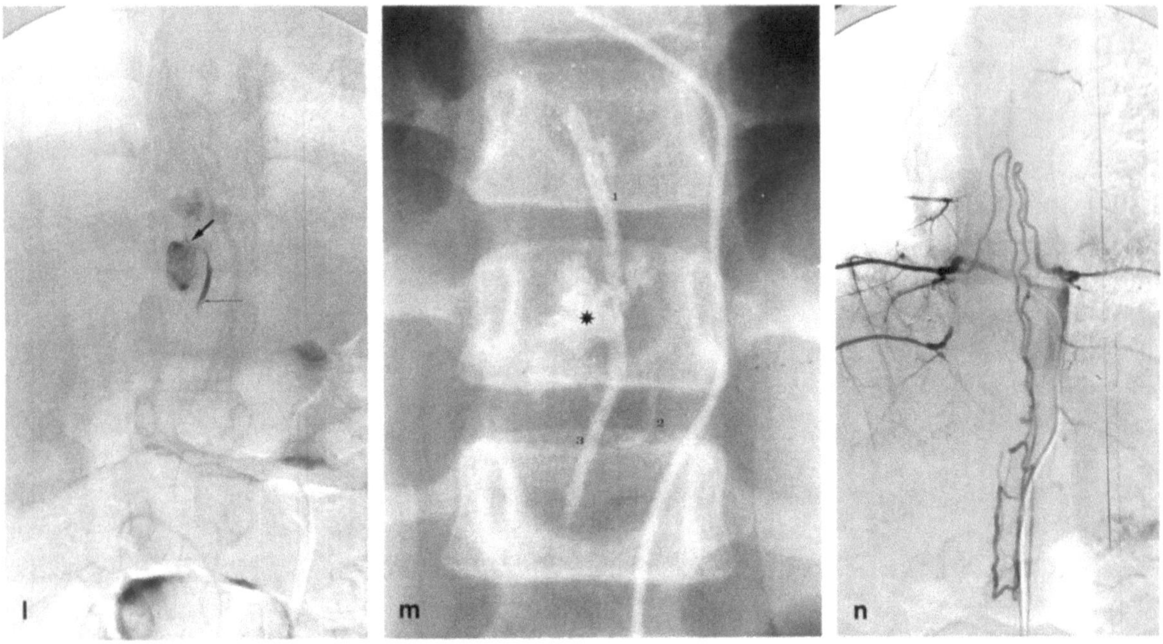

Fig. 9.1 (*continued*). An endovascular approach through the left T9 radiculopial artery (*arrow*) was decided upon. Through a Mini-torquer system, 0.4 ml of a 30% mixture of Histoacryl and Lipiodol, added to tantalum power, was injected (not shown). No changes in the child's neurologic examination were noted. **j** Control angiogram 7 months later, with injection into the anterior spinal axis, shows persistent filling of the AVF. **k** Selective injection into the third right lumbar artery shows a radiculopial artery (*small arrows*) reaching the same previously described fistulous point (*arrow*). Note the stenosis corresponding to the transdural passage of the artery (*asterisk*). **l** Superselective catheterization with a Mini-torquer system was carried out. The tip of the catheter (*long arrow*) was placed 1 cm below the fistula (*arrow*). **m** 0.4 ml of a 30% mixture of NBCA and Lipiodol added to tantalum powder was injected. Complete occlusion was obtained. Plain radiography of the dorsal region shows the casts of glue injected during the first (*1*), second (*2*), and third (*3*) sessions of embolization, as the pouch filled with NBCA (*asterisk*). **n** Final control angiogram: injection into the right T9 intercostal artery. The AVF is totally cured. Radiculopial arteries are still patent but do not fill any arteriovenous shunt. Neurologic status remained normal except for the previously noted lower limb spasticity

AAs) (Fig. 9.2). The hemodynamic conditions are indeed the same in the intracranial, cervical, and upper thoracic localizations. Of the 23 AVMs located in the cervical area, nine presented AAs (39%).

In contrast, SCAVMs situated in the thoracolumbar region are subjected to different hemodynamic conditions. AAs in this location are usually dysplastic and often associated with a recognized arterial dysplastic condition (e.g., Klippel-Trenaunay syndrome) (Fig. 10.3). Thirty-six AVMs in our series were located in the thoracolumbar region and only eight presented AAs (23%).

True isolated AAs at the spinal cord level are rare. They can be associated with aortic coarctation, dysplastic conditions (Kito et al. 1983; Saunders et al. 1987), infectious diseases (of mycotic origin), or special hemodynamic conditions caused by persistence of embryologic channels (Yonas et al. 1980). Most of the AAs reveal their presence by subarachnoid hemorrhage (Garcia et al. 1979; Kito et al. 1983; Saunders et al. 1987; Yonas et al. 1980), but some do so by spinal cord compression (Saunders et al. 1987). According to the literature (Garcia et al. 1979; Kito et al. 1983; Smith et al. 1986; Yonas et al. 1980), more than three-quarters of AAs arise on the anterior spinal axis (ASA). Review of most of these papers in fact confirms that these so-called ASA AAs are thrombosed ASA AVFs; and mechanical effects, related to venous pouches.

In our experience AAs associated with SCAVMs represent materialized weakness of the vasculature, explaining previous complications and suggesting future hazards. Of the 17 AVMs that presented AAs, eight were as-

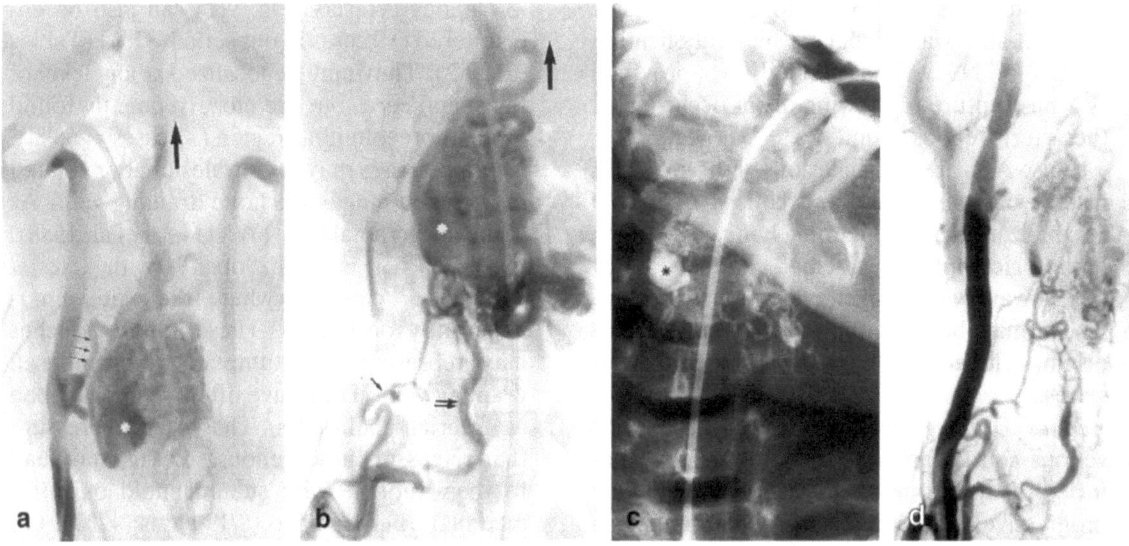

Fig. 9.2a–d. 29-year-old female presenting a slowly progressive myelopathy without any history of hemorrhage. Neurologic examination 11 years after the onset of symptoms showed: (1) left hemiparesis affecting predominantly the lower limb but also the face, (2) unstable atactic left hand, (3) left thermalgic hypoesthesia with an upper C1-2 level; (4) right hyperreflexia and impairment of the deep sensibility in the four limbs. Cervical myelography performed in 1985 showed large abnormal vascular structures in the midcervical region. Angiography of the cervical spinal cord demonstrates a large nidus-type AVM located at the C4 level and fed by a radiculo-medullary artery arising at C4 from the right vertebral artery (**a** *small arrows*). Other arterial feeders arose from the C5 and C6 anterior radiculopial arteries (**b** *single arrow and double arrow*) and from the right costocervical trunk. Additional supply came from the left cervical arteries (not shown). The venous drainage of the AVM is predominantly ascending (**a** and **b** *large arrow*). Arterial aneurysms are seen within the malformation (*asterisks*). Since they were considered as weak points of the angioarchitecture, they were embolized first with NBCA. **c** Plain radiography of the cervical spine shows the deposits of glue in the aneurysms and malformation (*asterisks*). **d** Control angiogram 2 years after the beginning of treatment and embolization of six vessels. A dramatic improvement in the symptomatology was noticed after endovascular management. Arterial aneurysms could no longer be detected and a frank decrease (more than 50%) could be observed in the size of the venous drainage (*large arrow*). No other embolization was performed because of the small size of the remaining vessels and the moderate morphologic result that would have been obtained. The patient is scheduled for further control

sociated with a hemorrhagic presentation (47%) (Table 9.2). In practice we preferentially treat the lesions that harbor an AA proximal to the shunt, and primarily the feeders that carry it (Fig. 9.2). So far no patient with an SCAVM

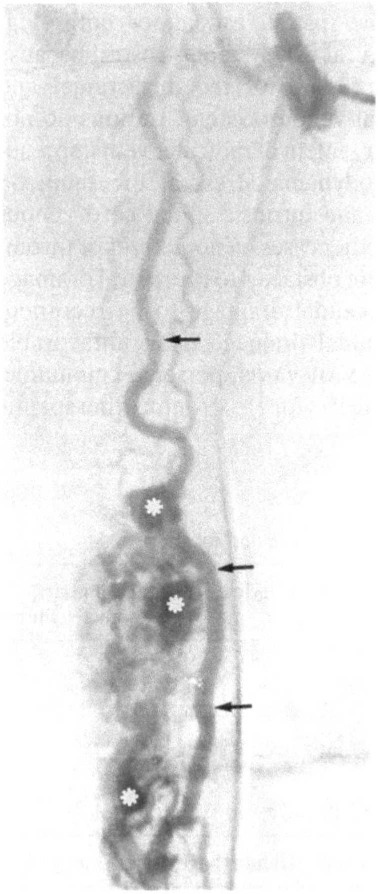

Fig. 9.3. Thoracolumbar spinal cord vascular malformation associated with Klippel-Trenaunay syndrome. Note the dysplastic aspect of the anterior spinal axis (*arrows*) and the associated arterial dysplastic aneurysms (*asterisks*). (By courtesy of R. Piske)

that had presented a previous hemorrhagic episode and was managed by embolization (IBCA or NBCA) has rebled. No proximal AA has ruptured following distal occlusion of the arteriovenous shunt.

False AAs are seen in lesions with a previous history of hemorrhage and consist of partial recanalization of a hematoma lying close to the pathologic ruptured vascular channels. They bear always witness of the hemorrhagic event, which may be of either arterial or venous origin. Three such cases were seen in our series.

3. *Venous Drainage and Related Features*. The venous constraints account for the great majority of symptoms. The symptoms may be progressive, being caused by extensive venous congestion leading to intrinsic disorders and myelopathy (e.g., Foix-Alajouanine syndrome) (CRISCUOLO et al. 1989), or acute following venous rupture or thrombosis. Drainage of the AVM may be rostral, caudal, or both (Fig. 9.2). The natural exit system is rostral because of the low pressure of the intracranial and upper cervical venous system. Lesions do not produce enlargement of radicular veins, spreading the hemodynamic stress of the shunt on the extrinsic and intrinsic spinal cord venous network. In other cases, venous kinks or thrombosis constitute obstacles to the rostral drainage and cause a caudal drainage to be recruited. Therefore caudal drainage is an unfavorable indicator (A. VALAVANIS, personal communication) and calls for a prompt therapeutic decision.

Venous ectasias (Fig. 9.1) can also be encountered (19 cases in our series: 32%) (Tables 9.1, 9.2). They may be localized at any level of the spinal cord, but are most frequently found in the thoracolumbar region (13 cases = 68%). These pouches may be intralesional or related to a kinked mega-dolichotic draining vein. As at the intracranial level (WILLINSKY et al. 1988), these ectasias may be "open" (with a distal outlet) or "closed" (where the exit vein is apparently occluded). These closed pouches may represent the stump of a thrombosed draining vein. They have often been described as arterial aneurysms. The arterial pressure that reigns in these venous ectasias may lead to their rupture with subarachnoid or intramedullary hemorrhage (8/19 cases: 42%). On the other hand, large pouches may compress the nervous parenchyma (Fig. 10.1b) and contribute to the progressive onset of neurologic symptoms. Primary treatment should then be targetted to the highest flow to decrease the venous drainage congestion and shrink the venous pouches.

4. *Dural vascularization and angiogenesis*. Like other AVMs, SCAVMs do not display any proliferative activity. However, angiogenetic activity can occur following ischemia or hemorrhage. Dural supply may follow either cause. Dural supply to an SCAVM is exceptional (one case in our series). It may develop as in intracranial AVMs, following superficial, sometimes infraclinical hemorrhages (WILLINSKY et al. 1988). As yet dural supply has never been demonstrated after incomplete embolizations.

Table 9.1. Angioarchitecture and locations

	Total	Cervical	Thoracolumbar (incl. conus + filum)
Aneurysms	17	9 (53%)	8 (47%)
Venous ectasias	19	6 (32%)	13 (68%)

Table 9.2. Angioarchitecture and symptomatology

	Total	Hemorrhage	Neurologic signs
Aneurysms	17	8 (47%)	9 (53%)
Venous ectasias	19[a]	8 (42%)	10 (53%)

[a] In one case the symptomatology could not be easily classified.

9.4 Semiology of SCAVMs

The locations of SCAVMs encountered in our series are listed in table 10.3. The symptoms caused by SCAVMs and the relationship between these symptoms and the location of the SCAVM are detailed in Tables 10.4 and 9.5, respectively.

Table 9.3. Location of SCAVMs

Cervical	23 (39%)
Thoracolumbar	31 (53%)
Conus	2 (3%)
Filum	3 (5%)
Total	59

Table 9.4. Symptoms of SCAVMs (based on data from DJINDJIAN, ROSENBLUM, YASARGIL, and BERENSTEIN and LASJAUNIAS). (BERENSTEIN and LASJAUNIAS 1992)

	Initial symptoms	Symptoms at diagnosis
Back and/or root pain	18%	6%
Paresis	32%	92%
Sensory changes	10%	74%
Impotence	4%	42%
Bowel and/or bladder disturbance	6%	80%
Bruit	–	8%
Hemorrhage	31%	51%

Table 9.5. Location and symptoms of the SCAVMs

Cervical ($n = 23$)	Hemorrhage	10 (44%)
	Neurologic signs	10 (44%)
	Fortuitous discovery	1 (4%)
	Unknown	2 (8%)
Thoracolumbar (+ conus and filum) ($n = 36$)	Hemorrhage	11 (31%)
	Neurologic signs	23 (64%)
	Doubt	2 (5%)

9.5 Embolization of SCAVMs

The therapeutic strategy that we use in brain AVMs also applies to SCAVMs, i.e.:

- A superselective endovascular approach
- Distal catheterization
- Use of bucrylate (NBCA)

A definitive and stable result is required and this can only reliably be achieved with liquid agents (BERENSTEIN and LASJAUNIAS 1992; BERENSTEIN and KRICHEFF 1979; LASJAUNIAS and BERENSTEIN 1987; MARGOLIS et al. 1979). Some teams have obtained satisfactory results with balloon occlusion (RICHE et al. 1983) or regularly use particles (HALL et al. 1989; HORTON et al. 1983, 1986; RICHE et al. 1983; THERON et al. 1986); in the great majority of cases the latter method leads to incomplete and transitory occlusions (BERENSTEIN and LASJAUNIAS 1992; BERENSTEIN and KRICHEFF 1979; LASJAUNIAS and BERENSTEIN 1987). It should therefore be reserved for exceptional situations or for flow redistribution.

Recognition of the weak points of the angioarchitecture is mandatory since this will serve as a basis for deciding upon the order in which vessels should be embolize. Total cure remains the ideal goal. However, partial treatment focused on the weak points will lead to clinical stabilization or improvement (Fig. 10.2).

Superselective distal catheterization is achieved with a 5F thin-walled guiding catheter and a variable stiffness microcatheter [Mini-torquer (Nycomed Ingenor) (Fig. 10.1e), Tracker (Target Therapeutics), or Magic (BALT)]. Superselective guidewires (Taper, Target Therapeutics) can be employed in order to facilitate the endovascular approach.

Of the 59 SCAVMs, 21 have been embolized by our team (35%). Of the remaining 38, four were operated on because of their location and two were inaccessible to embolization in safe conditions. Eleven were felt inaccessible to both surgery and embolization and were treated conservatively. In 17 further cases our advice was asked in respect of the most appropriate treatment; however, no follow-up could be obtained after our consultation. Finally four patients were embolized repeatedly by other teams (mainly with particles); one of them was operated on as secondary treatment.

Of the embolized population, 11 showed clinical improvement (52%) and six were unchanged (28%). Three transient complications (14%) occurred, and there were three permanent complications (14%) leading to neurologic incapacity. One patient was lost to follow-up after embolization (5%). Of the eight patients embolized only partially according to the angiographic protocol previously described, none have rebled till now, after a maximum follow-up of 5 years.

From an angioarchitectural point of view, total occlusion and anatomic cure was obtained in five patients (24%); two of these patients were worsened by embolization [one with a pure motor radicular syndrome with palsy of the deltoid and biceps muscles (Fig. 9.4) and one with right lower limb paresis]. In 13 patients (62%) a reduction of more than 50% in the size of the nidus and the flow into the SCAVM was achieved; an unsatisfactory result with a reduction of less than 50% was seen in only three patients (14%).

9.6 Special Considerations

9.6.1 SCAVMs in the Pediatric Population

In our series of 59 SCAVMs, ten (17%) were in children (less than 15 years old). Most of them (80%) were nidus-type AVMs, the remainder being direct AVFs. In one case, analysis of the

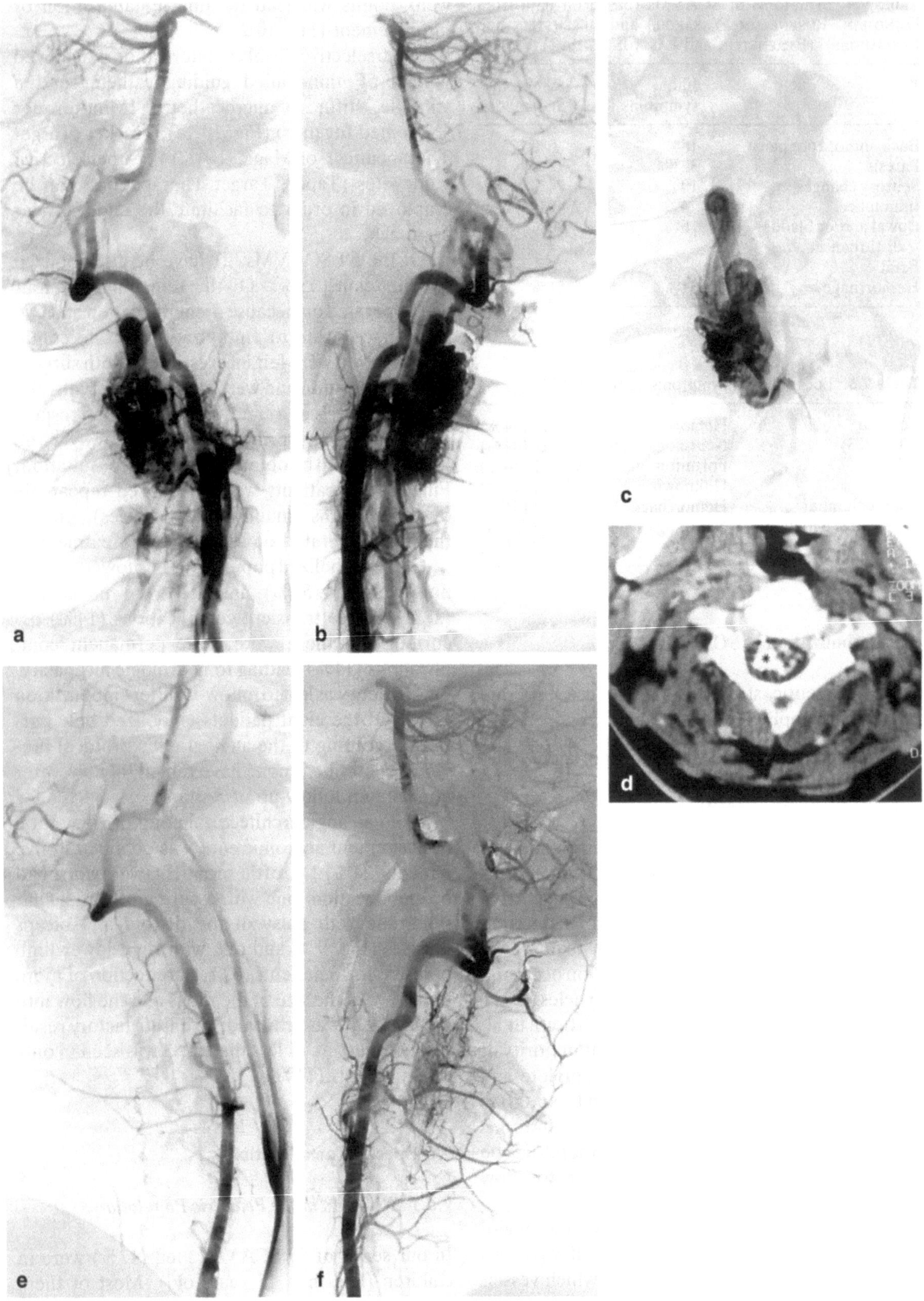

angioarchitecture showed an AVF buried in the AVM itself. No multiple lesions were found in our pediatric population.

No predominant localization was identified: 50% of lesions were situated in the cervical cord, 50% in the thoracic spinal cord. Most of the lesions (60%) revealed their presence by hemorrhage, but associated arterial aneurysms were only detected in one of these SCAVMs (17%). On the other hand, two venous ectasias were noted in the angioarchitecture of the SCAVMs that bled (34%). The vascular system in the pediatric population is usually flexible and absorbs most changes and constraint from hemodynamic conditions. However, symptomatic SCAVMs in children usually present with hemorrhage. The apparent aggressiveness of the disease is the same as in a similar adult case, and the early presentation reveals the weakness and the failure of the remaining vascular tree. Five of the pediatric cases were embolized by our team, all with bucrylate. Of the remaining five lesions, four (80%) were felt not to be safely embolizable. One patient was seen after previous embolization with particles by another team without a satisfactory anatomicoclinical result; one patient was lost to follow-up prior to any endovascular therapy.

Total occlusion and anatomic cure were achieved in one child with an AVF (20%) (Fig. 10.1). Control of more than half of the nidus was achieved in 40% of our patients, all with excellent clinical results. No complications, either transitory or permanent, have been observed. Sixty percent of our population showed frank neurologic improvement, even after partial treatment; two did not present any sequelae from their presenting episode and were unchanged after our procedure.

◁ **Fig. 9.4 a–f.** 24-year-old male presenting with an hemorrhagic accident from which he recovered totally. Cervical spinal cord angiography performed in 1982 reveals an intramedullary C3–C4 AVM and C3 spinal localization. Arterial feeders are represented by radiculomedullary arteries arising from the right (**a**) and left (**b**) vertebral arteries (lateral views). **c** Superselective injection via a open guidewire in the C3 branch opacifies a large portion of the AVM. Embolization was carried out with 0.2 ml of a 30% mixture of IBCA and Lipiodol added to tantalum powder. **d** A cervical nonenhanced CT scan of the third cervical vertebra after embolization of seven vessels in three therapeutic sessions shows the cast of glue projecting into the spinal cord (*asterisk*). **e**,**f** Control angiography: lateral views of the right (**e**) and left (**f**) vertebral arteries. The AVM has totally disappeared. This anatomic cure was followed by a permanent neurologic deficit (suspended pure motor radicular syndrome with paralysis of the deltoid and biceps muscles: anterior cornual syndrome, and partial anterior spinal artery syndrome)

9.6.2 Dural Arteriovenous Malformations (Fig. 9.5)

First described in 1977 by Kendall and Logue (1977), these lesions cannot be grouped with SCAVMs. They are acquired lesions affecting mainly male patients in their fifth decade. They can be suspected on the basis of their slowly progressive neurologic symptomatology. In these lesions the shunt is dural (intracanalar, extradural), being fed by radiculomeningeal arteries (Kendall and Logue 1977; Merland et al. 1980) and draining into congested radicular veins. Most often (in 96% of cases) the shunt is situated on the lateral outer surface of the lower thoracic or lumbar dura or on the dural extension of a nerve root sheath (Kendall and Logue 1977; Rosenblum et al. 1987). It may also be located at the sacral level (Berenstein and Lasjaunias 1992; Burguet et al. 1985; Kendall and Logue 1977). Cranial dural AVMs, near the foramen magnum or on the tentorium, draining secondarily into spinal cord veins may lead to a spinal cord symptomatology; such lesions are often included among spinal dural AVMs. Dural AVFs have never been reported in a cervical or upper thoracic location. As at the intracranial level, dural fistulas of the spinal cord may be multiple and coexist at different levels, being fed by different arteries and draining into different venous channels.

Spinal dural AVFs are different from their intracranial homologues in that they never bleed. This may be due to the anatomy and physiology of the venous system involved: the pressure in the dural cranial sinuses is low, or even negative, and a high pressure shunt here is more able to produce reflux into cortical veins. The normally high venous pressure in the lower thoracic and lumbar regions [74% of the systemic arterial pressure (Horton et al. 1986)] may partially counterbalance the output pressure of dural AVFs. Finally, the flow velocities in dural AVF vessels are not as high as those in other AVMs (Hutchings and Weller 1986; Rosenblum et al. 1987), and dural AVFs never produce flow-related arterial aneurysms or large venous ectasias, as are seen with SCAVMs (Rosenblum et al. 1987). It is nowadays widely recognized that it is the venous engorgement that is responsible for the clinical signs

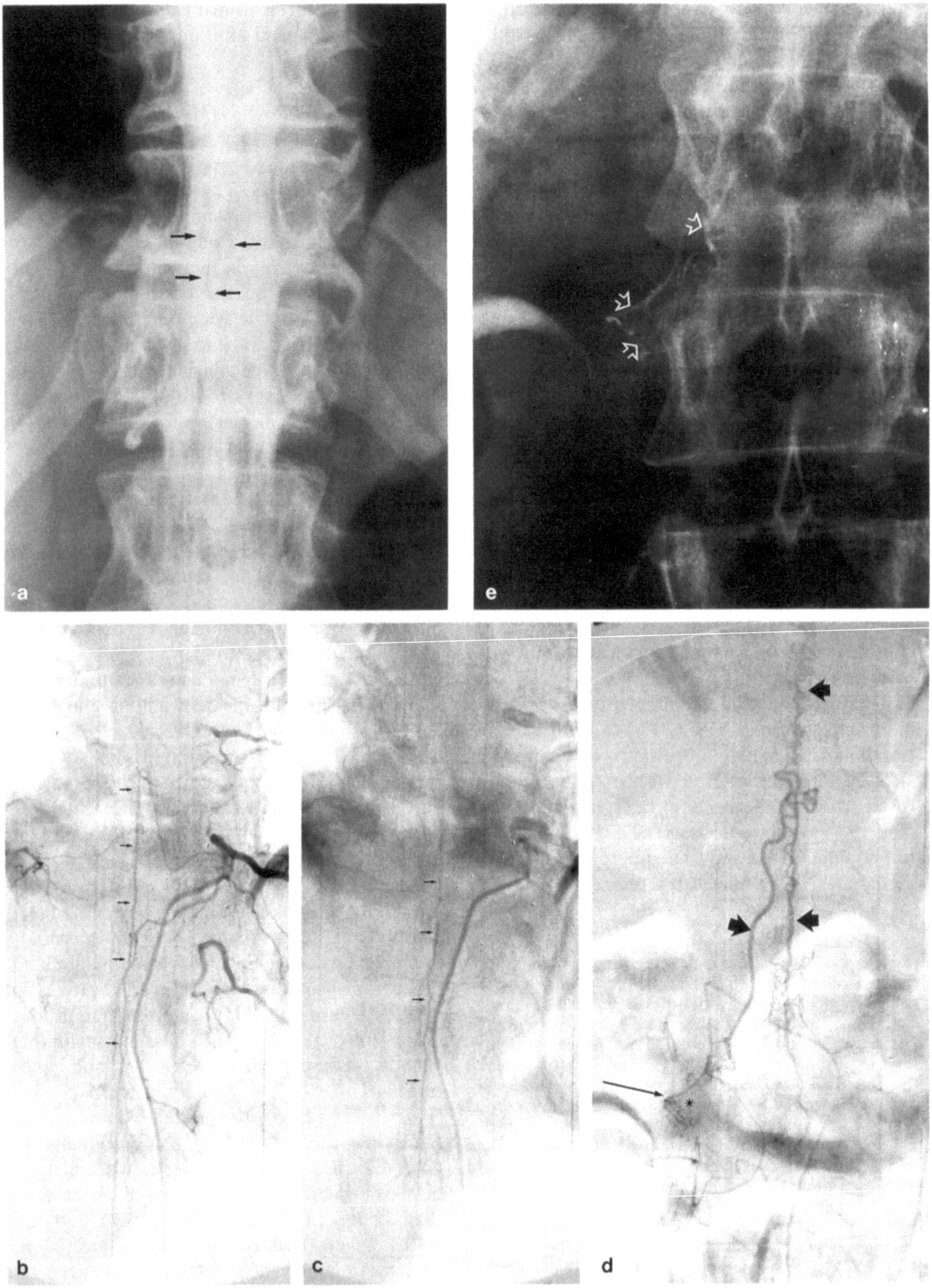
a
e
b
c
d

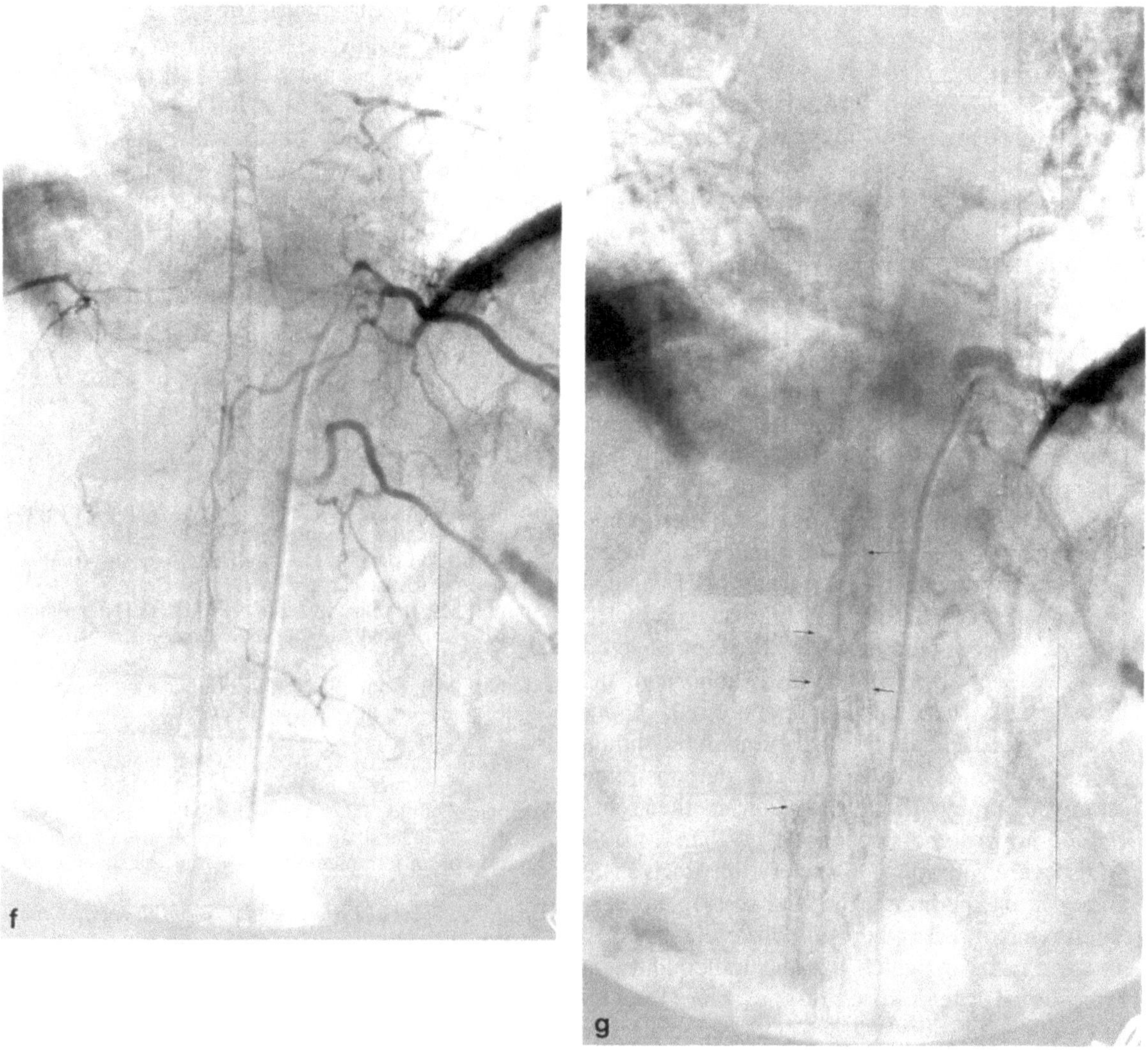

◁ **Fig. 9.5a–g.** 55-year-old male with a 3-month history of paresthesia and weakness of both lower limbs. Neurologic examination confirmed the paraparesis and showed bilateral absence of the Achilles tendon reflex, patellar hyperreflexia, and absence of cutaneous abdominal reflexes. CSF analysis revealed elevated protein levels. Myelography detected serpiginous images suggesting a vascular malformation (**a** *arrows*). Following the angiographic protocol, the radiculomedullary artery was first sought and found, arising from the left T10 intercostal artery (**b** *arrows*). At the 22nd second of the series, stagnation into the anterior spinal axis was observed (**c** *arrows*). **d** A dural AVM (*asterisk*) was found at the right L1 level, fed by dural arteries (*long arrow*) and draining into radicular and spinal cord veins (*large arrows*). Embolization was performed through the spinal cord catheter and the lesion occluded with 0.1 ml of a 50% mixture of NBCA, Lipiodol and tantalum powder (**e** *open arrows*). An immediate control angiogram at the left T10 level showed normal arterial opacification (**f**) and a now normalized venous phase (**g**) with detection of the spinal cord veins (*arrows*). The patient was able to walk within a few weeks after treatment

Table 9.6. Symptoms of spinal dural AVMs (based on data from DJINDJIAN, MERLAND, SYMON, ROSENBLUM, and BERENSTEIN and LASJAUNIAS). (BERENSTEIN and LASJAUNIAS 1992)

	Initial symptoms	Symptoms at diagnosis
Back and/or root pain	28%	37%
Paresis	40%	88%
Impotence	3%	43%
Bowel disturbance	4%	75%
Bladder disturbance	5%	85%
Hemorrhage	0%	0%

presented by the patients (CRISCUOLO et al. 1989; HASSLER et al. 1989; KENDALL and LOGUE 1977; MERLAND et al. 1980; ROSENBLUM et al. 1987; WILLINSKY et al. 1990). The symptomatology that may be encountered in these lesions is listed in Table 9.6.

When suspected clinically, dural AVFs are first looked for by myelography and/or MRI. While the former always shows the characteristic vermiform defects of the congested draining veins, the latter may be either normal or show the traditional hypointense vascular signals on T1- and T2-weighted images (WI) or hyperintense signals on T2-weighted images of the spinal cord parenchyma. It seems that these anomalies are mainly encountered in fistulas with a long history of evolution. Thus angiography should be performed when there is suspicion of a spinal dural fistula following myelography, even when MRI is negative. In our protocol a primary search is conducted for the venous drainage of the spinal cord (WILLINSKY et al. 1990). If this is abnormal, the fistula site is then sought. If a normal venous phase is visualized, the vessels demonstrated should correspond exactly to the defects demonstrated on myelography; the exploration is then considered normal and discontinued. When a fistula is discovered, primary consideration is given to endovascular methods in the same session. Surgery is reserved for cases where embolization has failed and for cases in which a radiculomedullary or radiculopial artery arises at the same level as the pathologic dural artery and superselective catheterization is not possible.

The fistulous points should be approached superselectively and occluded with a stable material (NBCA). This will close the shunt and instantaneously improve the circulation of the spinal cord vessels (HASSLER et al. 1989). A good outcome is usually reported in patients with dural AVFs after nidus obliterations (ROSENBLUM et al. 1987). However, it should be added that the best clinical results are obtained on recently symptomatic fistulas with no more than an 18- to 20-month history of evolution (BERENSTEIN and LASJAUNIAS 1992). Because of the irreversible damage caused by chronic venous congestion, long-term disease will give rise to severe myelopathy with associated necrosis and gliosis. No satisfactory neurologic improvement is seen in these cases even if the lesion is completely excluded. Indeed, occasionally some postoperative deterioration has been observed. Such deterioration was felt to be related to secondary thrombosis of spinal cord veins; aspirin and heparin treatments were employed in these cases with variable and unpredictable success. In some cases recurrence of symptoms necessitates further angiography to verify the quality of the result obtained, including confirmation of permanent thrombosis of the first few millimeters of radicular veins draining the shunt. Otherwise the same protocol as described above is applied to look for a second, undetected dural AVF.

References

Aminoff MJ, Logue V (1974a) Clinical features of spinal vascular malformations. Brain 97:197–210

Aminoff MJ, Logue V (1974b) The prognosis of patients with spinal vascular malformations. Brain 97:211–218

Aminoff MJ, Barnard LO, Logue V (1974) The pathophysiology of spinal vascular malformations. J Neurol Sci 23:255–263

Aminoff MJ, Gotin P, Norman D (1988) Unusual type of spinal arteriovenous malformation. Neurosurgery 22:589–591

Arseni C, Samitca DC (1959) Vascular malformations of the spinal cord. Acta Psychiatr scand 34:10–17

Ausman J, Gold GH, Tadavarthy SM, Amplatz K, Chou SN (1977) Intraparenchymal embolization for obliteration of an intramedullary AVM of the spinal cord. J Neurosurg 47:119–125

Bailey W, Sperl M (1969) Angiomas of the cervical spinal cord. J Neurosurg 30:560–568

Benhaiem-Sigaux N, Zerah M, Guerardi R, Bellot J, Hurth M, Poirier J (1985) A retromedullary arteriovenous fistula associated with the Klippel-Trenaunay-Weber syndrome. Acta Neuropathol (Berl) 66:318–324

Berenstein A, Kricheff I (1979) Catheter and material selection for transarterial embolization: technical considerations. II materials. Radiology 132:631–639

Berenstein A, Lasjaunias P (1992) Surgical neuroangiography, vol 5. Endovascular treatment of spine and spinal cord lesions. Springer, Berlin Heidelberg New York

Berenstein A, Young W, Ransohoff J, Benjamin V, Merrin H (1984) Somatosensory evoked potentials during spinal angiography and therapeutic transvascular embolization. J Neurosurg 60:777–785

Burguet JL, Dietemannn JL, Wackenheim A, Kehr P, Buchheit F (1985) Sacral meningeal arteriovenous fistula fed by branches of the hypogastric arteries and drained through medullary veins. Neuroradiology 27:232–237

Cogen P, Stein B (1983) Spinal cord arteriovenous malformations with significant intramedullary components. J Neurosurg 59:471–478

Criscuolo G, Oldfield EH, Doppman J (1989) Reversible acute and subacute myelopathy in patients with dural AV fistula. Foix-Alajouanine syndrome reconsidered. J Neurosurg 70:354–359

Di Chiro G, Doppmann J, Dwyer A et al. (1985) Tumors and arteriovenous malformations of the spinal cord: assessment using MR. Radiology 156:689–697

Djindjian R (1975) Embolization of angiomas of the spinal cord. Surg Neurol 4:411–420
Djindjian M (1976) Les malformations arterioveineuses de la moelle épinière et leur traitement à propos de 150 cas. Doctoral thesis, University of Paris VI
Djindjian R, Merland JJ (1978) Place de l'embolisation dans le traitement des malformations artério-veineuses médullaires. A propos de 38 cas. Neuroradiology 16:428–429
Doppman JL, Di Chiro G, Ommaya AK (1971) Percutaneous embolization in spinal cord AV malformations. J Neurosurg 84:48–55
Doppman J, Di Chiro G, Dwyer A, Franck J, Oldfield E (1987) Magnetic resonance imaging of spinal arteriovenous malformations. J Neurosurg 66:830–834
Garcia C, Dulcey S, Dulcey J (1979) Ruptured aneurysm of the spinal artery of Adamkiewicz during pregnancy. Neuroradiology 29:394–398
Garcia-Monaco R, Lasjaunias P (1990) Embolization of spinal AVMs and tumors. In: Kadir S (ed) Current practice of interventional radiology. Decker, Toronto, pp 154–161
Gross SW, Ralston BL (1959) Vascular malformations of the spinal cord. Surg Gynecol Obstet 108:673–678
Hall WA, Oldfield E, Doppmann JL (1989) Recanalization of spinal arteriovenous malformations following embolization. J Neurosurg 70:714–720
Hassler W, Thron A, Grote E (1989) Hemodynamics of spinal dural arteriovenous fistulas. An intraoperative study. J Neurosurg 70:360–370
Horton J, Marano GD, Kerber CW, Jenkins JJ, Davis S (1983) Polyvinyl alcohol-foam-Gelfoam for therapeutic embolization: a synergistic mixture. AJNR 4:143–147
Horton J, Latchaw R, Gold LH, Rang D (1986) Embolization of intramedullary arteriovenous malformations of the spinal cord. AJNR 7:113–118
Houdart R, Djindjian R, Hurth M (1974) Treatment of angiomas of the spinal cord. Surg Neurol 2:186–194
Hurth M, Houdart R, Djindjian R, Rey A, Djindjian M (1978) Arteriovenous malformations of the spinal cord. Prog Neurol Surg 9:238–266
Hutchings M, Weller OR (1986) Anatomical relationship of the pia mater to cerebral blood vessels in man. J Neurosurg 65:316–325
Kendall B, Logue V (1977) Spinal epidural angiomatous malformations draining into intrathecal veins. Neuroradiology 13:181–189
Kito K, Kobayashi N, Mori N, Kohno H (1983) Ruptured aneurysm of the anterior spinal artery associated with pseudoxanthoma elasticum. J Neurosurg 5:126–128
Krayenbuhl H, Yasargil MG, McClintock HG (1969) Treatment of spinal cord vascular malformations by surgical excision. J Neurosurg 30:427–435
Kunc Z, Bret J (1969) Diagnosis and treatment of vascular malformations of the spinal cord. J Neurosurg 30:436–445
Lasjaunias P, Berenstein A (1987) Surgical neuroangiography, vol 2. Endovascular treatment of craniofacial lesions. Springer, Berlin Heidelberg New York
Lasjaunias P, Berenstein A (1990) Surgical neuroangiography, vol 3. Functional vascular anatomy of brain, spinal cord and spine. Springer, Berlin Heidelberg New York
Lasjaunias P, Chiu M, Terbrugge K, Tolia A, Hurth M, Berenstein A (1986) Neurological manifestation of intracranial dural arteriovenous malformations. J Neurosurg 64:724–730
Lasjaunias P, Manelfe C, Chiu M (1986) Angiographic architecture of intracranial vascular malformations and fistulae. Therapeutic aspects. Neurosurg Rev 9:253–261
Latchaw RE, Gold LHA (1979) Polyvinyl foam embolization of vascular and neoplastic lesions of the head, neck and spine. Radiology 131:669–679
Maillot C (1991) Les espaces périmédullaires. Situation, organisation et relation avec le liquide céphalo-rachidien. J Neuroradiol (in press)
Malis LI (1979) Microsurgery for spinal cord arteriovenous malformation. Clin Neurosurg 26:543–555
Margolis MT, Birchfield RI (1974) Percutaneous embolization of a spinal cord arteriovenous malformation. Bull Mason Chir 28:87–93
Margolis MT, Freeny P, Kendrick M (1979) Cyanoacrylate occlusion of a spinal cord arteriovenous malformation. Case report. J Neurosurg 51:107–110
Masaryk T, Ross J, Modic M, Ruff R, Selman W, Ratcheson R (1987) Radiculomeningeal vascular malformation of the spine: MR imaging. Radiology 164:845–849
Merland JJ, Riche MC, Chiras J (1980) Les fistules artérioveineuses intra canalaires extramédullaires à drainage veineux médullaire. J Neuroradiol 7:271–320
Modik M, Masarik T, Ross J (1989) Magnetic resonance imaging of the spine. Year Book Medical, Chicago, pp 262–266
Morgan MK, Chaseling R, Johnston I, Desilva M (1986) Spinal arteriovenous malformation presenting at birth. Case report. Neurosurgery 19:637–640
Newton TH, Adams DE (1968) Angiographic demonstration and nonsurgical embolization of spinal cord angioma. Radiology 91:873–877
Nicholas D, Weller R (1988) The fine anatomy of the human spinal meninges. A light and scanning electron microscopy study. J Neurosurg 69:276–282
Ommaya AR, Di Chiro G, Doppman JL (1969) Ligation of arterial supply in the treatment of spinal cord arteriovenous malformations. J Neurosurg 30:670–692
Patterson RH Jr, Voorhies RM (1978) Surgical approaches to intracranial and intraspinal arteriovenous malformations. Clin Neurosurg 25:412–424
Riche MC, Melki JP, Merland JJ (1983) Embolization of spinal cord vascular malformations via the anterior spinal artery. AJNR 4:378–381
Riche MC, Scialfa G, Guegen B, Merland JJ (1983) Giant extramedullary arteriovenous fistula supplied by the anterior spinal artery: treatment by detachable balloons AJNR 4:391–394
Riche MC, Reizine D, Melki JP, Merland JJ (1985) Classification of spinal cord malformations. Radiat Med 3:17–24
Rodesch G, Berenstein A, Lasjaunias P (1991) Angioarchitecture of spinal cord arteriovenous malformations. In: Manelfe C (ed) Magnetic resonance imaging of spine and spinal cord. Raven, New York (in press)
Rosenblum B, Oldfield E, Doppmann J, Dichiro G (1987) Spinal arteriovenous malformations: a comparison of dural arteriovenous fistulas and intradural AVMs in 81 patients. J Neurosurg 67:795–802
Saunders F, Birchard D, Willner J (1987) Spinal artery aneurysm. Surg Neurol 27:269–272
Smith B, Penka C, Erickson LV, Matsuo F (1986) Subarachnoid hemorrhage due to anterior spinal artery aneurysm. Neurosurgery 18:217–219

Spetzler R, Zabramski J, Floh R (1989) Management of juvenile spinal AVMs by embolization and operative excision. Case report. J Neurosurg 70:628–632

Stein BM (1979) Surgery of intramedullary spinal cord tumors. Chir Neurosurg 25:529–542

Theron J, Cosgrove R, Melanson D, Ethier R (1986) Spinal arteriovenous malformations: advances in therapeutic embolization. Radiology 158:163–169

Tobin WD (1976) The diagnosis and natural history of spinal cord arteriovenous malformations. Mayo Clinic Proc 51:637–647

Willinsky R, Lasjaunias P, Terbrugge K, Pruvost P (1988) Brain arteriovenous malformations: analysis of the angioarchitecture in relationship to hemorrhage. J Neuroradiol 15:225–237

Willinsky R, Lasjaunias P, Terbrugge K, Hurth M (1990) Angiography in the investigation of spinal dural AV fistula. A protocol with application of the venous phase. Neuroradiology 32:114–116

Wyburn Mason R (1943) The vascular abnormalities and tumors of the spinal cord and its membranes. Kumpton, London

Yasargil MG, Delong WB, Guarnaschelli JM (1975) Complete microsurgical excision of cervical extramedullary and intramedullary vascular malformations. Surg Neurol 4:211–224

Yonas H, Patres S, White R (1980) Anterior spinal aneurysm. J Neurosurg 53:570–573

10 Superselective Therapy for Cerebral Gliomas

SAMUEL M. WOLPERT

CONTENTS

10.1 Introduction

The natural history of glioblastomas has been little altered by therapeutic attempts over the past 30 years. Surgical debulking and radiation therapy have had only a moderate effect on these patients (NEUWELT and DAHLBORG 1989), with the median survival being in the range of 7.5–9.5 months (EDWARDS et al. 1980; SHAPIRO and AUSMAN 1969). This dismal prognosis for patients with glioblastomas has stimulated the development of many alternative regimens, such as intra-arterial therapy and local high dose irradiation. This chapter will initially discuss the rationale behind the chemotherapy of brain tumors, the nature of the blood-brain barrier (BBB) and its significance in the treatment of patients with cerebral glioblastomas, and the problem with the BBB; it will conclude with a discussion on the intra-arterial delivery of chemotherapeutic agents.

10.2 Chemotherapy of Brain Tumors

The magnitude of the problem of treating malignant brain tumors with chemotherapy can be understood by considering the total tumor mass. The tumor burden must not exceed 1×10^5 cells if the body's immune system is expected to suppress and eventually kill the tumor (SHAPIRO 1986). Most patients present with neurologic symptoms when the tumors weigh 30–60 g ($3-6 \times 10^{10}$ cells). If 50% of the tumor burden is resected, the residual tumor is $1-5 \times 10^9$ cells. Radiation therapy might kill two additional logs of cells, reducing the tumor to about 1×10^7 cells. Intravenous chemotherapy usually produces a net kill of about 1 log, reducing the burden to 1×10^6 cells, unfortunately still larger than the burden of 1×10^5 cells. Thus the tumor grows despite the drug administration.

Many malignant gliomas contain fields of benign-appearing tumor, indicating the potential for progression from a slowly to a rapidly growing neoplasm. This heterogeneity is important in the chemotherapy of brain tumors, with rapidly growing cells being more sensitive to drugs than slower growing cells (YUNG et al. 1982). Chemotherapeutic agents are not only specific for tumors but unfortunately also affect normal cells. They may be cell cycle specific, i.e., effective during the cell's life cycle when DNA is synthesized, or cell cycle nonspecific, i.e., effective during both DNA synthesis and at other times during the cycle period (SHAPIRO and SHAPIRO 1986). Some drugs such as BCNU, although cell cycle nonspecific, are more effective during DNA synthesis (BARRANCO and HUMPHREY 1971). The efficiency of a cell cycle specific agent may be improved by modifying the growth fraction of a tumor through increasing the number of cells in active division with cell cycle nonspecific agents such as radiation or surgery (SHAPIRO and SHAPIRO 1986). These adjunctive techniques provide the rationale for combination chemotherapy, i.e., radiation followed by chemotherapy, or radiation and tumor debulking followed by chemotherapy. Most chemotherapeutic agents have been chosen because they cross the BBB (nitrosoureas, e.g., BCNU,

SAMUEL M. WOLPERT, M.B., B.Ch., Department of Radiology, Section of Neuroradiology, New England Medical Center Hospitals, 750 Washington Street, Boston, MA 0211, USA

CCNU, and methyl CCNU) or because they act directly in the brain (procarbazine, cisplatin, 5-fluorouracil, etc.) The nitrosoureas are lipid soluble whereas the other drugs mentioned above are water soluble but nevertheless readily cross the BBB. Unfortunately many lipophilic compounds do not dissolve readily in innocuous vehicles.

10.3 Problems with Delivery of Chemotherapeutic Agents to Brain Tumors

The unique biologic aspect of the BBB is an important focus when considering the therapy for brain tumors (Neuwelt and Barnett 1989). In patients with brain tumors, radioisotopes, radio contrast materials, and paramagnetic contrast agents usually cross the BBB into the tumor, paticularly with higher grade malignant lesions. It is clear, however, that the BBB is usually incompletely breached because water-soluble drugs found to be effective against tumors in extracranial sites in animals and man are much less effective when the tumor is in the CNS (Shapiro and Shapiro 1986). Furthermore the blood flow and hence the potential for the delivery of lipophilic and water-soluble drugs to brain tumors is often variable and frequently reduced. Also tumor cells which infiltrate the surrounding brain parenchyma are fed by capillaries of the normal brain which are minimally permeable to water-soluble drugs (Greig 1989a). All these factors prevent the delivery of tumoricidal drugs to the total volume of a brain tumor and hence have stimulated research into barrier breakdown prior to intra-arterial drug infusion.

10.4 Problem of the Blood-Brain Barrier

Important factors determining drug entry from blood into the CNS are molecular weight and lipid solubility. The BBB normally prevents the passage of ionized water-soluble drugs with a molecular weight of greater than 180 whereas most currently available and effective chemotherapeutic agents have molecular weights of 200–1200 (Mayhein and Heistod 1985). Thus on a molecular weight basis, the passage of many chemotherapeutic agents is impeded by the BBB. A linear correlation also exists between the octanol: water coefficient of chemotherapeutic agents and their cerebrovascular permeability. Methotrexate, with a relatively low octanol: water coefficient, is relatively impermeable. BCNU has a high and 5-fluorouracil an intermediate octanol: water coefficient (Greig 1989b).

10.5 Artificial Opening and Complications of Blood-Brain Barrier Disruption

The BBB can be opened by the administration of intracarotid hyperosmolar mannitol (Neuwelt et al. 1981). Markedly increased brain concentrations of methotrexate have been shown in animal studies with this technique but unfortunately considerable CNS toxicity results (Neuwelt et al. 1982, 1983). From a therapeutic point of view, BBB disruption must be reversible to be clinically useful. A reversible BBB disruption needs a sufficient infusion rate of hypertonic solution; too slow an infusion rate will result in a subthreshold event caused by dilution of the infusate from blood from the ipsilateral carotid artery or collateral flow from the circle of Willis (Neuwelt and Barnett 1989). Higher than necessary infusion rates may result in intravascular hypertension and permanent damage. The effect can be monitored by observing the extent of BBB breakdown by performing radionuclide brain scans with ^{99m}Tc-glucoheptonate. Neuwelt and Dahlborg (1989) showed that a regimen of reversible osmotic BBB modification following prior surgery and radiation together with a chemotherapy regimen of methotrexate, cytoxan, and procarbazine provided a median survival of 17.5 months for patients with glioblastomas, which is longer than that achieved by surgery and radiotherapy or surgery, radiotherapy, and systemic chemotherapy. Furthermore the combined BBB modification regimen resulted in a decrease in the size of many of the tumors. Age was found to be an important variable in survival, younger patients having improved survival over older patients.

Unfortunately the complications of BBB disruption are significant. Seizures may occur after mannitol-induced BBB disruption following the administration of intra-arterial methotrexate, and were found in 14% of the procedures carried out in patients treated for glioblastomas, leukemia, and metastases (Neuwelt and Dahlborg 1989). Transient exacerbation of the neurologic deficits lasting 48–72 h was seen in 60% of the patients with preexisting deficits. Other complications included stroke (5% of procedures), transient granulocytopenia, anemia, ocular toxicity, and transient increase in brain edema. For all these reasons many consider the risks of BBB disruption to be unacceptably high. Another drawback to the osmotic disruption of the BBB is that it results in only a modest increase in drug levels within the tumor compared to the large increase in drug levels in normal brain (NAKAGAWA et al. 1984). The lack of objective evidence that BBB disruption actually increases drug delivery to brain tumors indicates the need for further laboratory research since BBB disruption, if achievable, is an attractive means of enhancing drug delivery to brain tumors (GROOTHUIS et al. 1990).

Other substances such as leukotriene C4, a pharmacologically active compound that promotes vascular permeability, have been shown experimentally to selectively open the blood-tumor barrier, but to leave it intact after intracarotid injection (BLACK et al. 1990). Adenosine triphosphate, when injected through the carotid artery, also has been shown to selectively increase the blood flow in malignant gliomas, probably due to increased disruption of the blood-tumor barrier (BABA et al. 1990).

10.6 Intra-arterial Chemotherapy

Tumor cells subject to sublethal doses of cytotoxic drugs develop drug resistance. HIESIGER et al. (1984) however, found that the concentration × time exposure in a rat brain tumor doubled when the drug was administered via the carotid artery in comparison with the concentration after intravenous administration. Others have predicted a ten-fold greater drug concentration with intra-arterial as compared to intravenous administration (FENSTERMACHER and COWLES 1977). As a result of these findings the intracarotid infusion of chemotherapeutic agents has been proposed and implemented (BASHIR et al. 1988; GREENBERG et al. 1981; HOCHBERG et al. 1985; JOHNSON et al. 1987). Tumor size response to the intra-arterial regimens can easily be detected by computed tomography (CT) (Fig. 10.1) (BASHIR et al. 1988; CLAYMAN et al. 1989), and complete disappearance of the tumor has been reported in 22% of a series of 28 patients treated with BCNU, with partial disappearance in another 22% (BASHIR et al. 1988). We have similarly found a decrease in tumor size of up to 60% in 8 of 20 patients treated with subophthalmic BCNU (JOHNSON et al. 1987).

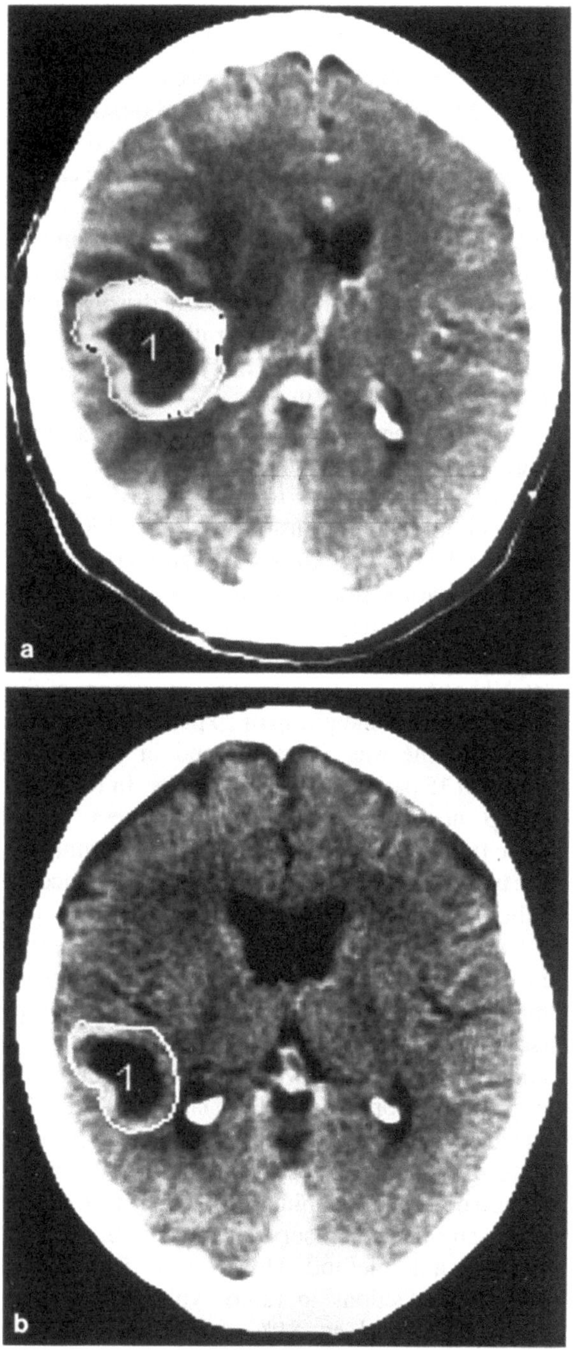

Fig. 10.1. a Contrast-enhanced CT scan before intra-arterial BCNU therapy. The total tumor volume (enhancement and central low density) was 40 cc. Note the midline shift of the ventricular system and the edema surrounding the tumor. **b** After one course of BCNU, the total tumor volume has decreased to 16 cc. There is no midline shift and the edema has almost completely resolved. (JOHNSON et al. 1987; by courtesy of Neurosurgery 20:577)

There are, however, two significant drawbacks to the intra-arterial delivery of BCNU; both eye toxicity and encephalopathy occur (Foo et al. 1985; MADAJEWICZ et al. 1981; SAFDARI et al. 1985). The eye toxicity can be obviated by the delivery of the drug above the ophthalmic carotid artery by microcatheter delivery techniques. The encephalopathy can be reduced by decreasing the dose of BCNU from 200 mg/m^2 to 100 mg/m^2 (SHAPIRO and GREEN 1987). Also dissolving the BCNU in dextrose in water rather than ethanol appears to reduce the toxicity (JOHNSON et al. 1987; LAYTON et al. 1984).

We have compared the overall medium survival time from operation to death or study conclusion in two groups of patients treated with BCNU: one with subophthalmic infusion at a dose of 150 mg/m^2 dissolved in 5% dextrose in water (D5W) and another with supraophthalmic and vertebral infusion at the same dose and with the same diluent (CLAYMAN et al. 1989). All the patients received BCNU at 6-week intervals for a maximum of five courses. In the first group of 20 patients, the mean survival time was 51 weeks and in the second group of 15 patients, it was 73 weeks. In this latter group, no patient experienced blindness, retinal toxicity, or leukoencephalopathy. Unfortunately, the two groups are strictly not comparable since the subophthalmic group commenced therapy upon CT evidence of tumor recurrence whereas the supraophthalmic group commenced therapy approximately 8 weeks after completion of radiotherapy (some members of the supraophthalmic group had also been treated with interstitial iridium 192 implantation or intra-arterial cisplatin). Ideally, survival estimate comparisons should be from the time of tumor diagnosis, and therapy variables should be kept to a minimum. We therefore cannot claim any benefit in survival times with the supraophthalmic method. However, in 6 of the 15 patients reductions in tumor volume occurred; one patient had an 84% reduction. Our data therefore indicate that intra-arterial selective supraophthalmic or posterior cerebral artery delivery of BCNU dissolved in D5W eliminates many of the complications found with subophthalmic infusions. Other agents such as 1-2-hydroxyethl-chloroethylnitrosourea (HECNU) have been infused in patients with malignant gliomas with good results (FAUCHON et al. 1990). With HECNU the toxicity appears to be less than with BCNU although cases of blindness and leukoencephalopathy have also been encountered (FAUCHON et al. 1990).

10.7 Techniques of Superselective Intra-arterial Chemotherapy

Different catheter systems have been described for selective arterial infusions. DOPPMAN et al. (1986) favor an everting or toposcopic catheter which they locate in the distal internal carotid artery. KAPP et al. (1985) have described a flexible, silicone rubber tube attached to a more rigid introducing catheter which they locate above the ophthalmic artery. CHARNSANGAVEJ et al. (1985) developed a flexible Gore-Tex sleeve which is attached to the end of a 3F angiographic catheter. METES et al. (1985) use a 2F jet-controlled microleak balloon catheter for supraophthalmic infusion. We favor using a 2F Tracker-18 catheter (Target Therapeutics, Inc., Los Angeles, California, USA) passed coaxially through a 5F catheter introduced into the internal carotid or vertebral artery (Fig. 10.2). After the vascularity of the tumor is assessed by standard angiography, the tip of the Tracker catheter is placed as close to the tumor in the appropriate artery as possible. Heparin is administered intravenously (5000 units) to prevent thrombus formation. Protamine sulfate

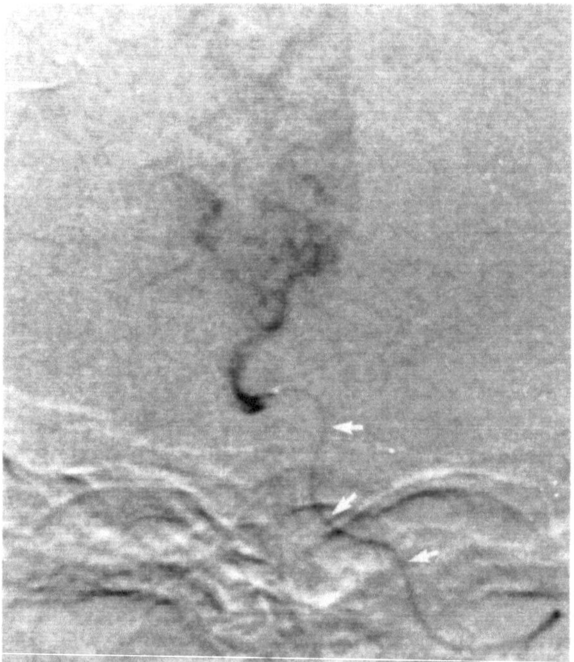

Fig. 10.2. Tracker catheter (*arrows*) is seen with its tip in the right posterior cerebral artery. The angiogram shows opacification of part of the posterior cerebral artery distribution to the occipital lobe. (CLAYMAN et al. 1989; by courtesy of AJNR 10:767)

is administered at the end of the procedure to reverse the anticoagulation (WOLPERT et al. 1988). The catheterization is not pain-free – presumably due to irritation of pain-sensitive fibers in the infused arteries.

Complications have been reported following the supraophthalmic infusion of chemotherapeutic agents. Spasm resulting in an infarct occurred in one of our 48 supraophthalmic infusion procedures (CLAYMAN et al. 1989). KAPP et al. (1985) carried out 48 supraophthalmic infusions of BCNU and cisplatin under general anesthesia following surgical exposure of the carotid artery and the insertion of a flexible catheter. The catheters were situated in the supraclinoid carotid arteries. In ten patients Marcus Gunn pupils developed, presumably secondary to anterior choroidal arterial infusion or direct tumor involvement of the optic tracts. In a follow-up study KAPP and SANFORD (1986) found that reducing the dose of cisplatin reduced the incidence of complications but also the efficacy of the treatment. CHARNSANGAVEJ et al. (1985) carried out 14 supraophthalmic infusions of BCNU and/or cisplatin with infusion catheters placed in the supraclinoid internal carotid arteries. Conjunctivitis developed in three patients, two of whom had retinal damage. METES and his coworkers (1985) used a microleak balloon catheter in six patients to perform 12 supraophthalmic infusions; three patients subsequently experienced permanent neurologic deficits, and one further patient treated with subophthalmic cisplatin became blind. BCNU (presumably dissolved in ethanol) was administered in 11 infusions, cisplatin in two. A high incidence of multifocal infarction has been documented on CT and positron emission tomographic studies in another series of patients treated for glioblastoma multiforme (DICHIRO et al. 1987). In clinical practice absolute alcohol is used to precipitate thrombosis and infarction in these patients (METES et al. 1985). We did not observe leukoencephalopathy in our patients treated with the supraophthalmic infusion of BCNU (CLAYMAN et al. 1989). This may reflect the lower dose of BCNU used (150 mg/m^2) as compared with that in some of the other studies [BCNU toxicity is dose related (LAYTON et al. 1984)], the use of dextrose in water rather than ethanol as the diluent, and the administration of BCNU weeks after completion of the radiation therapy rather than concurrently with the therapy.

Other authors have discussed the problem of streaming when slowly infused, concentrated chemotherapeutic agents are administered, relating this to the possible development of leukoencephalopathy (DOPPMAN et al. 1986; LUTZ et al. 1986). The rate of infusion influences streaming; an injection rate of not less than 15.0 ml/min (0.25–0.5 ml/s) prevents streaming (SILBERGLEIT et al. 1989). The location of the tip of the catheter also appears to influence streaming, which seems to be more likely with continuous supraophthalmic infusions than with subophthalmic infusions (SARIS et al. 1987, 1991). Intravascular streaming can be substantially reduced or eliminated by a diastole-phased infusion technique (SARIS et al. 1987).

Possibly the complications reported by CHARNSANGAVEJ et al. (1985) were due to too rapid an infusion of the chemotherapeutic agents or to the close proximity of the catheter tip to the ophthalmic arteries which would occur with supraclinoid, internal carotid artery infusion rather than middle cerebral artery infusion. Delivering the agents closer to the tumor site, i.e., in the middle cerebral artery, may prevent these problems. Furthermore we have observed that the tip of the Tracker catheter can slowly spontaneously retract from the artery during an infusion procedure and come to lie in a subophthalmic location. A more distal location of the catheter tip and frequent fluoroscopic checking during the infusion are therefore mandatory.

It is also important to realize that brain tumors may cross arterial territory and be in one, two, or three vascular distributions. Under such circumstances, separate infusions into each territory are necessary since we have seen cases in which perfused tumors regress, leaving unperfused tumors to simultaneously increase in size (JOHNSON et al. 1987).

10.8 Conclusion

The intra-arterial delivery of chemotherapeutic agents to patients with brain tumors is practical and can be carried out with an acceptably low incidence of complications. Whereas it is not yet established whether flooding a cerebral hemisphere containing a glioma with an increased concentration of a drug can achieve an improvement in quality of life, or an increase in life expectancy, the selective delivery of drugs closer to the tumor site shows promise. Any single treatment is bound to have a limited effect on tumor growth because the balance of tumor cell proliferation and tumor cell loss is usually only moderately altered. Under most circumstances, stabilization of the disease or a partial tumor response is all that can be expected. As yet no studies have been carried out using supraophthalmic chemotherapy with a diastole-phased infusion technique after BBB breakdown utilizing newer agents such as leukotriene or adenosine diphosphate.

References

Baba T, Fukui M, Takeshita I et al. (1990) Selective enhancement of intratumoral blood flow in malignant gliomas using intra-arterial adenosine triphosphate. J Neurosurg 72:907–911

Barranco SC, Humphrey RM (1971) The effects of BCNU on survival and cell progression in Chinese hamster cells. Cancer Res 31:191–195

Bashir R, Hochberg FH, Linggood RM, Hottleman K (1988) Preirradiation internal carotid artery BCNU in treatment of glioblastoma multiforme. J Neurosurg 68:917–919

Black KL, King WA, Ikezaki K (1990) Selective opening of the blood-tumor barrier by intracarotid infusion of leukotriene C4. J Neurosurg 72:912–916

Charnsangavej C, Lee Y, Carrasco CH et al. (1985) Supraclinoid intracarotid chemotherapy using a flow-directed soft-tipped catheter. Radiology 155:655–657

Clayman DA, Wolpert SM, Heros DO (1989) Superselective arterial BCNU infusion in the treatment of patients with malignant gliomas. AJNR 10:767–771

DiChiro G, Oldfield E, Wright DC et al. (1987) Cerebral necrosis after radiotherapy and/or intra-arterial chemotherapy for brain tumors: PET and neuropathologic studies. AJNR 8:1083–1091

Doppman JL, Dedrick RL, Shook DR et al. (1986) Glioblastoma: catheter techniques for isolated chemotherapy perfusion. Radiology 159:477–483

Edwards MS, Levin VA, Wilson CB (1980) Brain tumor chemotherapy: an evaluation of agents in current use for phase II and III trials. Cancer Treat Rep 64:1179–1205

Fauchon F, Davila L, Chatellier G et al. (1990) Treatment of malignant gliomas with surgery, intra-arterial infusions of 1-(2-hydroxyethyl) chloroethylnitrosourea, and radiation therapy: a phase II study. Neurosurgery 27:231–234

Fenstermacher JD, Cowles AL (1977) Theoretic limitations of intracarotid infusions in brain tumor chemotherapy. Cancer Treat Rep 61:519–526

Foo SH, Ransohoff J, Choi IS et al. (1985) Experience with supraophthalmic intra-arterial BCNU infusion in malignant glioma (abstr). Neurology 35 [Suppl]:114

Greenberg HS, Ensminger WD, Seeger JF et al. (1981) Intra-arterial BCNU chemotherapy for the treatment of malignant gliomas of the central nervous system: a preliminary report. Cancer Treat Rep 65:803–810

Greig NH (1989a) Drug delivery to the brain by blood-brain barrier circumvention and drug modification. In: Neuwelt EA (ed) Implications of the blood-brain barrier barrier barrier and its manipulations. Plenum Medical, New York, pp 311–367

Greig NH (1989b) Brain tumors and the blood-tumor barrier. In: Neuwelt EA (ed) Implications of the blood-brain barrier and its manipulation. Plenum Medical, New York, pp 77–106

Groothuis DR, Warkne PC, Molnar P et al. (1990) Effect of hyperosmotic blood-brain barrier disruption on transcapillary transport in canine brain tumors. J Neurosurg 72:441–449

Hiesiger EM, Voorhies R, Basler GA et al. (1984) Comparison of ^{14}C-methotrexate (^{14}C-MTX) delivery by intravenous vs. intracarotid (IC) route without or with IC mannitol in experimental rat brain tumors as measured by quantitative autoradiography (QAR). Proc Am Assoc Cancer 25:363

Hochberg FH, Pruitt AA, Beck DO et al. (1985) The rationale and methodology for intra-arterial chemotherapy with BCNU as treatment for glioblastoma. J Neurosurg 63:876–889

Johnson DW, Parkinson D, Wolpert SM et al. (1987) Intracarotid chemotherapy with 1,3-bis-(2-chloroethyl)-1-nitrosourea (BCNU) in 5% dextrose in water in the treatment of malignant glioma. Neurosurgery 20: 577–583

Kapp JP, Sanford RA (1986) Neurologic deficit after carotid infusion of cisplatinum and 1-3-bis (2-choroethyl-1-nitrosourea (BCNU) for malignant glioma: An analysis of risk factors. Neurosurgery 19:779–783

Kapp JP, Parker JL, Tucker EM (1985) Supra-ophthalmic carotid infusion for brain chemotherapy. J Neurosurg 62:823–825

Layton PB, Greenberg HS, Stetson PL et al. (1984) BCNU solubility and toxicity in the treatment of maligant astrocytomas. J Neurosurg 60:1134–1137

Lutz RL, Dedrick RL, Boretos JW et al. (1986) Mixing studies during intracarotid infusions in an in vitro model. J Neurosurg 64:277–283

Madajewicz S, West CR, Park HC et al. (1981) Phase II study – intra-arterial BCNU therapy for metastatic brain tumors. Cancer 47:653–657

Mayhein WG, Heistod DD (1985) Permeability of blood-brain barrier to various sized molecules. Am J Physiol 235:H712–H718

Metes JJ, Lazo A, Wilner HI et al. (1985) Supra-ophthalmic placement of microleak balloon catheters for intracranial chemotherapy infusion: complications and results of therapy. AJNR 6:948–952

Nakagawa H, Groothius D, Blasberg RG (1984) The effect of graded hypertonic intracarotid infusions on drug delivery to experimental RG-2 gliomas. Neurology 34:1571–1581

Neuwelt EA, Barnett PA (1989) Blood-brain barrier disruption in the treatment of brain tumors: animal studies. In: Neuwelt EA (ed) Implications of the blood-brain barrier and its manipulation. Plenum Medical, New York, pp 107–193

Neuwelt EA, Dahlborg SA (1989) Blood-brain barrier disruption in the treatment of brain tumors: clinical implications. In: Neuwelt EA (ed) Implications of the blood-brain barrier and its manipulation. Plenum Medical, New York, pp 195–261

Neuwelt EA, Diehl JD, Vu LH et al. (1981) Monitoring of methotrexate delivery in patients with malignant brain tumors after osmotic blood-brain barrier disruption. Ann Intern Med 94:449–454

Neuwelt EA, Barnett PA, Bigner DD, Frenkel EP (1982) Effects of adrenal cortical steroids and osmotic blood-brain barrier opening on methotrexate delivery to

gliomas in the rodent: the factor of the blood-brain barrier. Proc Natl Acad Sci USA 79:4420–4423
Neuwelt EA, Glasberg M, Frenkel E, Barnett P (1983) Neurotoxicity of chemotherapeutic agents after blood-brain barrier modification: neuropathological studies. Ann Neurol 14:316–324
Safdari H, Mompeon B, Dubois JB, Gros C (1985) Intra-arterial 1,3-bis(2-chloroethyl)-1-nitrosourea chemotherapy for the treatment of malignant gliomas of the brain: a preliminary report. Surg Neurol 24:490–497
Saris SC, Blasberg RG, Carson RE et al. (1991) Intravascular streaming during carotid artery infusions: demonstration in humans and reduction using diastole-phased, pulsatile administration. J Neurosurg 74:763–772
Saris SC, Shook DR, Blasberg RG et al. (1987) Carotid artery mixing with diastole phased pulsed drug infusion. J Neurosurg 67:721–725
Shapiro WR (1986) Therapy of adult malignant brain tumors: What have the clinical trials taught us? Semin Oncol 13(1):38–45
Shapiro WR, Ausman JI (1969) The chemotherapy of brain tumors: a clinical and experimental review. In: Plum F (ed) Recent advances in neurology. FA Davis, Philadelphia, pp 150–235
Shapiro WR, Green SB (1987) Letter to the editor: Re-evaluating the efficacy of intra-arterial BCNU. J Neurosurg 66:313–315
Shapiro WR, Shapiro JR (1986) Principles of brain tumor chemotherapy. Semin Oncol 13(1):56–69
Shapiro JR, Yung WK-A, Shapiro WR (1981) Isolation, karyotype and clonal growth of heterogeneous subpopulations of human malignant glioma. Cancer Res 51:2349–2359
Silbergleit R, Steffey DJ, DeFilipp GJ et al. (1989) Cerebral distribution of contrast medium during slow intracarotid infusion. AJNR 10:1061–1064
Wolpert SM, Kwan ESK, Heros D et al. (1988) Selective delivery of chemotherapeutic agents with a new catheter system. Radiology 166:547–549
Yung W-KA, Shapiro WR, Shapiro JR (1982) Heterogeneous chemosensitivities of subpopulations of human glioma cells in culture. Cancer Res 42:992–998

11 Local Intra-arterial Fibrinolysis in the Vertebrobasilar and Carotid Territories

HERMANN ZEUMER and F. ZANELLA

CONTENTS

11.1 Introduction

Thromboembolic occlusion of the large pial vessels is a major cause of cerebral ischemic stroke. Recanalization of such occluded vessels seems to be the most reasonable therapeutic strategy in stroke patients. However, after the introduction of streptokinase as an effective fibrinolytic agent in the 1960s, early trials to ascertain its efficacy in stroke-prone patients failed to demonstrate a reasonable benefit to risk ratio (DEL ZOPPO et al. 1986). On the other hand, local fibrinolysis with the aim of coronary artery recanalization proved effective in providing high recanalization rates with less systemic hemorrhagic effects. In the cerebral arteries local intra-arterial fibrinolytic (LIF) therapy has been applied primarily in those patients commonly displaying progression of stroke, usually with a lethal outcome, e.g., patients with acute vertebrobasilar occlusion (AVBO). The prognosis of patients suffering from AVBO was shown by HACKE et al. (1988) to be improved significantly using this treatment.

Middle cerebral artery (MCA) strokes, however, are much more frequent than AVBO. Following the availability of tissue plasminogen activator (tPA), an intravenously administrable, fibrinolytic agent with high fibrin specificity, several trials have been started to investigate its use in the MCA territory. Not all of these studies have been completed, but in our view the results are not convincing, especially with regard to the recanalization rate. Meanwhile more sophisticated microcatheter systems have been developed and we have therefore again started to use LIF in the MCA territory. Our results now demonstrate reasonable recanalization rates of about 80%. Heparinization is an excellent treatment in patients suffering from sinus thrombosis, but in certain cases fibrinolysis may be an important alternative. Until now, all therapeutic regimens trying to avoid blindness due to central retinal artery occlusion have failed. Recent results employing LIF in the ophthalmic artery demonstrate excellent clinical success (SCHMIDT et al. 1991; SCHUMACHER and SCHMIDT 1991).

HERMANN ZEUMER, M.D., Professor; F. ZANELLA, M.D., Professor; Abteilung für Neuroradiologie, Radiologische Klinik, Universitätskrankenhaus Eppendorf, Universität Hamburg, Martinistraße 52, W-2000 Hamburg 20, FRG

11.2 General Considerations

The death of neurons occurs within a few minutes after complete anoxia. However, daily observation of the natural course of stroke and the very heterogeneous outcome, especially in cases of MCA occlusion, taught us that almost all strokes have a progressive course. This progression seems to be the most reasonable therapeutic window for successful LIF therapy. But as we now know, the duration of the progression varies and is much longer than formerly estimated. Progression is influenced especially by the following five factors:

1. Type of occlusion
2. Collateralization
3. The ischemic penumbra
4. Secondary thrombi
5. Intrinsic/extrinsic fibrinolysis

Each of these factors is discussed in turn below.

11.2.1 Type of Occlusion

Up to 80% of MCA occlusions are considered to be embolic in origin. This includes cardiac emboli as well as arterio-arterial emboli deriving from arteriosclerotic lesions of the carotid bifurcation or the intracranial segment of the vertebral artery. It is well accepted that thrombi arising at the site of arteriosclerotic lesions may grow and thus lead to continuous worsening of the clinical symptomatology (ARCHER and HORENSTEIN 1977; CAPLAN 1983; DEL ZOPPO et al. 1986). From our clinical observations and superselective angiographic studies, we learned that progressive clinical deterioration also frequently occurs in the case of embolic occlusions of cerebral arteries. We regularly observed that emboli in the intracranial vessels did not occlude the vascular lumen completely (SIEPMANN et al. 1991; ZEUMER et al. 1989). Usually it is possible to pass the embolus by using a microcatheter, thereby reaching the distal end of the embolus. Angiographic studies revealed that the catheter does not penetrate the embolus but passes between the embolus and the vessel wall. This leads to the conclusion that there is persistence of very small and angiographically invisible channels which provide minimal residual blood flow. However, this fact alone cannot explain brain survival for a prolonged period.

11.2.2 Collateralization

With the exception of some functional terminal supply areas, e.g., the territory of the lenticulostriate arteries, the intracranial vessels are collaterally connected not only by means of the circle of Willis but also by numerous collateral leptomeningeal channels. In this context the basilar artery is a unique vessel, because it has four pedicles (both vertebral and both posterior communicating arteries), which may act as in- or outflow channels if necessary, providing strong collateral flow even in the presence of severe basilar vertebral obstruction.

11.2.3 Ischemic Penumbra

From animal experiments it is known that in the area surrounding completely anoxic brain, neurons may survive structurally although they have already lost their function (ASTRUP et al. 1981). With improved oxygenation neurons may survive and regain their function, but otherwise they will die due to metabolic disturbances. Furthermore, it is generally accepted that ischemic cellular dysfunction correlates strongly with the dysregulation of the energy-dependent cellular calcium metabolism (GELMERS and HENNERICI 1990; TRIGGLE 1990). Animal experiments have shown that brain ischemia is much better tolerated if calcium channel blockers have been administered in advance of ischemia. Thus the progression but potential reversibility of stroke-related deficits is a strong argument for the administration of calcium channel blockers in the early stage of stroke, particularly if reoxygenation is possible by means of LIF-induced recanalization. This view is supported by recent clinical studies (GELMERS and HENNERICI 1990).

11.2.4 Secondary Thrombi

Secondary (stagnation) thrombi may play an important role in the progression of stroke not only in the case of atherothrombotic growing lesions but also in that of embolic vascular occlusions. Using the microcatheter technique for superselective angiography we were able to demonstrate that emboli treated at an early stage are only locally adherent and can be passed (SIEPMANN et al. 1991; ZEUMER et al. 1989). However, if emboli are treated after lodging for several hours intravascularly, fibrinolysis may demonstrate the original embolus only after lysis of surrounding clots. We now believe that morphologic stroke progression is influenced at least as much by secondary thrombi occluding small collateral channels as by the breakdown of the ischemic penumbra due to metabolic processes.

11.2.5 Intrinsic/Extrinsic Fibrinolysis

Spontaneous recanalization of embolic vascular occlusion is not rare and is organized by the intrinsic fibrinolytic system; but usually it does not work as fast as is necessary to avoid severe stroke-related damage. It is well known that large lentiform nucleus infarctions are very often due to transient (or chronic) occlusion of the MCA at the level of the M1 segment (ADAMS et al. 1983; BLADIN and BERKOVIC 1984; FIESCHI and BOZZAO 1969; RINGELSTEIN et al. 1991; WEILLER et al. 1990; ZEUMER et al. 1981). Limitation of the infarction area to the lentiform (or the caudate) nucleus only occurs when there is well-established collateralization of the distal MCA but definite infarction in the functional terminal supply area due to occlusion of the lenticulostriate arteries. RINGELSTEIN et al. (1991) recently demonstrated that pure lentiform nucleus infarction usually appeared in those individuals in whom recanalization occurred on average within 3.8 h after embolic occlusion of the M1 segment. The intention of LIF is to mimic and enhance this spontaneous course.

11.2.6 Follow-up Problems

With respect to the basilar territory, the extremely bad prognosis of untreated AVBO is well known (ARCHER and HORENSTEIN 1977; BRÜCKMANN et al. 1986; FERBERT et al. 1990; KUBIK and ADAMS 1946). Any reduction of mortality or extreme disability ("locked-in syndrome") to below 90% has to be regarded as a success. The situation in respect of carotid territory strokes is different. Angiologically very similar MCA occlusions may lead to tremendously different types of brain lesions and functional deficits (RINGELSTEIN et al. 1991). Moreover, even extensive brain damage and initial functional deficit may be compensated by means of effective rehabilitation measures.

11.2.7 General Conclusions

Anticipating that stroke will be a progressive event pathophysiologically, and in view of the features of early stroke mechanisms outlined above, it is imperative that:

1. The obstructing thrombotic material is removed by means of fibrinolysis
2. Secondary thrombosis is avoided by administering heparin as early as possible, though only for as long as necessary (i.e., until recanalization is achieved)
3. Brain protection is ensured to the maximum extent currently possible, using the available calcium channel blockers

11.3 Clinical and Angiologic Findings

11.3.1 Vertebrobasilar Territory

The clinical features of proven basilar artery occlusion have been described by various authors (BRÜCKMANN et al. 1986; CAPLAN 1980, 1983; FERBERT et al. 1990; FISHER 1988). Two-thirds of acute basilar occlusions occur with progression over hours, and initially brain stem dysfunction is not always obvious. Especially lesions at the pontine level may initially present with monoparesis (FISHER 1988) which subsequently progresses to tetraplegia. Oculomotor disturbances and impaired consciousness with tetraparesis are indicative of a "top of the basilar" territory lesion (Fig. 11.1). However, one-third of patients initially present only with deep coma. Vertigo, vomiting, horizontal gaze palsy, and lower cranial nerve dysfunction are highly indicative of bilateral vertebral basilar occlusion. The period between the appearance of the first prodromal symptoms and the endpoint of deep coma and automatic stretch and flexion movements covers a variable time span lasting up to 24 h. In most patients with embolic occlusions, clinical progression takes place over a period of about 6 h.

Atherothrombotic occlusions are found more frequently in the intracranial vertebrobasilar system than in the MCA. The patient 60–70 years of age with longstanding hypertension and diabetes who initially presents with symptoms at the pontine level will often demonstrate an arteriosclerotic basilar stenosis with secondary thrombi (Fig. 11.2a). The subsequent clinical signs and symp-

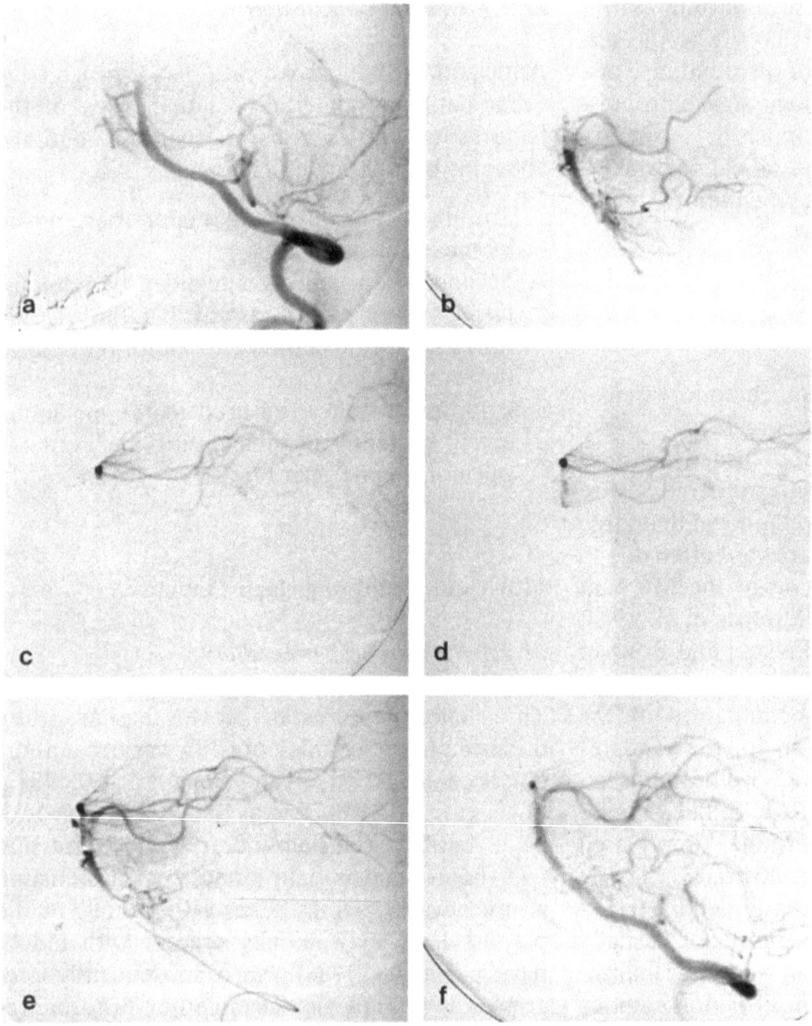

△

Fig. 11.1a–f. "Top of the basilar" embolic occlusion. **a** Vertebral angiography. **b** Superselective angiography demonstrating small residual channels around the embolus. **c** Angiogram distal to the embolus. **d** Tip of the catheter in between vessel wall and embolus. **e** Progressing lysis. **f** Full recanalization. Clinically good recovery after initial tetraparesis

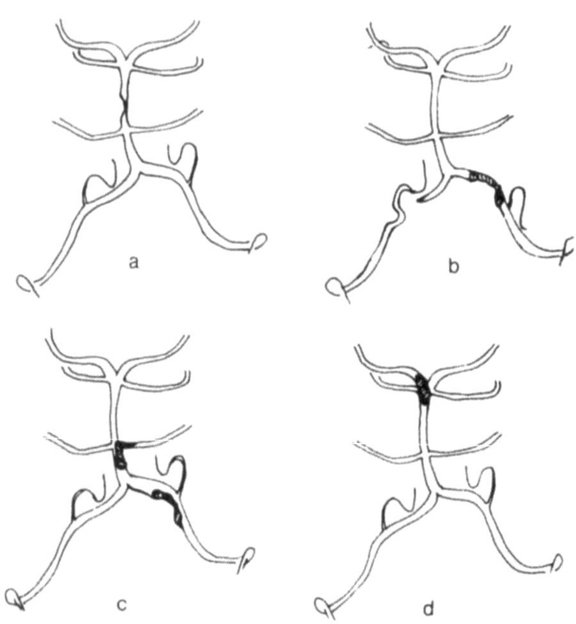

Fig. 11.2a–d. Types of vertebrobasilar occlusion. **a** Arteriosclerotic basilar stenosis with secondary thrombi. **b** Bilateral vertebrobasilar occlusion. **c** Embolus at mid-basilar region. **d** Embolus at top of basilar artery

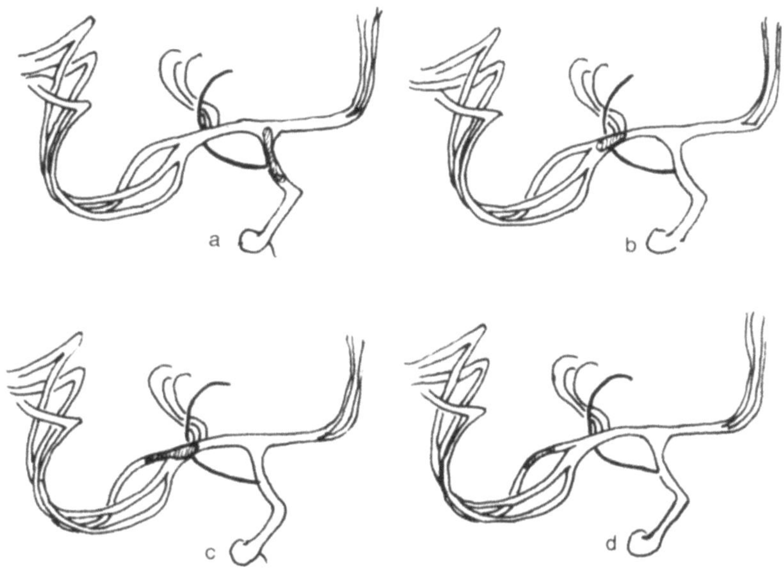

Fig. 11.3a–d. Embolic occlusion in the carotid territory: a–d, types I–IV respectively (see text for explanation of types)

toms depend on the major direction of the extension of the secondary thrombi. In the case of bilateral vertebrobasilar occlusion (Fig. 11.2b) one vertebral artery usually is obliterated at the intracranial level over a long period. On the other hand, fresh thrombi are detectable angiographically and usually present with clinical signs and symptoms contralateral to the initial hemiparesis. Concomitant impairment of consciousness indicates either that a secondary embolus has already occurred to the top of the basilar artery or that there are no communicating posterior cerebral arteries. If it is not treated, the thrombus will advance from the vertebral artery to the basilar artery, with the development of corresponding clinical signs and symptoms.

Embolic occlusions of the basilar artery very frequently occur due to arterio-arterial embolization. An atheroma of the intracranial segment of the vertebral artery will often prove to be the source of the embolus. The embolus may stop at the midbasilar region (Fig. 12.2c) or may ascend to the top of the basilar artery (Fig. 11.2d). Very large emboli often immediately lead to deep coma and complete loss of function of the brain stem. However, the clinical signs are regularly multiterritorial and involve more sites of function than, for example, a lacunar stroke. Progression of clinical symptoms is accordance with expansion of the embolus is frequently observed. For these reasons it is crucial that decisions concerning angiography and therapy be made as soon as multiterritorial brain stem dysfunction and clinical progress are ascertained by careful clinical observation. Results of treatment have been published in detail (Brückmann et al. 1986; Hacke et al. 1991; Hacke and Hirschberg 1990; Karnik et al. 1985, 1986; von Kummer et al. 1988; Lehmann et al. 1989; Möbius et al. 1989; Mori et al. 1988; Nenci et al. 1983; Zeumer 1985; Zeumer et al. 1982, 1983a,b) and taken overall show a 60% improvement in survival.

11.3.2 Carotid Territory

Carotid occlusion below the level of the anterior choroidal artery leads to hemodynamically induced strokes only if the circle of Willis is incomplete or other brain supplying arteries are also obstructed. Using a superselective angiographic technique we were able to identify more distal types of occlusion (Fig. 11.3). Occlusion of the internal carotid artery (ICA) at the level of the anterior choroidal artery – type I – usually leads to sensory motor hemiplegia. This type is a rare finding (Fig. 11.3a). Early recanalization usually provides excellent recovery. An embolic occlusion at the level of the M1 segment of the MCA – type II (Fig. 11.3b) – usually provokes dense hemiplegia due to the occlusion of the lenticulostriate arteries. In the event of successful recanalization, the

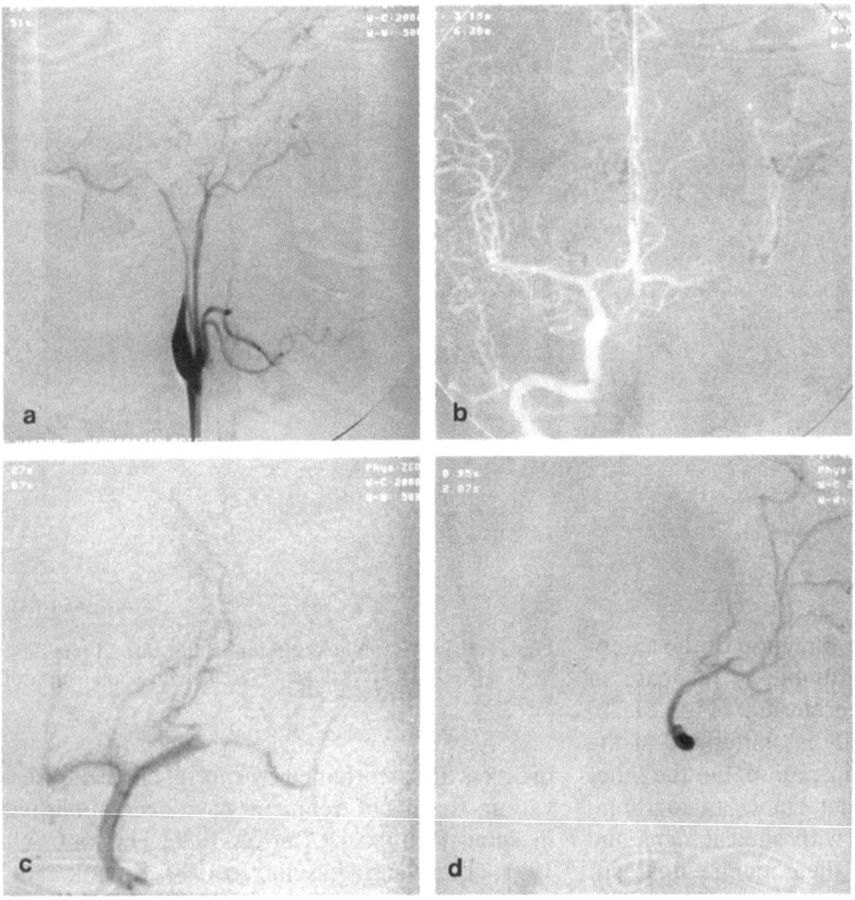

Fig. 11.4a–d. ICA dissection with secondary embolic occlusion of the MCA, type III. **a** Dissected ICA. **b** Cross-flow angiogram of the occluded left MCA. **c** Superselective angiogram demonstrating the embolus in the M1 segment of the MCA. **d** Control angiogram demonstrates M1 segment recanalization. Despite residual occlusion of the anterior main branch of the MCA, complete recovery occurred after initial hemiplegia and aphasia. The patient was a physician who was back at work 6 months later

extent of lentiform nucleus infarction depends on how many and which of the lenticulostriate arteries have been occluded for more than a few minutes.

In some cases of MCA occlusion the top of the embolus has entered one of the major branches – type III (Fig. 11.3c). Recanalization is usually possible in the M1 segment. However, if the tip of the catheter cannot be advanced beyond the top of the embolus, the embolus is often cut at the level of the trifurcation and residual embolic material occludes one of the major branches of the MCA persistently. In such cases the extent of brain damage depends on the capacity of the collateral pathways to the territory of the persistently occluded branch (Fig. 11.4).

Small emboli may enter one of the major branches of the MCA more or less distally – type IV (Fig. 12.3d). Clinical deficits depend on the site of occlusion and the extent of collateralization. Sometimes multiple emboli enter the carotid artery and are floated into the MCA and anterior cerebral artery (ACA) as well or are captured in the ICA siphon, which has been a bad prognostic sign in the limited number of cases that we have observed. Even if parts of the emboli can be lysed by LIF, major damage or death may occur. In general we might conclude from our experience that the clinical results of successful recanalization after MCA strokes are better, the more proximal a single occlusion site is found (Siepmann et al. 1991).

One further major aspect has to be considered with regard to LIF in the MCA territory: On the basis of the clinical experience described in the literature, the results of animal experiments, and our own early experiences with fibrinolysis, we have to propose a clear – cut time limit of 6 h after stroke for LIF in the MCA territory. Hemorrhagic transformation in necrotic brain areas after stroke is very frequently found on CT and MRI subsequent to intrinsic or extrinsic fibrinolysis (DEL ZOPPO et al. 1986; HACKE et al. 1988; STURM and ZEUMER 1983). The risk of cerebral hemorrhage with a space-occupying hematoma increases significantly if fibrinolytic treatment has been performed beyond the time limit of 6 h (POERSCH 1989). In our view the most probable reason for this observation is the anoxic damage to the lenticulostriate arteries, which may not resist the normal blood pressure beyond this time limit. Furthermore, animal stroke models have shown that secondary metabolic disturbances due to ischemia regularly show severe progression by this time. Clinically this observation is supported by the observations of RINGELSTEIN et al. (1991), who found that the extent of brain damage increases with the time lapse, prior to spontaneous recanalization.

Results of MCA recanalization have been described in detail by various authors (DEL ZOPPO et al. 1987; SIEPMANN et al. 1991; THERON et al. 1989; ZEUMER et al. 1983c, 1984). The results demonstrate the possibility of recanalization with a tolerable risk, but they have not yet provided evidence of clinical efficacy.

11.3.3 Ophthalmic Artery

In the past numerous therapeutic attempts have been made to avoid blindness following occlusion of the central retinal artery. They have all failed. However, SCHUMACHER and co-workers recently reported on six patients who regained partial or complete vision following LIF of the ophthalmic artery (SCHMIDT et al. 1991; SCHUMACHER and SCHMIDT 1991); we have now had similar experiences. A very promising aspect of our observations is the finding that even treatment 24 h after acute monocular blindness provides at least partial vision (Fig. 11.5). Earlier treatment would probably lead to even better results in respect of vision.

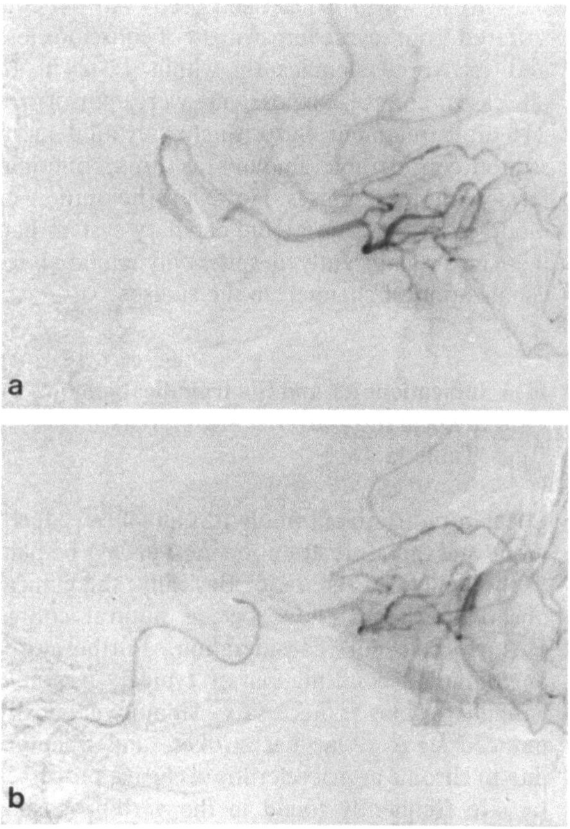

Fig. 11.5 a,b. Angiographic findings in patient with acute loss of vision in the left eye 34 h previously. **a** Ophthalmic artery shows only minimal ophthalmic retinal blush. **b** Almost normal ophthalmic blush is seen 90 min later after reappearance of vision, which began after 30 min

11.3.4 Sinus Thrombosis

Severe headache, epileptic seizures, and focal neurologic deficits due to congestive cerebral hemorrhage usually lead to the diagnosis of sinus thrombosis. In the less complicated cases full heparinization provides excellent success in avoiding further progression of the thrombosis while intrinsic fibrinolysis is removing the clot. However, in rare cases patients with extensive sinus thrombosis present with severely impaired consciousness due to brain swelling. Systemic fibrinolysis seems to be dangerous, especially in patients in whom congestive hemorrhage has already occurred. In such a situation, when extreme brain swelling will inevitably result in death, treatment has to be undertaken urgently. The number of our LIF treatments is very small in comparison to all the sinus thromboses we have seen; however, as yet LIF has proved successful in all the cases

($n = 6$) in which it has been used. All patients suffered from severe impairment of consciousness and recovered significantly within 12–24 h. In all cases control angiograms were performed 24 h after treatment. Surprisingly they all demonstrated considerable amounts of thrombotic material within the sinuses. However, the outflow of blood from the arterial and capillary system had increased significantly despite only minimal recanalization of channels in the sinuses.

11.4 Indications for and Contraindications to Local Intra-arterial Fibrinolysis (Table 11.1)

Local intra-arterial fibrinolysis is an invasive technique and therefore attention must always be paid to the benefit to risk ratio. Basically, the clinical observations and the expected natural course must receive full consideration. Furthermore, angiographic confirmation of typical, treatable vascular lesions is necessary. Hemodynamically induced strokes, lacunar strokes, and ischemia due to chronic arteriosclerotic occlusive processes (as are frequently found in the vertebrobasilar territory with a relatively benign prognosis) must not be treated by LIF. We believe that conventional angiographic devices should no longer be used for such interventional procedures. Digital subtraction angiography (DSA) allows faster diagnosis, more detailed imaging, better assistance for superselective catheterization, and the use of isosmotic contrast media. General contraindications to LIF are diseases or conditions involving impaired hemostasis or a high risk of hemorrhage, e.g., cerebral aneurysms, cerebral AVMs, recent cerebral infarction already visible on computed tomography, pregnancy, and the first 10 days after surgery.

11.4.1 Vertebrobasilar Territory

In our opinion LIF in the vertebrobasilar system is contraindicated (a) when there is unilateral vertebral artery occlusion only, and (b) in patients with chronic, well collateralized atheriosclerotic occlusions of the vertebral or basilar artery. Either the prognosis is not that bad or arteriosclerotic lesions cannot be adequately treated by means of LIF. When deep coma and longstanding severe brain stem deficits (e.g., tetraplegia and automatic movements) are present, the prognosis often cannot be improved by LIF. This is a relative contraindication, however, because LIF in any case offers the last chance for survival. At least two of our own patients would not have survived if we had taken the above-mentioned criterion as absolute. Although we cannot draw upon statistically significant data to support our conclusions, we would recommend that LIF be tried especially in young and middle-aged individuals with embolic basilar occlusion; it cannot be recommended in the elderly with extensive secondary thrombosis due to atherosclerotic lesions within the vertebrobasilar system. Extended hypodense brain stem lesions also are a striking contraindication to LIF. Treatment is absolutely indicated in any state of *progressive* vertebrobasilar stroke due to an appropriate (Fig. 11.1) vascular lesion (see Sect. 11.3.1). Further delay carries a higher risk than diagnostic angiography anyway. Due to the variability in the progress of clinical signs and symptoms in the course of AVBO we do not recommend any upper time limit for treatment in such patients; there is a realistic chance of achieving at least partial functional recovery after successful recanalization as long as any residual brain stem function is observed. In addition, as is known from the natural course and from the observations of those who have treated patients with LIF, the frequency of secondary hemorrhage

Table 11.1. Local intra-arterial fibrinolytic therapy: clinical and angiologic criteria

Contraindications	Questionable	Indications
Deep coma lasting more than 6 h Decerebrate rigidity	Deep coma lasting less than 6 h with tetraparesis	Basilar territory stroke in progress Incomplete deficit of brain stem function, regardless of the onset of symptoms
or	*and/or*	*and*
Well collateralized, chronic occlusion	Atherothrombotic midbasilar occlusion	Basilar embolism or acute bilateral intracranial verte-brobasilar occlusion

into the brain stem is lower than in the MCA territory.

11.4.2 Embolic Occlusion of the MCA

Dense hemiplegia with other signs of hemispheric ischemia and transcranial Doppler ultrasonographic or angiographic findings of the types of occlusion depicted in Fig. 11.3 are strong indications for LIF, if these observations are made before 4 h (or at most 5 h) have elapsed since stroke. At least 1 h should be left for treatment before the definitive endpoint of 6 h after stroke is reached. A "dense middle cerebral artery sign" on CT may be helpful. It is necessary to look closely at the CT scan because unrecognized, more advanced stroke events may sometimes have occurred. Low density areas represent a contraindication to LIF; however, usually they are not seen earlier than 6 h after stroke even with advanced CT devices.

11.4.3 Central Retinal Artery Occlusion

Acute monocular blindness and ophthalmoscopically demonstrated retinal ischemia are readily available criteria for the use of LIF. Neurologic examination and cerebral CT examination should be performed in advance of diagnostic and therapeutic angiography since unnoticed emboli may have occurred into the brain. Selective carotid angiography using DSA usually reveals no ocular blush, which reappears after successful fibrinolysis.

Time limits for LIF are not yet quite clear. Treatment seems to be reasonable up to 24–36 h.

11.4.4 Sinus Thrombosis

As pointed out above, LIF is not recommended generally in cases of sinus thrombosis. However, severe impairment of consciousness (especially) represents a prognostically bad sign and can develop to a life-threatening state. In these cases LIF should be taken into consideration. In all our own cases and in those that have come to our knowledge, intracerebral hemorrhage had already occurred. We did not observe any significant progression of hematomas with the proposed treatment regimen. Nevertheless, because the number of cases is as yet too small to allow significant conclusions, we recommend LIF only in those cases in which it is thought likely to be a life-saving measure.

11.5 Hamburg Acute Stroke Treatment (HAST) Protocol

11.5.1 In the Emergency Room

1. Evaluation of the patient's history in respect of onset of symptoms and the development of signs.
2. Neurologic examination (ophthalmologic).
3. If available, transcranial doppler ultrasonography.
4. If a stable, circumscribed brain stem deficit can be pinpointed or if there is hemispheric infarction with overrun of the above-mentioned time limits, the patient should be taken to the ward for further observation and conservative treatment.
5. Alarm neuroradiologists if this is warranted by the clinical findings.
6. Place central venous catheter and take a blood sample for laboratory analysis (cell count, fibrinogen, thrombin time, partial thromboplastin time, electrolytes, blood sugar, urea).
7. CT: Rule out hemorrhage or advanced ischemic infarction. Possibly demonstrate dense middle cerebral artery or basilar artery sign or severe calcifications of the vertebral or basilar artery.
8. Obtain the informed consent of the patient, or that of his relatives if the patient is unable to make decisions.
9. Bolus injection of 5000 units of heparin and infusion of 1000 units of heparin continuously unless it is known that the patient has been receiving platelet inhibitors. The combination of this medication carries a significantly increased risk of hemorrhage, especially when LIF is performed.
10. 30 mg nimodipine orally. We are aware that oral administration is not the optimal treatment; however, intravenous administration of nimodipine may lead to severe blood pressure problems. Calcium antagonists with a lesser effect on blood pressure but a greater effect on brain protection are currently in preparation. Use them when they become available.

11. Each uncooperative patient should undergo intubation in order to make angiography and superselective catheterization, as well as the placement of the microcatheter, fast, safe, and easy.
12. If hematocrit exceeds 50%, perform isovolemic hemodilution.
Proceed to the angiography suite.

11.5.2 In the Angiography Suite

1. Check laboratory results to be in the normal range. If they are not, consult the hematologist for assistance.
2. Prepare saline infusion containing 1000 units of heparin per 100 ml for flushing the coaxial catheter system with 100 ml/h. Do not forget to remove the intravenous heparin infusion before this measure.
3. Place a sheath set (6F) in the groin.
4. Prepare microcatheter (Tracker 18/10) with "J"-shape microwire and "Y"-shaped hemostatic valve connected to flush infusion.
5. A 5F Schneider Softip may be used for coaxial guidance but not for coaxial dye injection. A 6F introducer catheter allows both control angiography and microcatheter application.
6. Prepare two 50 ml syringes containing 0.9% saline and 10 mg tPA (Actilyse). (Alternatively, 500 IU urokinase per 50 ml may be administered.) An infusion pump (Perfusor, Braun-Melsungen) should be available and set on 50 ml/h. Ask the company for a device which allows higher pressure than usual (small and long microcatheters have a high flow resistance!).

   20 mg tPA (1 000 000 IU urokinase) is the maximum dose to be administered during a period of 2 h.
7. Use isosmotic contrast medium (Ultravist 150) for superselective angiography.

   Injections for superselective control angiography should be done gently under DSA control in order to avoid migration of thrombotic material. In the event of stagnation of the dye distal to an occlusion site, reaspirate the dye to avoid involuntary toxic effects of the dye. For the same reason, control angiography should be performed via the coaxial catheter whenever possible.

11.5.3 Vertebrobasilar Territory

1. Diagnostic angiography should demonstrate the occlusion site and possible collateral vessels (e.g., posterior communicating arteries, anterior spinal arteries, cerebellar arteries).
2. The patient's age and history as well as the site of the occlusion (lower basilar artery, midportion of the intracranial vertebral artery) may provide some clues as to underlying atherothrombotic disease. In the presence of such disease, coaxial superselective catheterization of the vertebral/basilar artery is not usually possible beyond the occlusion site. In this case the tip of the catheter should be placed as close as possible to the end of the vessel lumen, and in particular as far distal as possible to any branching vessels. In this situation it must be borne in mind that thrombotic material distal to the atherothrombotic stenosis may have a greater influence on the clinical outcome than thrombotic material proximal to or at the site of the atherothrombotic lesion. This is especially true in the case of a secondary "top of the basilar" embolism distal to an atherothrombotic lesion in the intracranial vertebral artery. Successful treatment is then usually possible only if the contralateral vertebral artery can be passed in order to lyse the most distal embolus.
3. In the case of basilar embolisms it is typically possible to bypass the embolus with the microguidewire and the microcatheter. The catheter tip is placed into the slit between the wall of the basilar artery and the thrombus in order to achieve the highest concentration of fibrinolytic agent at the surface of the embolus. Recently microcatheters with sideholes became available, and they will have to be tested for this purpose.
4. Never exceed 2 h of treatment (20 mg tPA).

11.5.4 Carotid Territory

1. Characteristic angiographic findings are depicted diagrammatically in Fig. 11.3. Embolic occlusions are much more frequent than in the basilar territory; therefore bypass of the catheter beyond the occlusion site is regularly possible:
2. Try to place the tip of the catheter close to the top of the embolus, which is usually possible in

the case of type II occlusions. In type III occlusions the catheter tip can be advanced easily to the trifurcation level. This may lead to cutting of the thrombus at this level, with some remaining thrombotic material in one MCA branch. Repeated control angiograms every 20–30 min at the occlusion site may lead to contrast transudation into the lentiform nucleus by way of the damaged lenticulostriate arteries and dye overload. Resulting hyperdensity on CT is not space occupying, in contrast to hemorrhage.

3. Lysis time varies significantly, from 30 to 120 min.
4. *Never* commence LIF in the MCA territory later than 5 h after stroke, never exceed 6 h after stroke with treatment, and *never* treat for more than a total of 2 h.
5. Even the treatment of arterio-arterial emboli has to be considered. If secondary MCA occlusion in the case of a seemingly occluded ipsilateral ICA has been demonstrated by collateral flow, try to get through the stump of the occluded – but usually only collapsed – ICA using the microguidewire. This is worthwhile because frequently the ICA can be passed easily at the occlusion site and the MCA can be entered by the microcatheter. We would not propose percutaneous transluminal angioplasty (PTA) of the ICA in these cases, except in the desperate situation of absence of collaterals to the appropriate hemisphere. Even in cases of spontaneous carotid dissection the microguidewire sometimes passes the stenosis caused by subintimal hematomas. Upon reaching the MCA, a secondary embolus may be lysed (Fig. 11.4).

11.5.5 Central Retinal Artery Occlusion

Central retinal artery occlusion is easily assessed by clinical means. Selective angiography of the ICA usually demonstrates no delineation of the ophthalmic artery at all or, at the least, absence of the physiologic ophthalmic blush. If possible to ophthalmic artery should be catheterized superselectively. We do not exceed the usual LIF time of 2 h (20 mg tPA). Reappearance of ophthalmic blush and improving vision seem to occur simultaneously. If the ophthalmic artery is no longer visible, a frontal branch of the temporal artery may be catheterized superselectively in order to perform the treatment by using the regularly collateralizing angular artery.

11.5.6 Sinus Thrombosis

The central goal of the treatment is to improve venous outflow as soon as possible. To be successful it is not necessary to remove all clots from the sinuses; for this reason we do not believe in venous catheterization and lysis. However, the administration of a fibrinolytic agent into the ICA causes it to accumulate in the sinuses, especially in those severe cases in which the fibrinolytic agent cannot escape in any way.

Fibrinolysis should be discontinued after 2 h even if there is no obvious recanalization. Clinical improvement will occur even if extended thrombi are present within the sinuses on late control angiography.

11.6 Treatment After Local Intra-arterial Fibrinolysis

Generally, if the treatment time of 2 h has expired, heparinization should be stopped in all cases of complete recanalization after embolization, in order to avoid hemorrhagic transformation of any infarctions. If, however, an atherothrombotic occlusion has been recanalized, full heparinization (1000 units per hour) has to be performed continuously in order to avoid reocclusion. It may be necessary to control the residual lumen of the stenotic vessel after a few days. If only a tiny lumen is present, it may be necessary to place the patient under a coumarin regimen. In the case of sinus thrombosis, continuation of heparinization is crucial. We usually keep the patient under heparin for at least 8 days and then switch to a coumarin regimen for 3 months.

It would be desirable to use a calcium antagonist with less impact on blood pressure but more impact on brain protection; however, such an agent is not yet commercially available. Thus we turn to an intravenous nimodipine regimen, similar to that used in patients with subarachnoid hemorrhage, as soon as we know that blood pressure is under control at any time.

After LIF the sheath set is left in place and the patient is taken to the intensive care unit. Another blood sample is taken to rule out systemic effects of fibrinolytic therapy. Although we have observed no serious disturbances of the hemostatic system using the above-described regimen, we only remove the sheath set if the partial thromboplastin time is not beyond twice the normal level in our laboratory.

A short time after fibrinolysis almost all patients reveal severe functional neurologic deficits. In our view, the avoidance of complications and the early implementation of rehabilitation measures are as important for the final outcome as successful recanalization initially.

11.7 Complications

Streptokinase, urokinase, and tPA are well known as potent fibrinolytic agents. Among these, tPA shows the highest fibrin specificity in the cascade of fibrinolytic processes. Furthermore this fibrin-specific substance shows the shortest half-life (3 min) and has the least influence on the hemostatic system in general (DEL ZOPPO et al. 1986; HACKE et al. 1987; SEIFRIED 1988). Nevertheless, owing to the tremendous heterogeneity of factors that influence the recanalization process in different ways in different individuals, at present we can only suppose that tPA is the safest fibrinolytic agent and the easiest to handle; moreover, we recently found that tPA is not in fact superior to urokinase in terms of recanalization time, as had been expected.

With the regimen mentioned above we have as yet observed no instances of clinically relevant hemorrhage. Furthermore, even when other regimens (streptokinase, urokinase) formerly employed are taken into account, cerebral hemorrhage only occurred when strict treatment guidelines (Table 12.2) were disregarded. In a total of 89 treatments, four cases of serious bleeding occurred either due to already visible brain stem infarction on CT or because time limits in the carotid territory were exceeded. Hemorrhage at the puncture site and hemorrhagic transformation of infarctions occur more frequently 24–36 h after treatment in those patients who are kept on heparin.

In our view the complication of major concern is the propagation of secondary emboli. Especially if large thrombi are adherent to an atherosclerotic lesion, rough injections during control angiography may cause thrombus fragments to move into the periphery. We have seen this once in our 89 cases. In the case in question embolic material was displaced from the intracranial vertebral artery to the top of the basilar artery. Despite complete removal of the embolic material within 10 min, serious and irreversible deterioration occurred.

Another potential risk is related to the contrast medium. Highly concentrated and slow flowing contrast medium has at least a transient toxic effect on brain tissue. Therefore superselective angiography must be avoided in territories without outflow, as are found regularly distal to an embolus within the MCA. Since, however, the correct catheter position has to be verified, we gently inject very small amounts of dye using DSA control and then reaspirate it if there is absence of outflow. In the basilar territory there is usually some in- and outflow distal to the occlusion due to the posterior communicating cerebral arteries. Nevertheless, serious deterioration occurred in one case after recanalization of a midbasilar atherothrombotic stenosis. Entering the distal basilar artery, we found lots of thrombotic material in this vascular segment due to insufficient outflow.

Using microcatheters with microguidewires there is a risk of vasodissection and perforation. To avoid this it is necessary to move the tip of the microguidewire at least 3–4 cm beyond the tip

Table 11.2. Local intra-arterial fibrinolysis: general guidelines

	Carotid territory	Basilar territory
1. Clinical signs	Dense hemiplegia	Incomplete loss of brain stem function
2. Occlusion site	Carotid siphon Proximal MCA	Bilateral vertebral occlusion Basilar embolism
3. Beginning	As early as possible but not after 5th hour	At any time
4. Dose (max 2 h)	20 mg tPA 5000 units heparin bolus 1000 units/h infusion	20 mg tPA 5000 units heparin bolus 1000 units/h infusion
5. End	Not after 6th hour	After 2 h

of the microcatheter during superselective catheterization. Only by using this configuration is it impossible to apply as much force to the tip of the microguidewire as is necessary for perforation or dissection. With this configuration the tip of the microguidewire will be deflected even by minimal resistance and will only enter preformed channels.

11.8 Future Aspects

The results of dose-finding and pilot studies concerning LIF in the brain-supplying arteries have been reported by a number of other groups and by ourselves. We nevertheless know from personal communications that there is much more experience with this technique than has been published. In the case of central retinal artery occlusion, up to now all therapeutic regimens have failed; on the basis of our initial results, however, it seems reasonable to anticipate that open prospective studies will prove the effectiveness of LIF. The fatal prognosis of strokes due to AVBO has been demonstrated repeatedly and the benefit of LIF is obvious (HACKE et al. 1988, 1991). This fact was demonstrated even in our first cohort, in which the results have been subject to bias caused by dose-finding problems and inaccurately defined evaluative criteria. Better results could subsequently be demonstrated in another cohort following the adoption of rigid inclusion criteria, as predominantly patients with embolic AVBO have been treated (MÖBLUS et al. 1989). We believe that a double-blind or randomized study is ethically unacceptable in patients with a more than 90% risk of lethal outcome, if a treatment is available that may reduce mortality and severe disability rates to 50% or less. Much more of an effort should be made to draw the attention of clinical neurologists to the typical course of AVBO and the possibility that treatment will be successful if it is performed as soon as possible.

In the carotid territory the problem is much more delicate. It is generally accepted that the final outcome following embolization in the internal carotid territory varies tremendously. Thus the outcome in patients with seemingly identical angiograms will range from death to survival with minimal residual deficits. Furthermore, there are no prognostically valuable tests in the early stage of embolic stroke. Thus it would be naive to believe that recanalization in the MCA territory means that prognosis will be generally improved. It has been demonstrated that LIF can be safely applied in the MCA territory, with an 80% recanalization rate and without major hemorrhagic complications. However, it is not known whether the clinical outcome is better in patients undergoing LIF or receiving intravenous tPA than in those who receive conservative treatment. Questions concerning indications and contraindications, technique, and dosage in respect of LIF now can be clearly answered, which, in our opinion, provides a basis for further prospective studies. However, we believe that such studies cannot be double blind in design because it would be unethical and dangerous to put a microcatheter into the MCA and then to infuse saline only. Thus we now need to organize a randomized study that will take into account the initial clinical and angiologic findings, sex, age, risk factors, etc. and examine the final outcome, including rehabilitation, after 1 year.

In our view the thesis to be tested is as follows: Patients who have been treated by means of LIF will have less severe deficits and will be rehabilitated earlier than those who have been treated conservatively.

References

Adams HP, Damasio HC, Putman SF, Damasio AR (1983) Middle cerebral artery occlusion as a cause of isolated subcortical infarction. Stroke 14:948–951

Archer CR, Horenstein S (1977) Basilar artery occlusion. Clinical and radiological correlation. Stroke 8:383–390

Astrup J, Siesjö B, Symon L (1981) Thresholds in cerebral ischemia: the ischemic penumbra. Stroke 12:723–725

Bladin PF, Berkovic SF (1984) Striatocapsular infarction: large infarcts in the lenticulostriate arterial territory. Neurology 34:1423–1430

Brückmann H, Ferbert A, del Zoppo GJ, Hacke W, Zeumer H (1986) The acute vertebral-basilar thrombosis. Angiological-clinical comparison and therapeutic implications. Acta Radiol [Suppl] 369:38–42

Caplan LR (1980) "Top of the basilar artery" syndrome. Neurology 30:72–79

Caplan LR (1983) Bilateral distal vertebral artery occlusion. Neurology 33:552–558

del Zoppo GJ, Zeumer H, Harker LA (1986) Thrombolytic therapy in stroke. Possibilities and hazards. Stroke 17:595–607

del Zoppo GJ, Ferbert A, Otis S et al. (1987) Local intra-arterial fibrinolytic therapy in acute carotid territory stroke. Stroke 19:307–313

Ferbert A, Brückmann H, Drummen R (1990) Clinical features of proven basilar artery occlusion. Stroke 21:1135–1142

Fieschi C, Bozzao L (1969) Transient embolic occlusion of the middle cerebral and internal carotid arteries in cerebral apoplexy. J Neurol Neurosurg Psychiatry 32:236–240

Fisher CM (1988) The "Herald hemiparesis" of basilar artery occlusion. Arch Neurol 45:1301–1303

Gelmers HJ, Hennerici M (1990) Effect of nimodipine on acute ischemic stroke. Pooled results from five randomized trials. Stroke 21:81–84

Hacke W, Hirschberg M (1990) Thrombolytic therapy in acute ischemic stroke – an update. Stroke Int 1:17–19

Hacke W, del Zoppo GJ, Harker LA (1987) Thrombosis and cerebrovascular disease. In: Poeck K, Ringelstein EB, Hacke W (eds) New trends in diagnosis and management of stroke. Springer, Berlin Heidelberg New York, pp 59–74

Hacke W, Zeumer H, Ferbert A, Brückmann H, del Zoppo GJ (1988) Intra-arterial thrombolytic therapy improves outcome in patients with acute vertebrobasilar occlusive disease. Stroke 19:1216–1222

Hacke W, del Zoppo GJ, Hirschberg M (1991) Thrombolytic therapy in acute ischemic stroke. Springer, Berlin Heidelberg New York

Hart RG, Easton JD (1986) Hemorrhagic infarcts. Stroke 17:586–589

Karnik R, Slany J, Perneczky G, Ammerer HP, Brenner H, Leitner H (1985) Regionale Fibrinolyse akuter Verschlüsse intracerebraler Gefäße. Intensivmedizin 22:31–34

Karnik R, Ammerer HP, Perneczky G, Slany J, Brenner H (1986) Akute Verschlüsse im vertebrobasilären Stromgebiet bei Kindern und jüngeren Erwachsenen. Dtsch Med Wochenschr 111:616–621

Kubik CS, Adams RD (1946) Occlusion of the basilar artery – a clinical and pathological study. Brain 69: 73–121

Lehmann R, Zschenderlein R, Gromnica-Ihle E, Ziemer S (1989) Lokale intravasale Fibrinolyse (LIF) bei akuten zerebrovaskulären Verschlüssen. Radiol Diagn (Berl) 30:481–488

Möbius E, Berg-Dammer E, Kühne D, Kunitsch G, Nahser HC (1989) Lokale intraarterielle Fibrinolyse: Therapie der Wahl bei A. Basilarisverschluß mit progredientem Hirnstamminfarkt. Aktuelle Neurologie 16:184–190

Mori E, Tabuchi M, Yoshida T, Yamadori A (1988) Intracarotid urokinase with thromboembolic occlusion of the middle cerebral artery. Stroke 19:802–812

Nenci GG, Gresele P, Taramelli M, Agnelli G, Signorini E (1983) Thrombolytic therapy for thromboembolism of vertebrobasilar artery. Angiology 34:561–571

Poersch M (1989) Lokale intraarterielle Fibrinolyse. Ergebnisse unterschiedlicher Therapiekonzepte. Inauguraldissertation, Med. Fakultät RWTH Aachen

Ringelstein EB, Biniek R, Weiller C, Ameling B, Nolte P, Thron A (1991) Type and extent of hemispheric brain infarctions and clinical outcome in early and delayed middle cerebral artery recanalisation. Neurology 42: 289–298

Schmidt D, Schumacher M, Wakhloo AK (1991) Catheter fibrinolytic therapy with urokinase in central retinal artery occlusion. Am J Ophthalmol (in press)

Schumacher M, Schmidt D (1991) Intraarterial thrombolysis in occlusion of the central retinal artery. Presented at: WIN Meeting, val d'Isere 12.1.91–19.1.91

Seifried E (1988) Klinische und biochemische Zielsetzungen bei der Thrombolysetherapie mit Neothrombolytika speziell mit Gewebeplasminogenaktivator, Prourokinase und deren Kombinationen. Hämostaseologie 8:199–213

Siepmann G, Müller-Jensen M, Goossens H, Lachenmayer L, Zeumer H (1991) Local intraarterial fibrinolysis in acute middle cerebral artery occlusion. (in press)

Sturm KW, Zeumer H (1983) Local intraarterial fibrinolysis therapy in the vertebrobasilar system: preliminary post mortem findings. Acta Neurol Scand 68:201

Theron J, Courtheoux P, Casasco A, Alachkar F, Notari F, Ganem F, Maiza D (1989) Local intraarterial fibrinolysis in carotid territory. AJNR 10:753–756

Triggle DJ (1990) Calcium antagonists. History and perspective. Stroke 21:49–58

von Kummer R, Hutschenreuter M, Krieger D, Wildemann B, Wilder-Smith E, Runkehl R, Hacke W (1988) Thrombolyse mit rt-PA bei akuten Verschlüssen intrakranieller Arterien. Intensivmedizin 25:345

Weiller C, Ringelstein EB, Reiche W, Thron A, Buell U (1990) The large striatocapsular infarct. A clinical and pathophysiological entity. Arch Neurol 47:1085–1091

Wise RJS, Bernardi S, Frackowiak RSJ, Legg NJ, Jones T (1983) Serial observations on the pathophysiology of acute stroke. Brain 106:197–222

Zeumer H (1985) Vascular recanalising techniques in interventional neuroradiology. J Neurol 231:287–294

Zeumer H, Ringelstein EB, Klose FC (1981) Lakunäre Infarkte im Computertomogramm. Differentialdiagnose, klinische und angiographische Befunde. Fortschr Röntgenstr 134:488–494

Zeumer H, Hacke W, Kolmann HL, Poeck K (1982) Lokale Fibrinolysetherapie bei Basilaristhrombose. Dtsch Med Wochenschr 107:728–731

Zeumer H, Hacke W, Ringelstein EB (1983a) Local intraarterial thrombolysis in vertebrobasilar thromboembolic disease. AJNR 4:401–404

Zeumer H, Ringelstein EB, Hacke W (1983b) Gefäßrekanalisierende Verfahren der interventionellen Neuroradiologie. ROFO 139:467–475

Zeumer H, Ringelstein EB, Hassel M, Poeck K (1983c) Lokale Fibrinolysetherapie bei subtotaler Stenose der A. cerebri media. Dtsch Med Wochenschr 108:1103–1105

Zeumer H, Hündgen R, Ferbert A, Ringelstein EB (1984) Local intraarterial fibrinolytic therapy in inaccessible internal carotid occlusion. Neuroradiology 26:315–317

Zeumer H, Freitag H-J, Grzyska U, Neunzig H-P (1989) Local intraarterial fibrinolysis in acute vertebrobasilar occlusion. Technical developments and recent results. Neuroradiology 31:336–340

12 Percutaneous Diskectomy and Chemonucleolysis

MARCO LEONARDI, GIULIANO FABRIS, and ANTONIO LAVARONI

CONTENTS

The degree of reliability and standardization of percutaneous diskectomy and chemonucleolysis achieved over the last few years has led these techniques to occupy a distinct and important position in the range of therapeutic options that can be employed to treat lumbar disk herniation. The role played by the neuroradiologist has furthermore gradually superseded that of the orthopedist or neurosurgeon in carrying out the basic manual procedure, namely puncture of the intervertebral disk under fluoroscopic monitoring. This procedure, though relatively simple, requires not only precise anatomic knowledge but also the so-called radiologic mentality that is indispensable for optimum exploitation of the equipment and superior orientation when using fluoroscopy. In effect, as we shall see below, close collaboration between clinicians and radiologists is indispensable for good results, but the percutaneous treatment of the herniated disk may rightfully be considered the domain of therapeutic neuroradiology (or interventional neuroradiology, as it may be called).

We also feel that it is right to present the two techniques of percutaneous diskectomy and chemonucleolysis together because, while they are extremely different in nature, they are directed in an almost complementary manner towards the same kind of patient, i.e., those with non-fragmented small to medium sized hernias. Percutaneous diskectomy is indicated chiefly in the treatment of minor lesions in which the posterior longitudinal ligament is intact, while chemonucleolysis allows larger hernias to be treated, provided that the contiguity between the nucleus pulposus and the herniated part has been readily ascertained by diskography.

While percutaneous diskectomy may be performed on an outpatient basis, chemonucleolysis requires more thorough preparation of the patient with desensitization treatment, as well as the constant presence of an anesthesiologist during the procedure itself.

Our experience, based on 790 patients (643 treated with chemonucleolysis and 147 with percutaneous diskectomy), was obtained over a 5-year period of hospital practice, working exclusively with inpatients.

The originality of our experience lies in the central role reserved for diskography. The patient first goes through a clinical selection procedure, which is fundamental, and then undergoes neuroradiologic selection on the basis of standard x-rays, computed tomography (CT), and magnetic resonance imaging (MRI). However, the definitive decision as to the treatment to be undertaken – chemonucleolysis or percutaneous diskectomy – is dependent upon diskography, being based on the morphologic characteristics of the hernia.

MARCO LEONARDI, M.D., Servizio di Neuroradiologia, IRCCS – Ospedale Maggiore, Via Francesco Sforza 35, 20122 Milano, Italy

GIULIANO FABRIS, M.D.; ANTONIO LAVARONI, M.D.; Servizio di Neuroradiologia, Unita'Sanitaria Locale N. 7 "Udinese", Stabilimento Ospedaliero S. Maria della Misericordia, 33100 Udine, Italy

We feel that the above routine is mandatory, but find it interesting to evaluate the influence of such a selection process. In this presentation, after providing a brief clinical and historical perspective, we shall first deal with the techniques themselves – diskography, chemonucleolysis, and percutaneous diskectomy – and afterwards with the problem of the drugs employed in chemonucleolysis and in the preparation of the patients. We shall then present our personal clinical experience and conclude with an analysis of both the patient selection indications and the results.

12.1 Lumbar Disk Herniation

We see no need to deal here with the clinical aspects or problems relating to lumbar disk herniation. Several absolutely essential points must, however, be mentioned:

- Lumbar disk herniation is one, and only one, of the "simplest" causes of sciatica.
- The further we study this pathology in depth, the more we realize how important it is that the spine be considered as a functional, organic tract which is in effect more unknown than known.
- The vast majority of the population has suffered, suffers, or will suffer from this pathology, even if in diverse ways.
- Experience indicates that at least half of the patients can recover simply by resting.

12.2 Historical Aspects

12.2.1 Percutaneous Diskectomy

The most widespread method today, to be described below, was proposed by G. Onik in 1984; utilizing an aspiration and cutting probe inserted in the nucleus pulposus, it enables the same to be partially removed. After studies on pigs and cadavers, the probe was used on man, initially only at levels L3–L4 and L4–L5, then at level L5–S1 as well, with the help of a curved probe that facilitated its penetration. The probe, produced by Surgical Dynamics, is presently available with a 2 mm or 2.5 mm diameter.

The Onik probe is the latest, most successful, and most opportunely conceived achievement in the way of percutaneous treatment that is essentially mechanical; its originality lies in its automated suction/cutting mechanism and in the greatly reduced diameter of the probe itself.

Other authors [in particular Hijikata (1975) and Kambin (1983)] had previously proposed the removal of the nucleus pulposus by means of manually operated pincers, using a percutaneous approach with the insertion of larger cannulas. These authors, too, designed a complete line of instrumentation.

12.2.2 Chemonucleolysis

The first attempts at enzymatic lysis with chymopapain were made in the 1960s by L. Smith, who also took part in the development and commercialization of purified chymopapain, Chymodiacttin, approved by the American FDA.

The results of the first attempts at chemonucleolysis therapy were extremely controversial, with neurologic complications and even deaths. The American Orthopedic and Neurosurgical Associations took differing stands, for and against the procedure. On the basis of our present experience, we believe that these unsatisfactory results and the risks which emerged at the time may be interpreted as due in part to the great difference in patient selection criteria and in part to technical differences.

In the 1960s and 1970s, patients were chosen exclusively on the basis of clinical findings or, at most, lumbar myelography. It must be observed that the injection of the enzyme shortly after lumbar puncture (myelography) exposes the patient to a greater risk of intrathecal passage of the enzyme; this can cause subarachnoid hemorrhage due to the toxic and sometimes fatal effect of the enzyme on arachnoid microvascularization. Today CT and MRI data allow for accurate selection of patients and identification of the level to be treated, which was unthinkable 20 years ago. Furthermore, the standard procedure now calls for diskography prior to injection of the enzyme, thus making possible decisive verification not only of the needle position but also of the accuracy of the indication. We are therefore surprised neither by the improvement in the results that may be achieved today nor by the difficulties encountered by those first pioneers.

The commercialization and use of the purified form of chymopapain (Chymodiactin) was only authorized by the FDA in 1982, while Discase was authorized in 1983. Since then many tens of thousands of patients have been treated all around the world, with results that are essentially homogeneous.

12.2.2.1 Notes on Chymopapain Action

Chemonucleolysis exploits the enzymatic activity of papain, extracted from the papaya, *Carica papaya* L, which acts on the proteoglycans, breaking up their protein "core." This results in depolymerization of the large molecules, with the liberation of the polysaccharide groups and consequent loss of water content: the nucleus pulposus thus loses its hydrophilia. The chymopapain – protein fragments – glycosaminoglycan complex is then eliminated in the blood and urine. The nucleus pulposus elimination process takes place over 15–20 days, with macroscopic evidence of the reduction in the height of the disk space, which may be verified radiologically about 30 days after the injection. After 20–30 days, repair work begins and leads to the formation of a "normal" nucleus within 5–6 months.

The toxicity of the enzyme is related to the hydrolysis of the mucopolysaccharides of the endothelial cells in the arachnoid capillaries. In the case of intrathecal injection, the effect can be fatal because of the toxic action of the enzyme on arachnoid and medullary vascularization, with hemorrhage. An intradural injection is easily avoided by employing the proper puncture technique and diskographic monitoring. At the doses normally administered, the enzyme acts neither on the collagen nor on the nervous tissue; in particular, the enzyme may be injected in cases in which diskography has revealed an epidural leak.

Chymopapain may, however, give rise to allergic and anaphylactic reactions, which in effect represent the one real risk of this treatment.

12.2.2.2 Notes on the Drugs Used for Chemonucleolysis

Discase, no longer available on the market in Italy, was produced by the Travenol laboratories; every bottle contains 12.5 nKat (the unit of measurement of sterile lyophilized chymopapain). As a reducing agent, it contains sodium cysteinate to keep the sulfur in its sulfide state -SH; sodium edetate (EDTA) is contained as an activator. Before the procedure, the enzyme is dissolved in 5 ml of sterile distiled water. The maximum dose per patient is 12.5 nKat, equal to 10 000 units. The dose normally used by us was 2000 or 4000 units, equal to 1 or 2 ml (4 or 8 mg).

Lekopain, produced by the LEK pharmaceutical industry in Ljubljana (Yugoslavia), comprises three proteolytic enzymes with analogous structures: chymopapain (43.5%), papain (12.4%), and proteinase X (26.7%). A mucolytic enzyme, lysozyme (17.4%), is combined with them and acts on the polysaccharide chains of the glycosaminoglycans. Besides these enzymes, there are activating and stabilizing substances: 18 mg NaCl, 0.2 mg cysteine, and 0.025 mg EDTA. It is marketed in bottles of 35 and 70 FIP units. The solution is made up immediately prior to the procedure with 2 ml of water. The usual dose employed by us, depending on the diskographic findings (degree of degeneration) and the height of the disk, is 0.5 or 0.25 ml.

Chymodiactin, produced by Smith Laboratories in the United States, is a proteolytic enzyme (chymopapain) containing sodium cysteinate as a reducing agent to keep the sulfur in its sulfide state -SH; it is not marketed in Italy.

12.3 Diskography Technique

12.3.1 Preliminaries

Diskography always precedes the treatment (to be discussed below); the insertion of the needle in the nucleus pulposus is furthermore the technical basis for all of the percutaneous procedures.

The patient preliminarily undergoes a CT scan in the prone position at target level. The unenlarged reconstruction of this section will serve as a means of checking the position of the intestinal loops and retroperitoneal structures. The risk of perforating a markedly posteriorized retropsoic loop is rare: we ourselves identified one risky position in about 1200 scans. The preliminary scan is also useful because it supplies two fundamental measurements: the angle of incidence on the sagittal plane and the distance of the penetration point from the midline. This information is basically sufficient for the approach to disks L2–5, which is effected on the same plane as the disk. The approach to L5–S1, however, is conditioned by the deep-lying position of the same, as access to the disk is masked by the iliac

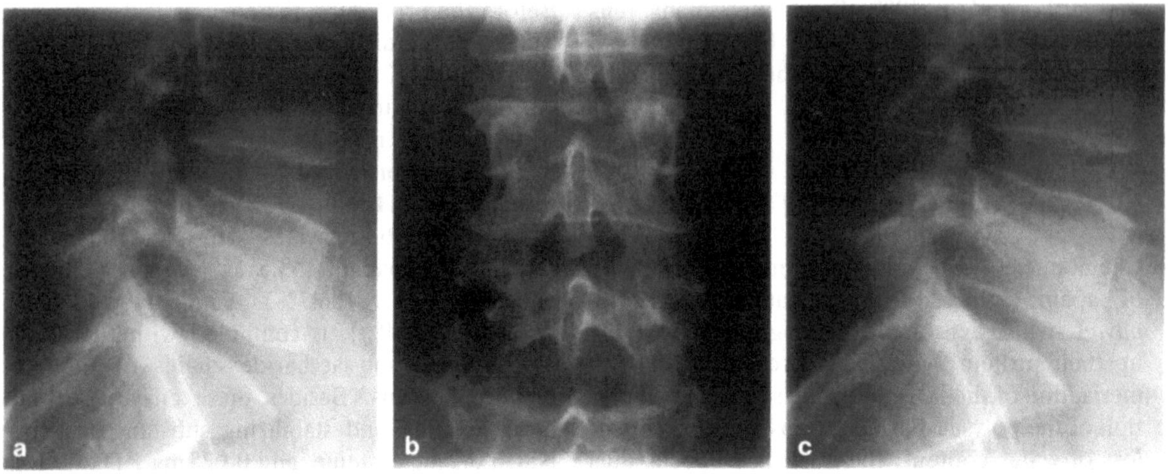

Fig. 12.1a–c. Proper delimitation of the x-ray beam. a In the lateral projection the boundaries of the disk and vertebral body are clearly delineated. b In the anteroposterior projection the pedicles are parallel and the spinous processes are well aligned. c The needle used to introduce local anesthetic in the muscle strata serves as a directional point of reference

wings. A second craniocaudal angle is therefore necessary in this instance; though not visible on axial scans, it may be provided by standard x-rays and was obtained by us by means of fluoroscopy at the moment of puncture.

12.3.2 Needle Penetration

The patient is positioned on the x-ray table (G.E. Omnitome), lying on the side opposite to the symptomatic one. The spine must be aligned as nearly as possible on a horizontal plane, for which purpose an inflatable balloon is placed under the patient's flank. He is strapped into position with his legs flexed at 60–80° by means of two maintenance straps. During the procedure, both blood pressure (by Dinamap) and cardiac activity are monitored, and an IV needle is always ready and positioned. The needle employed is generally a Becton-Dickinson, 18G or 22G.

After careful asepsis of the part, the patient is covered with a sterile sheet, the opening of which is centered around the needle penetration point. Local anesthesia is then performed at skin level, and infiltrated into the muscular parts along the pathway.

The target is centered (according to Troisier) by exploiting the isocentricity of the G.E. Omnitome system, but this can obviously also be achieved with an ordinary portable system; with fluoroscopy (of good quality), or with an angiographic system. The central rotation point of the axis of the tube–amplifier complex is centered on the nucleus pulposus: in the anteroposterior projection on the midline and in the lateral projection in correspondence with the passage between the middle and posterior thirds of the targeted vertebral body interspace.

The tube–amplifier complex is then rotated according to the angle determined on the CT scan (usually about 40°) on the median sagittal plane, in a direction from posterolateral towards the center of the target. The skin entry point must correspond with the CT scan findings and be situated at about 8–10 cm from the midline (Figs. 12.1–12.4).

12.3.2.1 Disk Puncture at L2–L3, L3–L4, and L4–L5

With the system in this position, the central beam traverses the pathway the needle will have to follow towards the center of the nucleus pulposus. Using fluoroscopy, at L2–L3, L3–L4, and L4–L5 the disk space is identified as being limited posteriorly by the edge of the inferior articular process: the cartilaginous plates must be parallel. In certain cases, it may be useful to impart a further slight inclination (cranial for the proximal levels and caudal for the distal one).

The needle is then brought to the skin penetration point and inserted, and its entry is checked

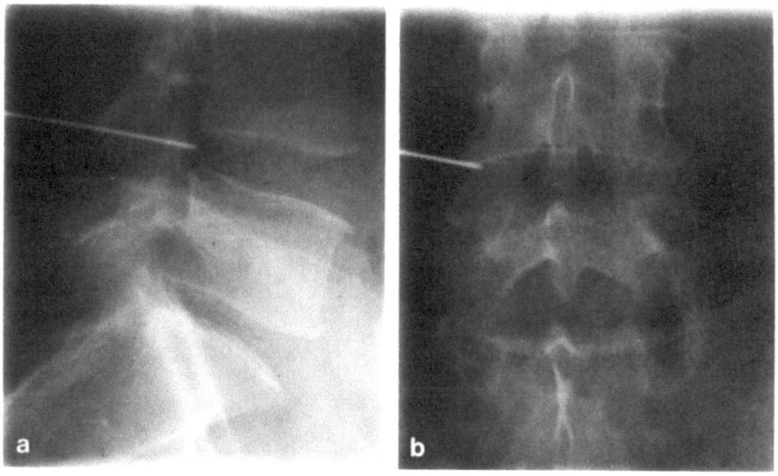

Fig. 12.2a,b. Intradiskal puncture needle (18G, B.D.) inserted employing an extradural, posterolateral approach. **a** In the lateral projection the needle corresponds to the posterior profile of the anulus. **b** In the anteroposterior projection the needle must be lateral to the midline of the pedicles

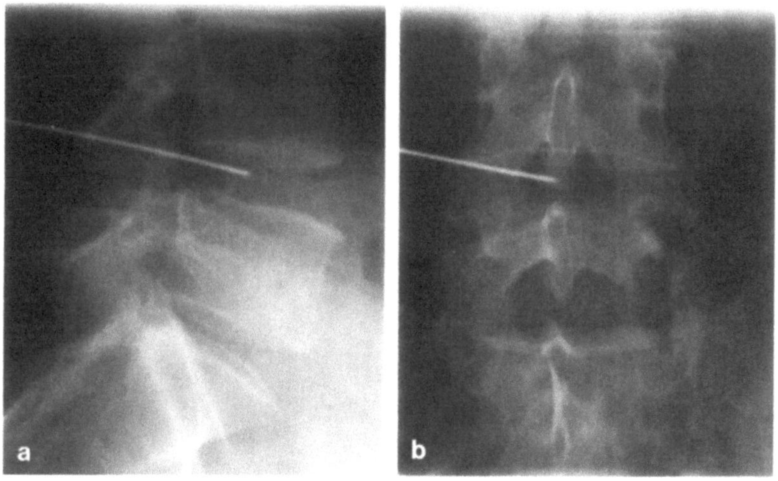

Fig. 12.3a,b. Penetration of the needle into the nucleus pulposus. **a** In the lateral projection the needle is between the middle and posterior thirds of the vertebral body interspace **b** In the anteroposterior projection the needle must not project beyond the midline of the spinous process

fluoroscopically; the needle must appear perfectly in cross-section. Needle penetration into the anulus is perceived as a slight, tough-elastic resistance.

12.3.2.2 Disk Puncture at L5–S1

To reach L5–S1, which is deeper lying and covered by the iliac wings, it is necessary to resort to a further craniocaudal inclination of the tube–amplifier complex (of about 30°), which may be accurately evaluated fluoroscopically: it is correctly centered when the edge of the iliac wing (on the puncture side) moves downwards (due to the upward inclination of the "U" complex) until it is superimposed over the edge of the superior cartilaginous plate of the inferior vertebra (S1).

Needle insertion takes place as at the other levels, under fluoroscopic monitoring: since the beam is centered on the directrix to be traversed, the needle will appear in cross-section.

The insertion of the needle, like the rest of the therapy, takes place with the collaboration of the patient in a state of neuroleptanalgesia: it is thus possible to recognize a possible erroneous puncture of the nerve root, the typical pain of which is felt by the patient. In this case, it is obviously mandatory that the needle pathway be slightly modified.

12.3.2.3 Posterolateral Extradural Approach (Lateral Projection)

Besides the puncture technique in the oblique projection (Troisier), we will describe the pos-

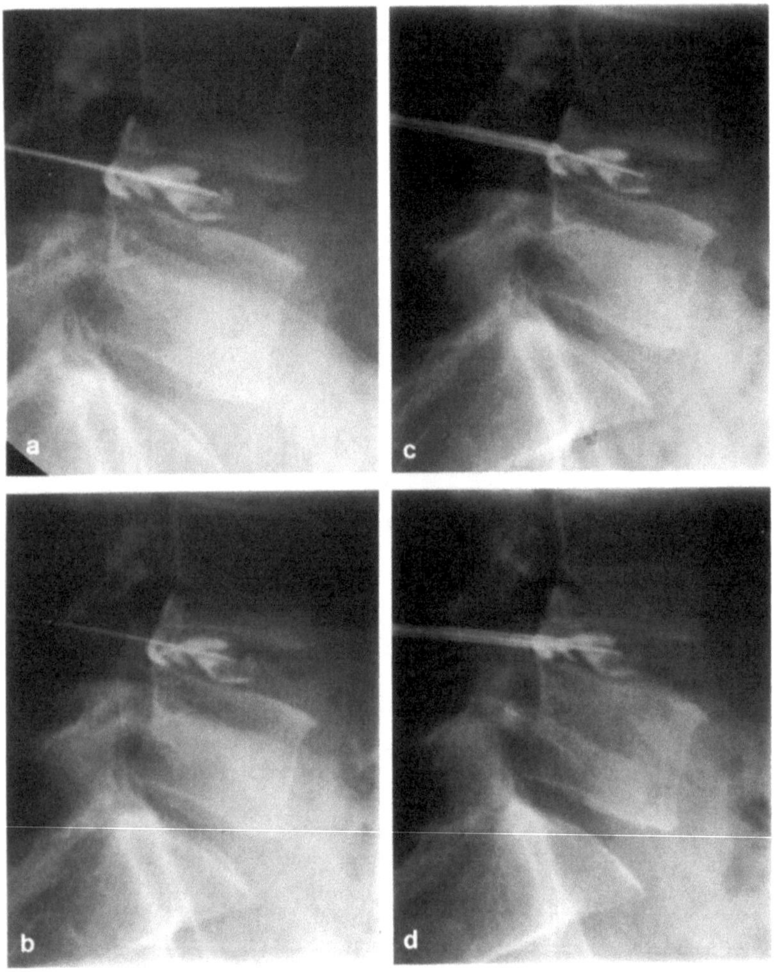

Fig. 12.4. **a** Diskography: clear demonstration of needle at center of nucleus pulposus; degenerate disk with a small posterior subligamentous (contained) hernia. The examination served as the basis for the choice of percutaneous procedure. In this case, treatment with the Onik probe was preferred. **b** Insertion of Kirschner's wire and removal of diskography needle. **c** Insertion of Onik instrumentation: cannula with dilator resting against anulus. **d** Removal of cannula with dilator and insertion of trephine

terolateral extradural approach with the customary technique. The patient is positioned laterally, with his symptomatic side upwards, and three fundamental points of reference are marked on his skin with a dermographic pencil:

- The spinous process line
- The outline of the iliac crest
- A line parallel to that of the spinous processes, the distance from which is determined by the panoramic CT scan and generally measures between 8 and 10 cm. This line represents the needle pathway to the target.

The placement of the needle varies with the disk to be treated: for the levels between L1–L2 and L4–L5, the needle has an inclination of about 45–55° on the sagittal plane (this measurement may be obtained with a goniometer from the tomogram of the panoramic CT scan). For levels L1–L2 and L2–L3, a caudocranial inclination is necessary on the frontal plane. For level L5–S1, besides the inclination on the sagittal plane, a craniocaudal inclination is fundamental to avoid the iliac crest; the inclination on the craniocaudal plane varies with the relationship between the iliac crest and the interdiskal space, which is generally about 30°.

The obstacles encountered most frequently are bony: superficially, the iliac crest; medium to deep lying, the transverse process, isthmus, and posterior articular process. When a bony obstacle presents itself, the needle must be withdrawn and the approach or inclination modified. Penetration is impossible (a) when the vertebral body interspace is excessively narrow, (b) in severe cases of osteophytosis, (c) in diskal caudal dystopia with high iliac wings, and (d) in severe hypertrophy of the transverse process, isthmus, or articular process.

12.3.3 Diskography

Needle placement is verified in the lateral, anteroposterior, and quasiaxial projections. In the lateral projection, the needle tip must be equidistant from the somatic borders of the vertebral body and situated between the middle and posterior thirds, while in the anteroposterior projection it must be lateral to the line connecting the median part of the pedicles (corresponding to the external profile of the dural sac) and must not project beyond the spinous process.

Diskography is carried out with the manual injection of nonionic iodinized contrast medium (Iopamidol 300) at low pressure, under fluoroscopic control. The quantity injected is between 0.5 and 1.5 ml, depending upon the resistance encountered and the fluoroscopic appearance.

A normal disk will logically offer marked resistance, while a degenerate one will present a resistance that decreases proportionately with its degree of degeneration; occasional cases in which it was impossible to perform the injection have been reported. The association of an interruption of the anulus with an interruption of the posterior longitudinal ligament, allowing the contrast to seep into the peridural space, would enable even larger quantities to be injected, although this would be of no diagnostic utility whatsoever.

The diskographic documentation is effected with standard x-rays in the lateral, anteroposterior, or posteroanterior projections; in addition, inclusion of a quasiaxial projection is useful, when this is possible.

If a percutaneous procedure of chemonucleolysis or diskectomy is decided upon, it is carried out immediately after diskography, utilizing, as we shall see, the needle inserted for the diskography itself.

Diskography performed for diagnostic purposes (for differential diagnosis between recurrent hernia and postoperative scarring in operated patients, or when there is a discrepancy between clinical findings and neuroradiologic examinations) is completed with CT (CT-diskography) that is performed 2 h after the diskography injection.

12.4 Chemonucleolysis Technique

When the diskographic findings confirm the suspected indication for therapy, we then inject the enzyme (chymopapain). The enzyme dose administered varies according to the product, the height of the vertebral body interspace, and the characteristics of the hernia. The drugs we use are Discase and Lekopain.

Chemonucleolysis consists in the injection of the enzyme, through the diskography needle, a few minutes after the diskography itself, without observing any particular time lapse. Shortly thereafter, under fluoroscopic control, the needle is withdrawn as far as the periradicular space, where infiltration with anti-inflammatory drugs and analgesics (Depomedrol and Marcaine) is carried out. The needle is then extracted and the procedure concluded.

12.5 Percutaneous Diskectomy Technique

The method adopted by us is the one proposed by Onik et al. (1985), utilizing the Surgical Dynamics Nucleotome. Two probes are available, with 2 and 2.5 mm diameters. They may be inserted in a connula with a straight or curved guide (the latter is designed for L5–S1, but we have never used it). The choice between the two diameters is made on the basis of the accessibility of the vertebral body interspace; the 2.5-mm probe has obviously proved more effective in the aspiration/removal of the disk material (Figs. 12.5, 12.6).

12.5.1 Constituent Elements of the System

- Needle guide (marketed separately).
- Trocar for the insertion of the cannula with an inner tapered dilator and trephine to cut the anulus.
- Control panel connected to a cylinder of nitrogen or compressed air to create the vacuum, with a collection bottle and three tubes hooked up to the flushing liquid (saline solution), the receptacle for the material aspirated, and the probe.
- Probe assembly for aspiration/cutting; this instrument has a to-and-fro mechanism controlled automatically by the control panel at the rhythm and aspiration force desired (maximum 180 cycles per minute). It activates a double probe: the outer one has a closed, rounded point presenting a small lateral aperture that is rhythmically closed, guillotine style, by the inner probe. The disk material drawn by the vacuum into the small aperture of the probe is thus cut

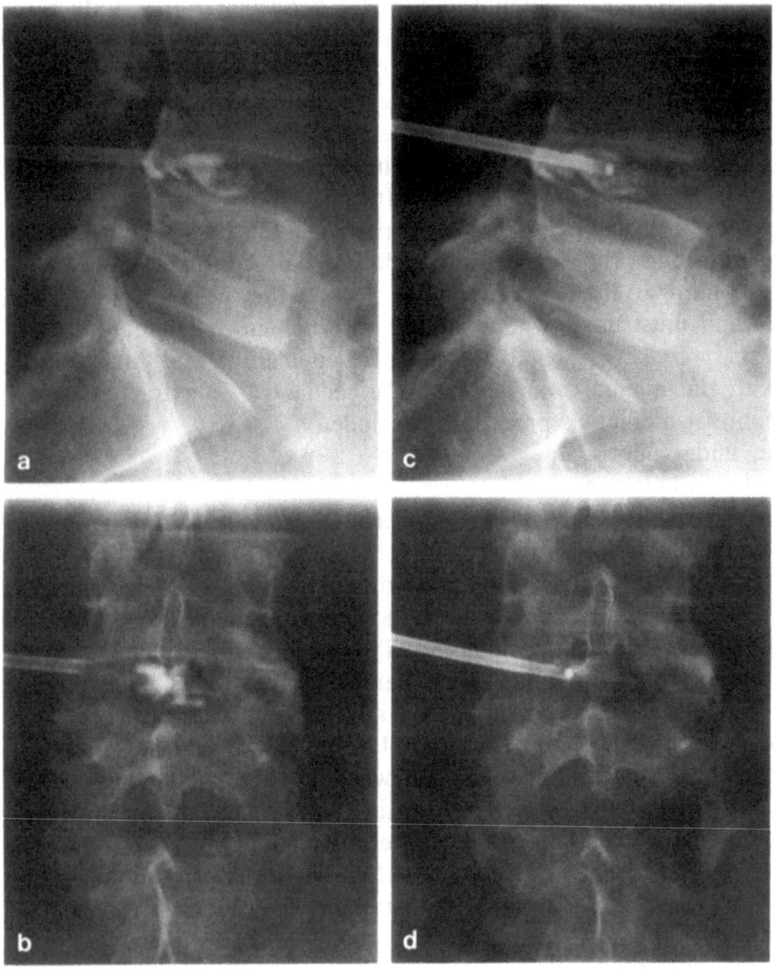

Fig. 12.5. a,b Clear visualization of cannula resting against anulus. **c,d** Insertion of Onik probe at center of nucleus pulposus

and aspirated (with a flushing system) into the bottle, where it is collected in a small filter that allows its quantity to be evaluated.

- As a wire guide we use a Kirschner's wire (0.8 mm in diameter), which in our experience has several considerable practical advantages over the trocar.

12.5.2 Method

Percutaneous diskectomy, too, is performed by us immediately after diskography. When the latter examination confirms the suspected indication, the Kirschner's wire is inserted through the diskography needle to serve as a guide, with its blunted apex in the nucleus pulposus. The needle is then withdrawn and, following further subcutaneous anesthetization around the wire, an incision is made with a pointed lancet, widening the hole to 3–4 mm in diameter and deepening it by 2–3 cm. The first cannula is then inserted with a slightly longer (2 mm) conical-tip dilator. The insertion of this complex along the Kirschner's wire is checked fluoroscopically up to the margin of the anulus, against which it must only rest, and care must be taken to avoid the nerve root; if the latter is touched this can only be recognized via the response of the patient, who experiences a shock-like pain along the nerve root.

Once the cannula has been positioned all the way up to the margin of the anulus, the tapered dilator is withdrawn and the trephine is inserted along the Kirschner's wire and inside the cannula; with its pressure and rotatory motion, it will enable the anulus to be cut. After removing the

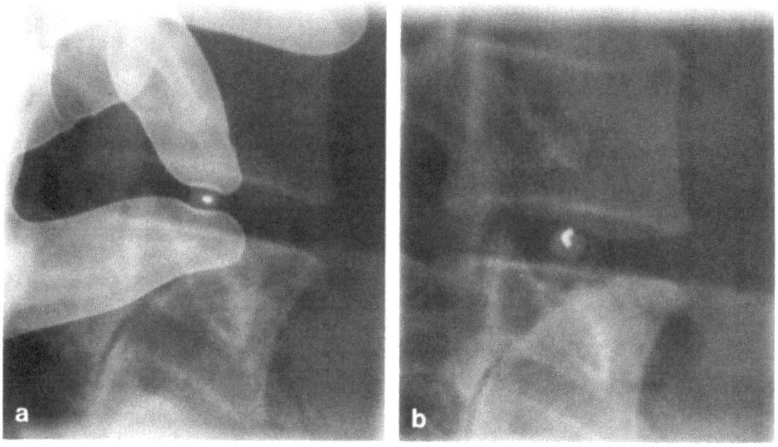

Fig. 12.6 a,b. Technique of oblique projection according to O. Troisier. **a** Operator inserts needle. **b** Ideal point of penetration and positioning of needle (needle seen in cross-section)

trephine and the Kirschner's wire, the cannula is fastened with an adjustable stop and the cutting/aspiration probe is inserted into the cannula. The probe is subjected to to-and-fro movement and rotation on its own axis to enable it to reach as much of the disk volume as possible. This aspiration procedure is performed for 10–15 min, until no further significant removal of disk material is seen to take place (such removal is clearly visible in the transparent tube connecting the handpiece to the bottle).

Upon conclusion of the procedure, all of the instrumentation is withdrawn and the skin is medicated, covering the cut with sterile strips; there is no need for sutures.

12.5.3 Criteria for the Selection of Patients Considered for Percutaneous Treatment

The percutaneous therapy approach has clear limits and its indication must therefore always be discussed within a specialized medicosurgical team. The criteria on which an indication for percutaneous treatment is based are both clinical and neuroradiologic in nature.

Table 12.1. Percutaneous procedures in lumbar disc herniation: general clinical indications

Failure of medical treatment and physical therapy
Specific clinical findings
Brief duration of symptomatology
Negative psychodiagnostic tests

Table 12.2. Influence of the intensity of the neurologic deficit on the choice of percutaneous treatment

Slight neurologic deficit: Percutaneous diskectomy
Slight to medium neurologic deficit: Chemonucleolysis

12.5.3.1 Clinical Criteria

The clinical selection of patients considered for percutaneous treatment must take place after medical therapy and physical therapy (undertaken for at least 2 months) have failed and must follow rigorous guidelines. There must be sciatica prevailing over lumbago with typical radicular irradiation, sometimes associated with paresthesia or hypesthesia in the area corresponding to the root involved. A brief duration of the symptomatology in patients with an athletic build and negative psychodiagnostic tests are parameters that contribute to an excellent result (Table 12.1).

The choice of the percutaneous treatment to be performed is influenced not only by general clinical criteria but also by the intensity of the neurologic deficit that may be present (Table 12.2; Figs. 12.7–12.9).

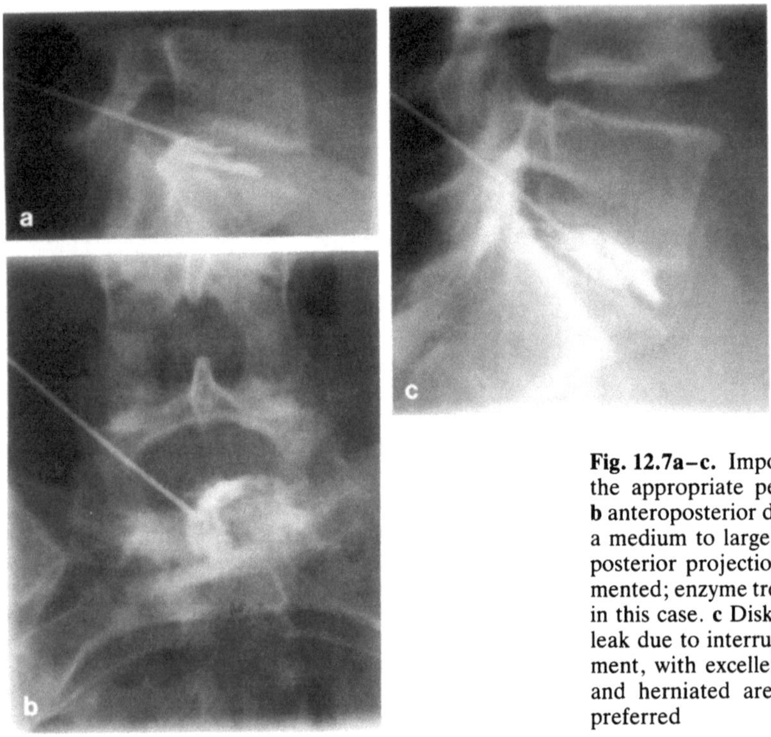

Fig. 12.7a–c. Importance of diskography in deciding upon the appropriate percutaneous procedure. **a** Lateral and **b** anteroposterior diskography with clear demonstration of a medium to large subligamentous hernia. In the anteroposterior projection the hernial pathway is clearly documented; enzyme treatment with chymopapain is preferable in this case. **c** Diskogram demonstrating massive epidural leak due to interruption of the posterior longitudinal ligament, with excellent visualization of the hernial pathway and herniated area. Enzyme treatment is again to be preferred

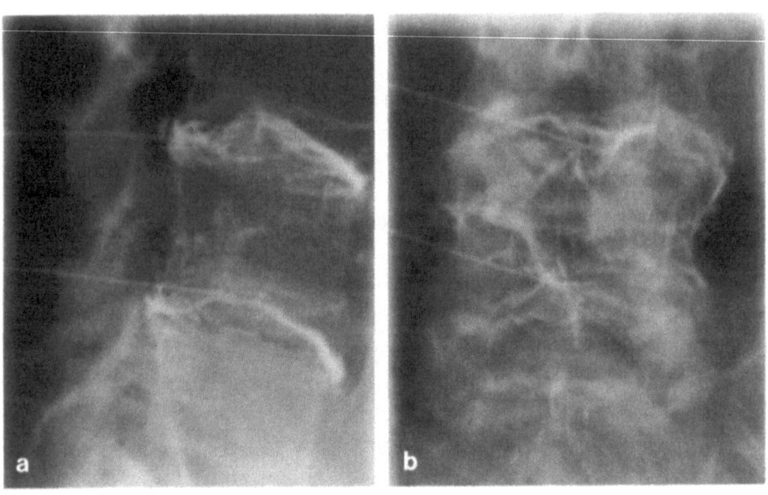

Fig. 12.8 a,b. Diskogram visualizing vascular leak at L4 level: contraindication to percutaneous procedures

12.5.3.2 Neuroradiologic Criteria

The neuroradiologic selection of patients suffering from lumbar disk herniation is based both on preoperative examinations (standard radiograms, CT or MRI, lumbar myelography) and intraoperative examinations (diskography, CT-diskography, diskomanometry). Standard radiographs allow the identification of cases in which diskography puncture will be difficult or impossible, or in which there are contraindications to percutaneous treatment (infections, tumors, malformations, stenosis of the spinal canal or radicular foramina, serious cases of arthrosis and vertebral instability).

The CT examination, or even better, MRI, is necessary to clear up the clinical doubt by permitting evaluation of the spinal canal and its

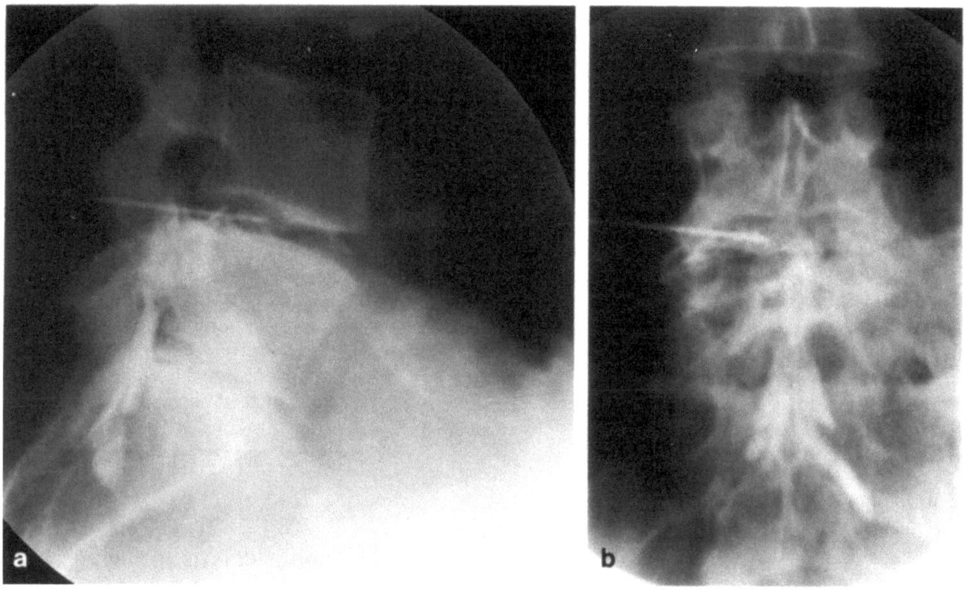

Fig. 12.9 a,b. Diskogram showing an almost empty disk with associated massive peridural leak: contraindication to percutaneous procedures

content, the radicular foramina, and the articular processes. Both diagnostic methods must define the morphologic characteristics (the integrity or interruption of the posterior longitudinal ligament) and the size of the hernia. The visualization of very small anatomic structures, such as the posterior longitudinal ligament, is difficult, and the distinction between subligamentous or contained hernias (i.e., hernias contiguous with the gelatinous pulp) and extraligamentous hernias is imprecise and sometimes impossible.

The CT scan with the patient in the prone position is a mandatory step which cannot be forgone if abnormalities in the position of colic loops (retro- or lateropsoic) or vessels are to be detected: these elements represent a risk during needle penetration. This examination is particularly advantageous in that it enables the distance of the skin penetration point from the midline and the needle angle to be determined accurately. Lumbar myelography is used rarely, in particular cases of marked discrepancy between CT and clinical findings. If chemonucleolysis is to be undertaken, it must be performed at least 7–8 days after myelography in order to avoid the toxic action of the enzyme on arachnoid microvascularization, the cause of very critical cases of subarachnoid hemorrhage.

Diskography is an indispensable intraoperative examination – a mandatory step for percutaneous treatment that documents the accurate positioning of the needle, the morphologic characteristics and enhancement of the hernial surface, and the contraindications to either percutaneous diskectomy or chemonucleolysis; furthermore by means of the pain response it indicates with precision the level to be treated in multiple-disk disorders. Because of the distinctive character of the data it provides – the morphologic aspect and the size and filling characteristics of the hernial surface – diskography plays a decisive role in the choice of treatment (percutaneous diskectomy or chemonucleolysis).

CT-diskography allows direct visualization of the hernial pathway and surface, with anatomic detail superior even to that provided by MRI, and differentiates between recurrent herniation and postoperative scarring with a high degree of reliability and accuracy.

When using diskomanometry certain difficulties of interpretation still persist, and the procedure cannot verify the positioning of the needle. It is most certainly an important examination in the evaluation of disk pathology, but needs further development.

The choice of the percutaneous treatment is influenced not only by clinical findings but also by neuroradiologic findings (Table 12.3). If percutaneous diskectomy is to be employed the hernia must be contained and the longitudinal ligament

Table 12.3. Influence of neuroradiologic findings on the choice of percutaneous treatment

Contained hernia of small to medium size, not displaced upwards or downwards: Percutaneous discectomy
Subligamentous or extraligamentous hernia, contiguous with the nucleus pulposus, of medium to large size: Chemonucleolysis

Table 12.4. Absolute contraindications (clinical and neuroradiologic) to percutaneous procedures in lumbar disk herniation

Paralyzing sciatica
Nondiskal sciatica or leg pain
Risky clinical situation
Degenerative arthrosis
Spondylolysis with spondylolisthesis
Major stenosis of the spinal canal or radicular foramina
Calcified hernia
Intradural hernia
Fragmented hernia
Diskographic contraindications (vascular leak, diskal incontinence, massive peridural leak, poor filling of the hernial surface)
Positive testing on psychodiagnostic examination
Symptoms reported for insurance or pension purposes

must be intact or, if detached, uninterrupted. The hernia must be small to medium in size and must be positioned medially or paramedially because the probe has very limited directionality and therefore cannot be used for the treatment of hernias in particular topographic situations, e.g., hernias positioned laterally or toward the foramina.

For chemonucleolysis to be used, the hernia must be contiguous with the gelatinous pulp, regardless of the integrity of the posterior longitudinal ligament.

12.6 Contraindications to Percutaneous Procedures

12.6.1 Absolute Contraindications

There are numerous contraindications (both absolute and relative, clinical and neuroradiologic) to the use of percutaneous procedures in lumbar disk herniation. These contraindications must be known and abided by.

Besides the absolute contraindications to percutaneous procedures listed in Table 12.4, we have extended the absolute contraindications to

Table 12.5. Absolute contraindications (clinical and neuroradiologic) to chemonucleolysis

Previous surgery
Hypersensitivity to papaya, contrast, or anesthetics
Previous chemonucleolysis
Presently taking β-blockers
Pregnancy

Table 12.6. Absolute contraindications (clinical and neuroradiologic) to percutaneous diskectomy

Lateral or foraminal hernia
Hernia displaced upwards or downwards
Large hernia

chemonucleolysis to include previous surgery, as the possibility of a dural tear represents a serious risk to the introduction of the enzyme (Table 12.5). We likewise do not use chemonucleolysis in patients who have already undergone this treatment owing to their greater risk of sensitization; this risk is also increased in patients being treated with β-blockers. We do not perform the procedure on pregnant women due to the possibility of teratogenesis posed by the enzyme.

The specific absolute contraindications to percutaneous diskectomy are shown in Table 12.6. The limited directionality of the Onik probe makes it inadvisable to undertake the treatment of hernias in particular topographic situations or of large hernias.

12.6.2 Relative Contraindications (Table 12.7)

We employed percutaneous procedures in several patients suffering from pure lumbago, carefully chosen from a clinical and neuroradiologic point of view, in whom the pathogenic momentum seemed to be due to a laceration of the outer fibers of the anulus, with stimulation of the algogenic receptors. We have also extended the indication for percutaneous therapy to patients with small hernias associated with minor stenosis of the spinal canal. We feel that wherever there is an alteration in the relationship between the containing structure and the structures contained, the presence of even a small hernia gives rise to significant algesic symptomatology that can benefit from chemonucleolysis or, even better, from percutaneous diskectomy. We also treated several patients who

Table 12.7. Relative contraindications (clinical and neuroradiologic) to percutaneous procedures in lumbar disk herniation

Chronic lumbago
Small hernias associated with minor stenosis of the spinal canal
Previous surgery[a]

[a] We have used only percutaneous diskectomy in such cases.

had previously undergone surgery and who presented clinical evidence of recurrent herniation associated with a small- to medium-sized hernia; in these cases we resorted exclusively to treatment with percutaneous diskectomy.

12.7 Treatment Data

In the period from 20 December 1985 to 31 December 1990, 948 patients underwent diskography, for a total of 1195 diskographic procedures. Subsequently 917 levels underwent percutaneous treatment with either chemonucleolysis (770) or percutaneous diskectomy (147) (Table 12.8). In the remaining 278 levels examined by diskography, the examination either contraindicated percutaneous therapy (vascular leak, diskal incontinence, massive epidural leak, poor filling of the hernial surface) or demonstrated situations of initial degeneration. In 36 cases, diskography was integrated with CT (CT-diskography) to discriminate, in operated patients, between recurrent herniation and postoperative scarring.

It is to be noted that 126 patients were treated with chemonucleolysis at two levels, while one patient was treated with chemonucleolysis at one level and percutaneous diskectomy at the other. When two levels are treated, we prefer enzyme therapy to percutaneous diskectomy because the more prolonged procedure of the latter causes greater discomfort to the patient.

12.8 Analysis of the Results

The evaluation of the results in patients who underwent percutaneous treatment was carried out by means of both (a) a questionnaire that reflected the subjective view of the patient and was filled in from 1 to 12 months after treatment, and (b) clinical follow-up examinations, in which the patient was seen 1, 3, and 6 months after therapy.

Table 12.8. Percutaneous procedures employed in the Departments of Neuroradiology and Neurosurgery in Udine, 20 December 1985 to 31 December 1990

Patients examined by diskography	948
Levels examined diskographically	1195
Patients treated with chemonucleolysis	643 (127 at two levels)
Levels treated with chemonucleolysis	770
Patients treated with percutaneous diskectomy (Onik procedure)	147
Levels treated with percutaneous diskectomy (Onik procedure)	147
Levels undergoing percutaneous treatment	917

Table 12.9. Assessment of the results of percutaneous treatment according to the modified McNab method

Success	
Excellent:	Disappearance of symptomatology Complete reintegration in occupational and sports activities
Good:	Occasional episodes of lumbago or sciatica No limitation of occupational activity
Fair:	Improvement of symptomatology Strenuous physical exercise given up
Failure	
Mediocre:	Insufficient improvement of symptomatology Periodic administration of drugs Limitation of physical exercise
No result:	No improvement Surgery required
Bad:	Worsening of clinical situation Surgery required

Different criteria have been proposed by various authors (MacNab, Cabot, Benoist, and Onik) for the evaluation of the results. We used MacNab's method, modified with a minimum follow-up period of at least 9 months (Table 12.9).

The first 329 patients treated with chemonucleolysis were analyzed, with a minimum follow-up period of more than 2 years and a maximum of 5 years. Success according to the MacNab criteria was achieved in 81.5%. We feel that an accurate analysis of the results requires the longest possible follow-up.

Between 1985 and 1990, two different drugs were used by us: Discase (from 20 December 1985 to 14 February 1989, in a total of 370 patients) and Lekopain (from 15 February 1989 to 31 December 1990, in a total of 273 patients). A review of the results in relation to the drug employed – Discase or Lekopain – revealed that the results obtained with Lekopain are more stable and superior to those obtained with Discase. This finding has been confirmed by a thorough analysis made by Bersi (1987).

Between 9 May 1988 and 31 December 1990, 147 patients underwent percutaneous diskectomy; of these, 111 were treated with the 2-mm probe and 36 with the 2.5-mm probe. In spite of the larger size of the latter, we encountered no technical difficulty with the procedure: the duration of the aspiration and therefore of the procedure is considerably shorter (on average, 10–12 min), with greater rapidity in the removal of the disk material and a larger amount of material removed.

After the 2.5-mm probe was made available, we treated only five patients out of 41 with the smaller 2-mm probe, which was called for by the limited vertebral body interspace involved.

Our statistical analysis on the first 100 patients treated with the 2-mm probe revealed a success rate of 70% (failure rate: 30%); there was no significant difference in results in the various grouping by age or sex with regard to the quantity of material removed and the duration of the aspiration, which must in any case be short so as to reduce not only the discomfort of the patient but also the possibility of complications such as diskitis. Young patients with athletic builds had shorter recovery times and better results.

Among the 36 patients treated by percutaneous diskectomy using the 2.5-mm probe, success was achieved in 30 (83.3%); moreover the failure rate of 16.7% included two patients in whom the result of diskectomy was unknown. These results, notwithstanding the limited number of patients treated and the brief follow-up documented before the end of the study, are particularly encouraging. We feel that the larger anulopulpal fenestration, by creating a locus minoris resistentiae (exhaust valve effect), allows for a more significant decompression of the disk and its adjacent structures. The subsequent removal of disk material reduces the pressure inside the disk and may enable the herniated part to be drawn back into the vertebral body interspace.

We analyzed the relationship between the number of patients undergoing chemonucleolysis and percutaneous diskectomy, choosing 1989 as the year of reference. The analysis showed that 72% underwent chemonucleolysis and only 28% percutaneous diskectomy. Among the neuroradiologic examinations, diskography proved decisive in the choice of the therapy to be performed.

We analyzed the relationship between the number of patients undergoing surgery and those undergoing percutaneous procedures: the percentage was obviously in favor of surgery (58.4% vs 41.6%). Chemonucleolysis and percutaneous diskectomy are not alternatives but supplements to surgery.

12.9 Complications

Over a period of more than 5 years, from 20 December 1985 to 31 December 1990, during which time 1195 diskographies and 917 percutaneous procedures were carried out, we registered two cases of spondylodiskitis, one following chemonucleolysis and the other following percutaneous diskectomy; both patients recovered with appropriate medical treatment.

Our case studies reveal very few complications: among the patients treated with chemonucleolysis (643), a skin rash was noted in 0.78% during the 24 h following the procedure, but disappeared in a few hours with appropriate treatment.

There were some cases (0.93%) of significant lowering of the vertebral body interspace, probably due to an overdose of enzyme, which required longer periods of hospitalization.

We did not encounter any other complications; in particular we saw no complications of a neurologic or anaphylactic order. We feel that the pharmaceutic prophylaxis implemented in the 3 days prior to chemonucleolysis proved effective in preventing the latter.

12.10 Comments

A patient who is to undergo percutaneous treatment is hospitalized in the Department of Neurosurgery. In the 3 days prior to the procedure, he receives H_1 and H_2 antagonists, antihistamines, and complement inhibitors. This pharmaceutic prophylaxis has shown itself to be effective in preventing complications of an anaphylactic order following the injection of the enzyme.

The percutaneous procedure is performed in the presence of an anesthesiologist: neuroleptanalgesia is the ideal choice for anesthesia. Rigorous asepsis and proper technique are essential to avoid complications.

Diskography is an integral part of the treatment; it ensures correct positioning of the needle and accurately evaluates the size and morphologic characteristics of the hernial surface, thereby assuming a decisive role in the choice of the percutaneous treatment to be employed. During the (on average) 3-day period of hospitalization following the procedure, the patients undergo a cycle of anti-inflammatory and analgesic drugs; they wear a type-B orthopedic corset (for a period of 15–25 days) and abstain from work (for 30 days). The final result builds up gradually and may be appraised after a period of 2 or 3 months.

The availability of more than one percutaneous therapeutic method enables us to extend our treatment options and, in the case of failure, to offer a more flexible range of therapy, leaving surgery as a last resort.

Percutaneous procedures have proved to be of extreme utility in the case of patients suffering from lumbar disk herniation who have tested positive for AIDS, as the risk represented by percutaneous treatment is lower than that of surgery.

With regard to the risk of radiation posed by these therapeutic procedures, we have evaluated the dose for chemonucleolysis and percutaneous diskectomy. The average effective dose equivalent is 0.5 mSv for chemonucleolysis and 1.2 mSv for percutaneous diskectomy. These values are 10–20 times lower than those for urography, gastrointestinal series, or barium enema. The benefit that these percutaneous procedures afford is much greater than the risk of radiation.

All of the patients undergoing percutaneous treatment for herniated disks undergo standard radiologic follow-up of the lumbosacral spine 1 month and 12 months afterwards. In particular, in our study we noted that with chemonucleolysis there was a lowering of the vertebral body interspace of about 30.5%, evidencing the lytic action of the drug. After 1–3 years, in the majority of the patients, we were able to ascertain disk reexpansion, with a recovery of about 70%. In the case of percutaneous diskectomy, no particular lowering of the vertebral body interspace was observed.

As for the CT follow-up in the medium (2–3 months) and long term (after 6 months), there was a discrepancy between the clinical findings and the CT examination: we noted that the CT image was unmodified in patients who presented a good clinical result. In the case of failure or recurrent herniation, a CT or MRI examination is warranted to search for a recurrent hernia, hernia fragment, hernia situated at another level, or other factors causing radicular compression.

12.11 Conclusions

Percutaneous diskectomy and chemonucleolysis complement surgical treatment and must be considered possible, but not mandatory, stages in the dynamic therapy of the patient. Conservative medical treatment is, in any case, to be scrupulously followed for a period of at least 2 months. The ideal patient is one suffering from lumbar disk herniation for whom the possibility of surgery has been advanced: a bad candidate for surgery is also a bad choice for percutaneous therapy.

The good results obtained with percutaneous procedures are the fruit of fine teamwork between the Departments of Neuroradiology and Neurosurgery, with rigorous, scrupulous selection of patients on the basis of clinical and neuroradiologic parameters.

The possibility of choosing from among physical therapy, percutaneous diskectomy, chemonucleolysis, and surgery is essential for balanced and optimal exploitation of the techniques. The availability of such a wide selection, in fact, makes it possible to adapt with ease to the actual requirements of the patient; in each case the technique most appropriate to the specific situation must be proposed, without any preconceived partiality for one technique or another.

Suggested Reading

Acampora S, Fabris G, Leonardi M, Troisi F (1987) Sulla nucleolisi enzimatica dell'ernia discale lombara. Moderna, Naples

Adams MA, Dolan P, Hutton WC (1986) The stages of disc degeneration as revealed by discograms. J Bone Joint Surg [Br] 68:36–41

Aubergé T, Chivrot R, Pallardy G (1985) Radiological aspects of chemonucleolysis. In: Sutton JC (ed) Current concepts in chemonucleolysis. The Royal Society of Medicine, London, pp 25–34

Benoist M (1984) Technique de la chimonucleolyse. In: Benoist M, Deburge A (eds) La Chimonucleolyse. Maestria, Levallois-Perret, pp 107–124

Benoist M, Deburge A, Busson J (1984) La chimonucleolyse dans le traitement des sciatiques par hernie discale. Presse Med 13:733–736

Benoist M, Deburge A, Chevrot A (1988) Bilan radiologique dans les radiculalgies post-operatoires. In: Mas-

sare C (ed) Rachis et moelle. L'imagerie, aujourd'hui. Vigot, Paris, pp 115–127
Bersi G (1985) Indicazioni e limiti della chemonucleolisi nel trattamento dell'ernia discale lombare. In: Dettori P, Leonardi M (eds) Attualita' in Neuroradiologia. Monduzzi, Bologna, pp 393–410
Bersi G (1987) La chemonucleolisi oggi. Libreria Cortina, Turin
Bocchi L, Ferrata P, Passarello F et al. (1989) La nucleoaspirazione secondo Onik nel trattamento dell'ernia discale lombare. Analisi multicentrica dei primi risultati su oltre 650 trattamenti. Riv Neuroradiol 2 [Suppl 1]:119–122
Bonneville JF (1985) Il punto sulla chemo-nucleolisi. In: Pistolesi GF, Bergamo Andreis IA (eds) L'imaging diagnostico del rachide. Libreria Cortina, Verona, pp 355–361
Bonneville JF (1986) Focus on chemonucleolysis. Springer, Berlin Heidelberg New York
Bonneville J-F, Clarisse J, Deramond H et al. (1989) Radiologie interventionnelle. In: Manelfe C (ed) Imagerie du rachis et et de la moelle. Vigot, Paris, pp 761–784
Brown BM, Stark EH, Dion G, Hiroisa O (1985) Computed tomography and chymopapain chemonucleolysis: preliminary findings. AJNR 6:51–54
Cauchoix PJ, Massare C, Benoist M, Deburge A, Hautiers S (1967) La discographie lombaire. Presse Med 75: 2751–2756
Chafetz NI, Lang P, Light KI, Norman D, Genant HK (1988) Correlation of MR and discography in lumbar intervertebral disc degeneration: treatment implications. Abstracts of VIIth Annual Meeting SMRM, San Francisco, 20–26 August 1988, p 92
Chevrot A, Vilgrain V, Pousse T et al. (1988) Incidence quasi-axiale descendante au cours de la discographie lombaire – evaluation clinique sur hernie avérée. J Radiol 69:223–226
Colhoun E, McCall IW, Williams L, Cassar Pullicino VN (1988) Provocation discography as a guide to planning operations on the spine. J Bone Joint Surg [Br] 70: 267–271
Collis JS, Gardner WJ (1961) Lumbar discography. JAMA 178:67–70
Collis JS, Gardner WJ (1962) Lumbar discography. An analysis of one thousand cases. J Neurol Surg 19:452–461
Crawshaw C (1985) Needle insertion techniques of chemonucleolysis. In: Sutton JC (ed) Current concepts in chemonucleolysis. The Royal Society of Medicine, London, pp 55–60
Davis GW (1989) Discography. In: APLD – International Symposium, Marbella, Spain, 1989, paper 7, pp 1–3
Decoulx MMP, Houlcke E, Razemon J-P, Lemerle P (1958) Anatomie pathologique de la hernie discale. Presse Med 66:899–902
De Nardi F, Cecotto C, Comelli L et al. (1988) La chemonucleolisi nell'ernia discale lombare. 1a parte: analisi clinica dei risultati. Riv Neuroradiol 1:53–62
Deutman R (1985) Anatomical considerations. In: Sutton JC (ed) Current concepts in chemonucleolysis. The Royal Society of Medicine, London, pp 35–40
Drouillard J, Lavignolle B, Philippe J-C et al. (1982) Scanographie et chémonucléolyse des hernies discales. J Radiol 63:267–272
Edholm P, Fernstrom I, Lindblom K (1967) Extradural lumbar disk puncture. Acta Radiol 6:322–328
Edwards WC, Orme TJ, Orr-Edwards G (1987) CT discography: prognostic value in the selection of patients for chhemonucleolysis. Spine 12:792–795
Erlacher PR (1952) Nucleography. J Bone Joint Surg [Br] 34:204–210
Fabris G, Penco T, Biasizzo E, Zappoli F, Lavaroni A, Leonardi M (1987) In: Calabrò A, Leonardi M (eds) Discography and chemonucleolysis. Computer aided neuroradiology. CIC, Rome, pp 453–458
Fabris G, Lavaroni A, De Nardi F et al. (1989) La chemonucleolisi dell'ernia discale lombare. 2a parte: analisi neuroradiologica dei risultati. Riv Neuroradiol 2 [Suppl 1]:93–102
Fabris G, Lavaroni A, Leonardi M (1991) Discography. Edizioni del Centauro, Udine
Feinberg SB (1964) The place of diskography in radiology as based on 2320 cases. AJR 92:1275–1281
Feldmann JL, Menkes CJ (1983) La chimonucléolyse. Le Concours Médicale 105:2387–2391
Folinais D, Frot B, David M, Bourgeois P, Benacerraf R (1987) La disco-tomodensitométrie, une nouvelle approche horizontale du disque. Presse Med 16:33
Fraser RD, Osti OL, Vernon-Roberts B (1987) Discitis after discography. J Bone Joint Surg [Br] 69:26–35
Friedman J, Goldner MZ (1955) Discography in evaluation of lumbar disk lesions. Radiology 65:653–662
Fuentes JM, Maupoux R, Bourbotte F et al. (1981) L'épidurographie. J Neuroradiol 8:21–34
Galligioni F (1980) Discografia. In: Galligioni F (ed) Neuroradiologia. Piccin Padua, p 605
Gandolfi M, Jucopilla N, Salvi V, Tomasso A (1987) Discografia. In: La sciatica vertebrale. Atti 18 Congresso Nazionale OTODI, Verona, 5–6 June 1987, pp 39–46
Gentry LR, Strother CM, Turski PA, Javid MJ, Sackett JF (1985a) Chymopapain chemonucleolysis: correlation of diagnostic radiographic factors and clinical outcome. AJNR 145:351–360
Gentry LR, Turski PA, Strother CM, Javid MJ, Sackett JF (1985b) Chymopapain chemonucleolysis: CT changes after treatment. AJNR 145:361–369
Gibson M, Buckley J, Mawhinney R, Worthington BS (1985) A comparison of discography and magnetic resonance imaging in the diagnosis of disc degeneration. Abstracts of XIII ESNR, Amsterdam, 11–15 Sept 1985, p 56
Gibson MJ, Buckley J, Mawhinney R, Mulholland RC, Worthington BS (1986a) Magnetic resonance imaging versus discography in the recognition of disc degeneration. J Bone Joint Surg [Br] 68:369–373
Gibson MJ, Buckley J, Mulholland RC, Worthington BS (1986b) The changes in the intervertebral disc after chemonucleolysis demonstrated by magnetic resonance imaging. J Bone Joint Surg [Br] 68:719–723
Gomori JM, Floman Y (1984) Chymopapain disk-injection therapy. Modified lumbar approach. Radiology 151: 245–246
Grenier N, Vital J-M, Greselle J-F et al. (1988) CT-diskography in the evaluation of the postoperative

lumbar spine. Preliminary results. Neuroradiology 30: 232–238
Grenier N, Greselle J-F, Vital J-M et al. (1989) Normal and disrupted lumbar longitudinal ligaments: correlative MR and anatomic study. Radiology 171:197–205
Grubb SA, Lipscomb HJ, Bonner Guilford W (1987) The relative value of lumbar roentgenograms, metrizamide myelography, and discography in the assessement of patients with chronic low-back syndrome. Spine 12: 282–286
Guillot M, Pionchon H, Pialat J, Bancel B, Galtier B (1988) Etude de l'innervation des ligaments du rachis lombaire chez l'homme. Rev Rhum Mal Osteoartic 55:421–423
Helms CA, Munk PL, Witt WS, Davis GW, Morris J, Onik G (1989) Retrorenal colon: implications for percutaneous diskectomy. Radiology 171:864–865
Hendry NGC (1958) The hydration of the nucleus pulposus and its relation to intervertebral disc derangement. J Bone Joint Surg [Br] 40:132–144
Hijikata S, Yamagishi M, Nakayama T, Oomori K (1975) Percutaneous diskectomy: a new treatment method for lumbar disk herniation. J Toden Hosp
Holt EP (1968) The question of lumbar discography. J Bone Joint Surg [Am] 50:720–726
Holtas S, Nordstrom C-H, Larsson E-M, Petterson H (1987) MR imaging of intradural disk herniation. JCAT 11:353–356
Hopper K, Sherman J, Luethke JM, Ghaed N (1987) The retrorenal colon in the supine and prone patient. Radiology 162:443–446
Houser OW, Onofrio BM, Forbes GS, Baker HL Jr (1986) Correlation of radiological features to failure of lumbar intervertebral disc chemonucleolysis. J Neurosurg 64:736–742
Huckman MS, Clark JW, McNeill TW et al. (1987) Chemonucleation and changes observed on lumbar MR scan: preliminary report. AJNR 8:1–4
Kambin P, Gellman H (1983) Percutaneous lateral diskectomy of the lumbar spine. Clin Orthop 174:127–132
Konings JG, Williams FJB, Deutman R (1984) The effects of chemonucleolysis as demonstrated by computerised tomography. J Bone Joint Surg [Br] 66:417–421
Kornberg M (1987) Computed tomography of the lumbar spine following discography. Spine 12:823–825
Kosteljanetz M, Bang F, Schmidt-Olsen S (1988) The clinical significance of straight-leg raising (Lasègue's Sign) in the diagnosis of prolapsed lumbar disc. Interobserver variation and correlation with surgical finding. Spine 13:393–395
Lewit K, Sereghy T (1975) Lumbar peridurography with special regard to the anatomy of the lumbar peridural space. Neuroradiology 8:233–240
Lindblom K (1944) Protrusion of disks and nerve compression in the lumbar region. Acta Radiol XXV:195–212
Lindblom K (1948) Diagnostic puncture of intervertebral disks in sciatica. Acta Orthop XVII:231–239
Luyendijk W, van Voorthuisen AE (1966) Contrast examination of the spinal epidural space. Acta Radiol Diagn 5:1051–1066
MacKinnon SE, Hudson AR, Llamas F, Dellon AL, Kline DG, Hunter DA (1984) Peripheral nerve injury by chymopapain injection. J Neurosurg 61:1–8
MacNab I (1973) Chemonucleolysis. Clin Neurosurg 20: 183–192
Maldague B, Malghem J (1985) La discografia. In: Pistolesi GF, Bergamo Andreis IA (eds) L'imaging diagnostico del rachide. Libreria Cortina, Verona, pp 331–355
Malmivaara A (1987) Disc degeneration in the thoracolumbar junctional region. Acta Radiol 28:755–760
Malmivaara A, Videman T, Kuosma E, Troup JDG (1987) Plain radiographic, discographic, and direct observations of Schmorl's nodes in the thoracolumbar junctional region of the cadaveric spine. Spine 12:453–457
Masaryk TJ, Boumphrey F, Modic MT, Tamborrello C, Ross JS, Brown MD (1986) Effects of chemonucleolysis demonstrated by NMR imaging. JCAT 10:917–923
Masaryk TJ, Ross JS, Modic MT, Boumphrey F, Bohlman H, Willber G (1988) High-resolution MR imaging of sequestered lumbar intervertebral disks. AJNR 9: 351–358
Massare C, Benoist M, Frot B, Bloch-Michel H (1969) La discographie lombaire son traitement dans le diagnostic et le traitement chirurgical des discopathies douloureuses lumbaires et lombo-sacrées. Bilan de 4 ans d'expérience. Rev Rhum Mal Osteoartic 36:312–317
Massare C (1971) Discographie. In: Fishgold H (ed) Traité de Radiodiagnostic, tome XV – Neuroradiologie. Masson, Paris, pp 39–49
Massare C (1973) Discographie lombaire. In: Encycl Méd Chir, Paris, Radio II, pp 30655 A10 and A20
Massare C, Benoist M, Cauchoix J (1973) Le diagnostic des hernies discales lombaires et lombo-sacrées. Intéret de la discographie. Rev Chir Orthop 59:61–67
Massare C, Bard M, Benoist M, Cauchoix J, Bloch-Michel H (1974) Renseignetments fournis par la discographie lombaire pour le diagnostic et le traitement chirurgical des discopathies douloureuses lombaires et lombosacrées. Rev Rhum 41:113–122
Matsui H, Tsuji H, Itoh T, Yashima S, Ichimura K (1987) Significance of tangential views in lumbar discography. Clin Orthop Rel Res 221:165–171
McCormick CC (1978) Radiology in low back pain and sciatica. An analysis of the relative efficacy of spinal venography, discography and epidurography in patients with a negative or equivocal myelogram. Clin Radiol 29:393–406
McCulloch JA (1977) Chemonucleolysis. J Bone Joint Surg [Br] 59:45–52
McCulloch JA, Waddell G (1978) Lateral lumbar discography. Br J Rad 51:498–502
McCulloch JA (1984) Alternatives in spinal surgery. Omnis Surgical, Akron
Menkes CJ, Feldmann JL, Ben Sedrine H et al. Traitement des hernies discales lombaires par chimionucléolyse. Rev Rhum 49:621–628
Miller JAA, Schmatz C, Schultz AB (1988) Lumbar disc degeneration: correlation with age, sex and spine level in 600 autopsy specimens. Spine 13:173–178
Modic MT, Masaryk TJ, Ross JS, Carter JR (1988) Imaging of degenerative disk disease. Radiology 168: 177–186
Moseley I (1986) Diagnostic imaging in neurological disease. Churchill Livingstone, London, pp 81–83
Moutounet J, Chevrot A, Vallée C, Wybier M, Gizes F, Pallardy G (1988) L'incidence quasi-axiale descendante du disque au cours de la discographie. J Radiol 69: 357–364
Nachemson A (1964) the influence of spinal movements on the lumbar intradiscal pressure and on the tensile

stresses in the annulus fibrosus. Acta Orthop XXXIII: 183–207
Naessens P (1989) Multilevel disc disease. In: APLD – International Symposium, Marbella, Spain, 1989, paper 12, pp 1–2
Naylor A (1982) The biophysical and biochemical aspects of intervertebral disc herniation and degeneration. Ann R Coll Surg Engl 31:91–114
Nazarian S (1985) Anatomical basis of intervertebral puncture with chemonucleolysis. Anat Clin 7:23–32
Nordin JY, Frot B (1988) Itinéraires d'imagerie dans les radiculalgies lombo-sacrées présumées d'origine discale. In: Massare C (ed) Rachis et moelle. L'imagerie, aujourd'hui, Vigot, Paris, pp 73–92
Onik G, Helms CA (eds) (1988) Automated percutaneous lumbar discectomy. Radiology Research and Educational Foundation, San Francisco
Onik G, Maroon JC (1989) Percutaneous automated discectomy. A less invasive alternative for the treatment of herniated lumbar discs. In: APLD – International Symposium, Marbella, Spain, 1989, paper 20, pp 1–10
Onik G, Helms CA, Ginsbourg L, Hooglund FT, Morris J (1985) Percutaneous lumbar diskectomy using a new aspiration probe. AJNR 6:290–293
Pech P, Haughton VM (1985) Lumbar intervertebral disk: correlative MR and anatomic study. Radiology 156: 699–701
Peyron J-G (1984) Anatomie et biochimie du disque intervertébral normal et pathologique. In: Benoist M, Deburge A (eds) La Chimonucléolyse. Maestria, Levallois-Perret, pp 15–26
Pon A, Seifert J, Schlegel KF (1986) Bedeutung der Diskographie und Kontrastmittel-Enzym-Interaktionen. Neurochirurgia (Stuttg) 29:134–137
Rabischong P (1989) L'ernia discale lombare. Basi anatomiche. Riv Neuroradiol 2 [Suppl 1]:5–14
Rabischong P, Louis R, Vignaud J, Massare C (1978) The intervertebral disc. Anat Clin 1:55–64
Ross JS, Modic MT, Masaryk TJ (1990) Tears of the anulus fibrosus: assessment with Gd-DTPA-enhanced MR imaging. AJNR 10:1251–1254
Sachs BL, Vanharanta H, Spivey MA et al. (1987) Dallas discogram description. A new classification of CT/ discography in low-back disorders. Spine 12:287–294
Schneiderman G, Flannigan B, Kingston S, Thomas J, Dillin WH, Watkins RG (1987) Magnetic resonance imaging in the diagnosis of disc degeneration: correlation with discography. Spine 12:276–281
Smith L (1964) Enzyme dissolution of the nucleus pulposus in humans. JAMA 11:137–140
Smith L, Brown E (1967) Treatment of lumbar intervertebral disc lesions by direct injection of chymopapain. J Bone Joint Surg [Br] 49:502–519
Smith L, Garvin PJ, Jennings RB (1963) Enzyme dissolution of the nucleus pulposus. Nature 198:1311–1312
Solini A (1989) Atlante della nuclectomia percutanea (secondo Onik). Aulo Gaggi, Bologna
Testut L (1942) Articolazioni della colonna vertebrale. In: Testut L (ed) Anatomia normale. UTET, Turin, pp 27–30
Théron J, Blais M, Casasco A et al. (1983) La Radiologie thérapeutique du rachia lombaire. J Neuroradiol 10: 209–230
Théron J (1989) Exploration of herniated lumbar discs with standard radiographs and CT. In: APLD – International Symposium, Marbella, Spain 1989, paper 5
Troisier O (1980) Indications des injections intradiscal d'enzymes protéolytiques (nucléolyses) dans le traitement des sciatiques discales. J Med Phys Rééducation 75–80
Troisier O (1982) Technique de la discographie extradurale. J Radiol 63:571–578
Troisier O (1983) La discographie dans les lumbagos a répétition et les lombalgies chroniques. In: Lombalgies et Médecine de Rééducation. Masson, Paris, pp 54–58
Troisier O (1984) Technique de la nucléolyse de l'Hopital Foch. In: Benoist M, Deburge A (eds) La Chimonucléolyse. Maestria, Levallois-Perret, France, pp 87–106
Troisier O, Cypel D (1986) Discography: an element of decision. Clin Orthop Rel Res 206:70–78
Troisier O, Cypel D (1987) Chirurgie ou Nucleolyse. La discographie est-elle un facteur de decision? Acta Orthop Belg 53:195–203
Urban JPG, McMullin JF (1988) Swelling pressure of the lumbar intervertebral discs: influence of age, spinal level, composition, and degeneration. Spine 13:179–187
Vallee C, Chevrot A, Gites F, Auberge T, Bellin MF, Pallardy G (1986) Méthodes radiologiques et pronostic de la nucléolyse dans le traitement des sciatiques par hernie discale. Ann Radiol 29:237–239
Vanharanta H, Sachs BL, Spivey A et al. (1987) The relationship of pain provocation to lumbar disc deterioration as seen by CT/discography. Spine 12:295–298
Vanharanta H, Sachs BL, Spivey A et al. (1988) A comparison of CT/discography, pain response and radiographic disc height. Spine 13:321–324
Videman T, Malmivaara A, Mooney V (1987) The value of the axial view in assessing discograms. An experimental study with cadavers. Spine 12:299–304
Waddell G (1983) Technique of chemonucleolysis. Acta Orthop Belg 49 [Suppl 1]:20–31
Wolkin J, Sachs MD, Hoke GH (1955) Comparative studies of discography and myelography. Radiology 64:704–713
Yu S, Haughton VM, Hops P, Sether LA, Wagner M, Ho KC (1988a) Progressive and regressive changes in the nucleus pulposus. Part II. The adult. Radiology 169: 93–97
Yu S, Sether LA, Hops P, Wagner M, Haughton VM (1988b) Tears of the anulus fibrosus: correlation between MR and pathologic findings in cadavers. AJNR 9:367–370
Yu S, Haughton VM, Sether LA, Wagner M (1989) Comparison of MR and diskography in detecting radial tears of the anulus: a postmortem study. AJNR 10: 1077–1081
Zimmer EA (1986) Colonna vertebrale. In: Zimmer EA (ed) Limiti del normale ed inizio del patologico nella diagnostica radiologica dello scheletro. Casa Ed Ambrosiana, Milano, pp 435–620

Subject Index

List of Contributors

HORTENSIA AVAREZ, M. D.
Unité de Neuroradiologie Vasculaire
Diagnostique et Thérapeutique
Hôpital Bicêtre
Université Paris Sud
78, Rue du Général Leclerc
94275 Kremlin-Bicêtre, France

ALEX BERENSTEIN, M. D.
Professor of Radiology and Neurosurgery
Department of Radiology
Surgical Neuroangiography Service
New York University Medical Center
560 First Avenue
New York, NY 10016, USA

IN SUP CHOI, M. D.
Radiology, Massachusetts General Hospital
Fruit Street
Boston, MA 02114, USA

GERARD M. DEBRUN, M. D.
Professor of Radiology and Neurological Surgery
Director of Interventional Neuroradiology
Department of Radiology
Neuroradiological Section
The Johns Hopkins University Medical Institutions
Meyer Building # 8-140
600 North Wolfe Street
Baltimore, MD 21205, USA

JOSEPH M. ESKRIDGE, M. D.
Associate Professor of Radiology
Department of Neurological Surgery RI-20
University of Washington Medical Center
1959 NE Pacific Street
Seattle, WA 98195, USA

GIULIANO FABRIS, M. D.
Servizio di Neuroradiologia
Unita'Sanitaria Locale N. 7 "Udinese"
Stabilimento Ospedaliero S. Maria della Misericordia
33100 Udine, Italy

RICARDO GARCIA-MONACO, M. D.
Unité de Neuroradiologie Vasculaire
Diagnostique et Thérapeutique
Hôpital Bicêtre
Université Paris Sud
78, Rue du Général Leclerc
94275 Kremlin-Bicêtre, France

GUIDO GUGLIELMI, M. D.
Department of Radiological Sciences
Service of Endovascular Therapy
UCLA Medical Center
10833 Le Conte Avenue
Los Angeles, CA 90024-1721, USA
and Department of Neurological Sciences
Service of Therapeutic Neuroangiography
University of Rome Medical School
Viale Dell'Universita'30/A
00185 Roma, Italy

VAN V. HALBACH, M. D.
Associate Professor of Radiology and Neurological Surgery
Neurointerventional Radiology Section
Department of Radiology
University of California
505 Parnassus Avenue
San Francisco, CA 94143-0628, USA

PIERRE LASJAUNIAS, M. D., Ph. D.
Professor of Radiology and Neurosurgery
Unité de Neuroradiologie Vasculaire
Diagnostique et Thérapeutique
Hôpital Bicêtre
Université Paris Sud
78, Rue du Général Leclerc
94275 Kremlin-Bicêtre, France

ANTONIO LAVARONI, M. D.
Servizio di Neuroradiologia
Unita'Sanitaria Locale N. 7 "Udinese"
Stabilimento Ospedaliero S. Maria della Misericordia
33100 Udine, Italy

MARCO LEONARDI, M. D.
Servizio di Neuroradiologia
IRCCS – Ospedale Maggiore
Via Francesco Sforza 35
20122 Milano, I

GEORGES RODESCH, M. D.
Unité de Neuroradiologie Vasculaire
Diagnostique et Thérapeutique
Hôpital Bicêtre
Université Paris Sud
78, Rue du Général Leclerc
94275 Kremlin-Bicêtre, France

AVI SETTON, M. D.
Department of Radiology
Surgical Neuroangiography Service
New York University Medical Center
550 First Avenue
New York, NY 10016, USA

ANTON VALAVANIS, M. D.
Professor of Neuroradiology
Abteilung für Neuroradiologie
Departement Medizinische Radiologie
Universitätsspital Zürich
Frauenklinikstrasse 10
8091 Zürich, Switzerland

SAMUEL M. WOLPERT, M. B., B. Ch.
Department of Radiology
Section of Neuroradiology
New England Medical Center Hospitals
750 Washington Street
Boston, MA 0211, USA

F. ZANELLA, M. D.
Professor
Abteilung für Neuroradiologie
Radiologische Klinik
Universitätskrankenhaus Eppendorf
Universität Hamburg
Martinistrasse 52
W-2000 Hamburg 20, FRG

HERMANN ZEUMER, M. D.
Professor
Abteilung für Neuroradiologie
Radiologische Klinik
Universitätskrankenhaus Eppendorf
Universität Hamburg
Martinistrasse 52
W-2000 Hamburg 20, FRG

Springer-Verlag and the Environment

We at Springer-Verlag firmly believe that an international science publisher has a special obligation to the environment, and our corporate policies consistently reflect this conviction.

We also expect our business partners – paper mills, printers, packaging manufacturers, etc. – to commit themselves to using environmentally friendly materials and production processes.

The paper in this book is made from low- or no-chlorine pulp and is acid free, in conformance with international standards for paper permanency.

MIX
Papier aus verantwortungsvollen Quellen
Paper from responsible sources
FSC® C105338

If you have any concerns about our products,
you can contact us on
ProductSafety@springernature.com

In case Publisher is established outside the EU,
the EU authorized representative is:
Springer Nature Customer Service Center GmbH
Europaplatz 3, 69115 Heidelberg, Germany

Printed by Libri Plureos GmbH
in Hamburg, Germany